AN INTRODUCTION TO

Medical Terminology for Health Care

For Elsevier:

Senior Commissioning Editor: Sarena Wolfaard
Associate Editor: Dinah Thom
Project Manager: David Fleming
Design Direction: George Ajayi
Illustration Manager: Bruce Hogarth
Illustrator: Jane Fallows

AN INTRODUCTION TO

Medical Terminology for Health Care

FOURTH EDITION

ANDREW R. HUTTON BSc MSc
Lecturer in Life Science, Edinburgh, UK

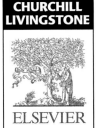

CHURCHILL LIVINGSTONE

ELSEVIER

EDINBURGH LONDON NEW YORK OXFORD PHILADELPHIA ST LOUIS SYDNEY TORONTO 2006

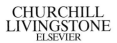

CHURCHILL
LIVINGSTONE
ELSEVIER

First published 1993
Second edition 1998
Third edition 2002
Fourth edition 2006
    Reprinted 2007

ISBN 10: 0 443 10075 6
ISBN 13: 9780 443 10075 8

British Library Cataloguing in Publication Data
A catalogue record for this book is available from the British Library

Library of Congress Cataloging in Publication Data
A catalogue record for this book is available from the Library of Congress

---

Notice

Knowledge and best practice in this field are constantly changing. As new research and experience broaden our knowledge, changes in practice, treatment and drug therapy may become necessary or appropriate. Readers are advised to check the most current information provided (i) on procedures featured or (ii) by the manufacturer of each product to be administered, to verify the recommended dose or formula, the method and duration of administration, and contraindications. It is the resposibility of the practitioner, relying on their own experience and knowledge of the patient, to make diagnoses, to determine dosages and the best treatment for each individual patient, and to take all appropriate safety precautions. To the fullest extent of the law, neither the publisher nor the author assumes any liability for any injury and/or damage to persons or property arising out or related to any use of the material contained in this book.

The Publisher

Working together to grow
libraries in developing countries

www.elsevier.com | www.bookaid.org | www.sabre.org

ELSEVIER   BOOK AID International   Sabre Foundation

ELSEVIER   your source for books, journals and multimedia in the health sciences

www.elsevierhealth.com

The publisher's policy is to use paper manufactured from sustainable forests

Printed in China

CONTENTS

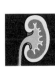
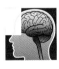

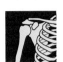

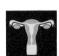

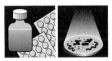

ABOUT THIS BOOK

This book is designed to introduce medical terms to students who have little prior knowledge of the language of medicine. Included in the text are simple, non technical descriptions of pathological conditions and symptoms, medical instruments and clinical procedures.

The medical terms are introduced within the context of a body system or medical specialty and each set of exercises provides the student with the opportunity to learn, review and assess new words. Each unit includes a case history exercise that outlines the presentation, diagnosis and treatment of a specific medical condition. Once complete, the exercises will form a valuable reference text.

No previous knowledge of medicine is required to follow the text and, to ensure ease of use, the more complex details of word origins and analysis have been omitted. The book will be of great value to anyone who needs to learn medical terms quickly and efficiently.

This edition gives the reader access to the evolve website containing interactive exercises that complement the written work in this book.

Edinburgh 2006
Andrew R. Hutton

Acknowledgements

The medical notes included in Units 2–17 were selected with reference to *Anatomy and Physiology* (fifth Edition) by Gary A. Thibodeau and Kevin T. Patton, published by Mosby, ISBN 0-323-01628-6

HOW TO USE THIS BOOK

Before you begin working through the units, read through the introduction which explains the basic principles of reading, writing and understanding medical terms.

Once you have understood the elementary rules of medical word building, complete Units 1–21, which are based on different medical topics. The units can be studied in sequence or independently.

For ease of use each unit has the same basic plan and is arranged into:

WORD EXERCISES

AN ANATOMY EXERCISE

A CASE HISTORY

MEDICAL NOTES

A WORD CHECK

SELF-ASSESSMENT

The word exercises should be completed using the Exercise Guide at the beginning of each unit or with knowledge acquired during the course of this study. Each word exercise is based on analysing and understanding medical terms associated with a specific word root. The answers to the word exercises are on p. 301.

The anatomy exercise enables you to relate the combining forms of medical roots to their position in the body. Check the meaning of the root words using the Quick Reference box. You can find help for these exercises and test your knowledge of body systems by logging onto the *evolve* website at the address given on the back cover of this book.

The case history presents a patient's medical history associated with a particular body system or medical speciality. The purpose of this exercise is to understand the medical terms associated with disease presentation, investigation, diagnosis and treatment. Some of the case histories may seem difficult to follow because of the terminology used when doctors write formal reports. To assist your understanding, a Word Help box is included with each case listing the meanings of difficult or unfamiliar words. For each case history try to gain an overall picture of the health care required for a successful treatment. Answers to the exercise that accompanies each case can be found with the answers to the word exercises on p. 301.

The medical notes act as a reference source providing additional information relating to symptoms, diseases and disorders associated with the body system being studied. Use this section for reference only.

The word check lists all prefixes, combining forms and suffixes in each unit. Try to write the meaning of each component from memory and then correct any errors you have made. Errors can be corrected using the Exercise Guide or the Quick Reference box that follows each Case History. The glossary on p. 347 can also be used.

The self-assessment at the end of each unit consists of a set of exercises that test your knowledge of the meaning of word components and their association with the anatomy or with a medical speciality. Aim to complete the assessment tests using knowledge gained from studying each unit and record your score in the box next to each test. Check your answers on p. 325. Unit 22 contains sixteen final self-assessment tests that enable you to test your knowledge of medical word components used throughout the package.

Note: All word exercises in this book can also be completed using *Pocket Medical Terminology* by A. R. Hutton published by Elsevier Churchill Livingstone (ISBN 0-443-07456-9). This conveniently sized compilation of medical terms and their definitions is arranged into a sequence that complements the exercises in this self-teaching package.

INTRODUCTION

OBJECTIVES

Once the introduction is complete you should be able to:

- name and identify components of medical words
- split medical words into their components
- build medical words using word components.

Students beginning any kind of medical or paramedical course are faced with a bewildering number of complex medical terms. Surprisingly it is possible to understand many medical terms and build new ones by learning relatively few words that can be combined in a variety of ways. Even the longest medical terms are easy to understand if you know the meaning of each component of the word. For example, you may never have heard of **laryngopharyngitis** but if you learn that **-itis** always means inflammation, **laryng/o** refers to the larynx or voice box and **pharyng/o** refers to the throat or pharynx, its meaning becomes apparent, i.e. inflammation of the pharynx and larynx. Laryngopharyngitis is an inflammation of the upper respiratory tract with symptoms of sore throat and loss of voice.

Doctors do not usually use precise medical terminology when conversing with patients as they may become worried rather than reassured by a complex description of their illness. However, precise medical terms are used when medical records and letters are completed. They are also used when doctors discuss a patient and when medical material is published.

The terms you will use in this book describe common diseases and disorders, instruments, diagnostic techniques and therapies.

The components of medical words

In this introduction you will learn how to split medical terms into their components and deduce their meanings. Skills developed here will enable you to derive the meanings of unfamiliar medical words and improve your ability to understand medical literature.

Let us begin by using a medical word associated with an organ with which you are familiar, the stomach:

Example 1 GASTROTOMY

First we can split the word and examine its individual components:

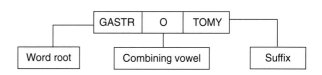

The word root

Roots are the basic medical words. Most are derived from Greek and Roman (Latin) words. Others have their origins in Arabic, Anglo-Saxon and German. Some early Greek words have been retained in their original form whilst others have been Latinized. In their migrations throughout Europe and America many words have changed their spelling, meaning and pronunciation.

In our first example we have used the root **gastr** which always means stomach.

The combining vowel

Combining vowels are added to word roots to aid pronunciation and to connect the root to the suffix. In our first example the combining vowel **o** has been added to join the root and suffix. All the combining vowels a, e, i, o and u are used but the most commonly used is o.

In our first example we have added the combining vowel **o** to the root **gastr**.

The suffix

The suffix follows the word root and is found at the end of the word. It also adds to or modifies the meaning of the word root.

In our first example we have used the suffix -**tomy** which always means to form an incision.

We can now fully understand the meaning of our first medical word:

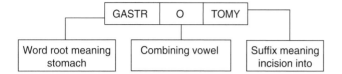

The meaning of gastrotomy is – incision into the stomach. Gastrotomy is a name used by surgeons to describe an operation in which a cut is made into the wall of the stomach.

The combining form

In our first example the root **gastr** can be combined with the vowel **o** to make **gastro**. This word component is called a **combining form** of a word root, i.e.

Word root + combining vowel = combining form
gastr + o = gastro

Most combining forms end in o and we will be using many of them in the exercises that follow.

Now we have learnt the meaning of our first root we can use it again with a new word component:

Example 2 EPIGASTRIC

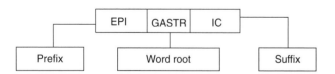

Here we have split the word into its components and we can see it begins with a prefix that appears before the root **gastr**.

The prefix

The prefix precedes the word root and changes its meaning. The prefix **epi-** means upon and so it modifies the word to mean upon or above the stomach. Prefixes, like roots and suffixes, are also derived from Greek and Latin words.

The suffix -**ic** meaning pertaining to was also used in our second example so we can now write the full meaning of epigastric:

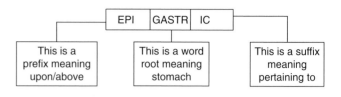

The full meaning of epigastric is – pertaining to above or upon the stomach.

> **Key Point**
> The components of medical words are:
> - prefixes
> - roots
> - suffixes
> - combining vowels
> - combining forms.

The use of prefixes, combining forms and suffixes

There are certain simple 'rules' that need to be applied when building and analysing medical words. To practise using these rules, some new combining forms are introduced. Don't worry about remembering their meanings at the moment, we will study them in a later unit.

Rule 1: Joining a combining form to a suffix

If we add the suffixes -**logy**, meaning study of, and -**algia**, meaning condition of pain, to the combining form gastr/o we can make two new words:

gastr/o + -logy = gastrology (study of the stomach)
gastr/o + -algia = gastralgia (condition of pain in the stomach)

Notice that in gastrology the combining vowel o has been left in place whilst in gastralgia it has been dropped. The o has been dropped in gastralgia because -algia begins with a, a vowel. Gastroalgia is not used and it would be more difficult to pronounce.

> **Key Point**
> When a combining form of a root is joined to a suffix, the combining vowel is left in place if the suffix begins with a letter other than a vowel.

Here are some more examples where the vowel is left in place because the suffix begins with a letter other than a vowel:

gastr/o + -tomy = gastrotomy (incision into the stomach)
gastr/o + -scope = gastroscope (instrument to view the stomach)

Here are some examples where the vowel is dropped:

gastr/o + -itis = gastritis (inflammation of the stomach)

gastr/o + -ectomy = gastrectomy (removal of the stomach)

WORD EXERCISE 1

Use Rule 1 to join the combining forms of word roots and suffixes to make medical words. The meanings of the words will be studied in following units. The first has been completed for you.

Combining form of word root	Suffix		Medical word
(a) gastr/o	+ -pathy	=	gastropathy
(b) gastr/o	+ -scopy	=	
(c) hepat/o	+ -itis	=	
(d) hepat/o	+ -megaly	=	
(e) hepat/o	+ -oma	=	

Rule 2: Joining the combining forms of two word roots

Some medical words contain two or more combining forms of roots, as in Example 3.

Example 3   GASTROENTEROLOGY

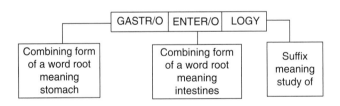

The full meaning of gastroenterology is the study of the intestines and stomach. Notice that the vowel between the two roots **gastr** and **enter** is left in place.

Key Point
When the combining forms of two roots are joined, the combining vowel of the first root is kept in place.

Here are some more examples:

pylor/o + gastr/o + ectomy = pylorogastrectomy
duoden/o + enter/o + stomy = duodenoenterostomy

WORD EXERCISE 2

Use Rules 1 and 2 to join the combining forms of two roots with suffixes to make medical words. The meanings of the words will be studied in following units. The first has been completed for you.

Combining form of word root	Combining form of word root	Suffix		Medical word
(a) duoden/o	+ jejun/o	+ -stomy	=	duodenoje-junostomy
(b) trache/o	+ bronch/o	+ -itis	=	
(c) gastr/o	+ enter/o	+ -stomy	=	
(d) laryng/o	+ pharyng/o	+ -ectomy	=	
(e) oste/o	+ arthro	+ -pathy	=	

Note. There are a few exceptions to this rule which are hyphenated, e.g. pharyngo-oral.

Rule 3: Joining a prefix to a root

When a prefix that ends in a vowel is added to a root that begins with a vowel or 'h', the vowel of the prefix is dropped.

Examine our second example **epigastric** again, notice the vowel 'i' of epi- was retained because the root **gastr** begins with 'g' which is not a vowel.

Consider another example, which may be familiar to you – **antacid**, a drug used to neutralize stomach acid. This word is made from:

anti + acid = antacid
(prefix meaning against) (root meaning acid)

The 'i' is dropped because acid begins with the vowel 'a'.

Here are some more examples, we will learn their meanings later.

Here the vowel of the prefix is retained:

hemi- + col/o + -ectomy = hemicolectomy

Here the vowel of the prefix is dropped:

endo- + arter/i + -ectomy = endarterectomy
anti- + helminth + -ic = anthelminthic (Here 'i' is dropped because helminth begins with 'h').

Note. Rule 3 is not a strict rule and there are many exceptions to it, e.g. periosteitis.

Key Point
When a prefix that ends in a vowel is joined to a root, the vowel of the prefix is dropped if the root begins with a vowel or 'h'.

WORD EXERCISE 3

Use the rules we have just described to join prefixes, combining forms of roots and suffixes to make medical words. The meanings of the words will be studied in following units. The first has been completed for you.

Prefix		Combining form of word root		Suffix	Medical word
(a) endo-	+	odont/o	+	-ic	= endodontic
(b) prostho-	+	odont/o	+	-ist	=
(c) para-	+	rect/o	+	-al	=
(d) mono-	+	ocul/o	+	-ar	=
(e) peri-	+	splen/o	+	-itis	=

Reading and understanding medical words

Now you have learnt the basic principle of building medical words, you should be able to deduce the meaning of an unfamiliar word from the meaning of its components. To illustrate this we will use two examples.

Example 1: Gastroenterology

First
Split the word into its components gastro/entero/logy.

Then
Think of or look up the meaning of these components.

Finally
Read the meaning of the word *beginning with the suffix and reading backwards*:

e.g. gastr/o[3], enter/o[2], -logy[1]

1 study of
2 the intestines and
3 the stomach.

We read the full meaning of gastroenterology as – the study of the intestines and stomach.

Example 2: Pararectal

Here the prefix *para-* has modified the meaning of the root *rect/* to mean beside the rectum.

First
Split the word into its components para/rect/al.

Then
Think of or look up the meaning of these components.

Finally
Read the meaning of the word *beginning with the suffix followed by the meaning of the modified root*

e.g. pararect[2],al[1]

1 pertaining to
2 beside the rectum.

We read the full meaning of pararectal as pertaining to beside the rectum.

Key Point
When deducing the meanings of compound medical words, begin with the meaning of the suffix followed by those of the root(s) or modified root (from right to left).

Once you have an understanding of these simple rules you should be able to complete the exercises in Units 1–22. Each unit introduces different medical terms associated with a body system or medical specialty. The units can be completed in an order that complements your studies in anatomy, physiology and health care.

UNIT 1
LEVELS OF ORGANIZATION

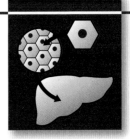

OBJECTIVES

Once you have completed Unit 1 you should be able to:

- understand the meaning of medical words relating to levels of organization

- build medical words relating to levels of organization

- understand medical abbreviations relating to cells and tissues.

EXERCISE GUIDE

Use this list of word components and their meanings to complete the word exercises in this unit.

Prefixes

micro-	small

Roots/Combining forms

bio-	life/living
chem/(istry)	chemicals (study of)
chondr/o	cartilage
erythr/o	red
fibr/o	fibre (Am.fiber)
granul/o	granule
haem/o	blood
hem/o (Am.)	blood
leuc/o	white
leuk/o (Am.)	white
lymph/o	lymph
melan/o	pigment/melanin
oo	egg/ovum
path/o	disease
spermat/o	sperm
tox/o	poisonous

Suffixes

-blast	germ cell/cell that forms . . . / embryonic or immature cell
-genic	pertaining to formation/genesis
-genesis	formation of
-ic	pertaining to
-ical	pertaining to
-ist	specialist
-logist	specialist who studies ...
-logy	study of
-lysis	breakdown/disintegration
-pathy	disease of
-scope	instrument to view/examine
-scopist	specialist who uses viewing instrument
-scopy	technique of viewing/examining
-trophic	pertaining to nourishing

Levels of organization

The human body consists of basic units of life known as **cells**. Groups of cells similar in appearance, function and origin join together to form **tissues**. Different tissues then interact with each other to form **organs**. Finally groups of organs interact to form body **systems**. Thus there are four levels of organization in the human body: cells, tissues, organs and systems. Let us begin by examining the first level of organization.

Cells

The cell is the basic unit of life and the bodies of all plants and animals are built up of cells. Your body consists of millions of very small specialized cells. It is interesting to note that all non-infectious disorders and diseases of the human body are really due to the abnormal behaviour of cells.

Body cells are all built on the same basic plan. Figure 1 represents a model cell.

Most cells have the same basic components as are shown in the model but they are all specialized to carry out particular functions within the body. In your studies you will come across many terms that relate to different types of cell. Now we will examine our first word root which refers to cells:

ROOT ────────────────

Cyt
*(From a Greek word **kytos**, meaning cell.)*

Combining forms **Cyt/o**, *also used as the suffix* **-cyte**

(Remember from our introduction that combining forms are made by adding a combining vowel to the word root.)

Here we have a word that contains the root **cyt**:

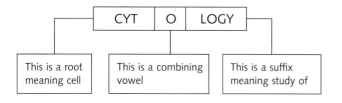

Reading from the suffix back, cytology means the study of cells.

(Remember when trying to understand medical words, first split the word into its components, then think of

the meaning of each component and finally write the meaning beginning with the suffix.)

Cytology is a very important topic in medicine as many diseases and disorders can be diagnosed by studying cells. Cells removed from patients are sent for cytological examination to a hospital cytology laboratory where they are examined with a microscope. (In the word cytological, *-ical* is a compound suffix meaning pertaining to or dealing with.)

The exercises that follow rely on the use of the Exercise Guide that appears at the beginning of this unit; use the guide to look up the meaning of path/o and -pathy and then try Word Exercise 1.

WORD EXERCISE 1

(a) Name the components of the word and give their meanings:

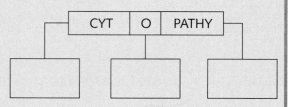

(b) Reading from the suffix back, the meaning of cytopathy is:

_____

The combining form **path/o** can be used at the beginning and in the middle of a compound word as in the next two examples. Write the meaning of these words:

(c) **path/o/logy** _____

(d) cyt/o/**path/o**/logy _____

Using the Exercise Guide again find the meaning of -ic, -logist, -lysis and tox/o, then write the meaning of the words below. Remember to read the meaning from the suffix back to the beginning of each word:

(e) **cyt/o**/lysis _____

(f) **cyt/o**/tox/ic _____

(g) **cyt/o**/logist _____

In (g) **cyt/** was used at the beginning of a word. It can also be used in combination with other roots at the end of words as in lymph/o/**cyt**e, its meaning remaining the same. As the word -cyte appears at the end of the word it is also acting as a suffix. Remember, when two roots are joined the combining vowel remains in place.

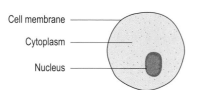

Cell membrane
Cytoplasm
Nucleus

Figure 1 A cell

WORD EXERCISE 2

Here we have an example of two roots joined to make a compound word:

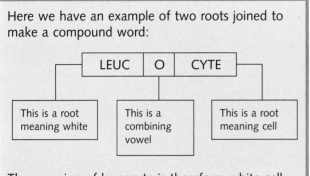

LEUC	O	CYTE
This is a root meaning white	This is a combining vowel	This is a root meaning cell

The meaning of leucocyte is therefore: white cell (actually a type of blood cell) (Am. leukocyte).

(a) Name the components of the following word and find the meaning of erythr/o using your Exercise Guide.

ERYTHR	O	CYTE

(b) The meaning of erythrocyte is: _____

WORD EXERCISE 3

Figure 2 and Figure 3 show two specialized cells, each one carrying out a different function.

(i) This cell produces the pigment melanin that gives the dark colour to black or brown skin.

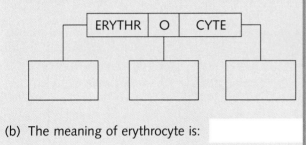

Melanin

Figure 2 A pigment cell

(ii) This cell produces white collagen fibres (Am. fibers) that give the skin strength.

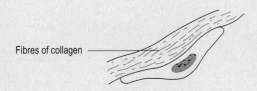

Fibres of collagen

Figure 3 A fibre cell (Am. fiber)

Use your Exercise Guide to find the combining forms of melanin and fibre, then build words that mean:

(a) A cell containing melanin _____

(b) A cell that produces fibres _____

(c) Complete the table by looking up the combining forms of the following roots in your Exercise Guide and building words that name the cell types.

Root	Combining form	Name of cell
oste	osteo	osteocyte (bone cell)
lymph		
spermat		
oo		
granul		
chondr		

All of the above examples show how the combining vowel is retained when the combining forms of two roots are joined.

Now we will examine another root that refers to a special type of cell:

ROOT _____

Blast
(A Greek word meaning bud or germ. Here blast/o means a cell that is forming something, a germ cell or an immature stage in cell development.)

Combining forms **Blast/o**, *also used as the suffix* **-blast**

WORD EXERCISE 4

Without using your Exercise Guide, write the meaning of:

(a) oste/o/**blast** _____

(b) fibr/o/**blast** _____

Using your Exercise Guide, write the meaning of:

(c) haem/o/cyt/o/blast _____

(Am. hem/o/cyt/o/**blast**)

Tissues

As cells become specialized, they form groups of cells known as tissues. A definition of a tissue is a group of cells similar in appearance, function and origin. There

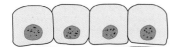

Figure 4 Cuboidal epithelium

are four basic types of tissue: epithelia, muscle, connective and nervous tissue; these form the second level of organization in the body. Figure 4 illustrates how cells associate to form a cuboidal epithelium in the kidney.

The study of tissues is known as histology, the combining form coming from a Greek word *histos* meaning web (web of cells). Histology is an important branch of biology and medicine because histological techniques are used to process and identify diseased tissues. The histology and cytology laboratories are usually sections of the pathology laboratory of a large hospital.

ROOT

Hist
(From a Greek word **histos**, *meaning web. Here hist/i/o means the tissues of the body.)*

Combining forms **Hist/i/o**

WORD EXERCISE 5

Using your Exercise Guide, find the meaning of:

(a) **hist/o**/chemistry

Without using your Exercise Guide, write the meaning of:

(b) **hist/o**/path/o/logy

(c) **hist/o**/logist

(d) **hist/o**/lysis

Cells and tissues are very small and can only be examined using an instrument known as a microscope.

WORD EXERCISE 6

Using your Exercise Guide, find the meaning of:

(a) **micro-**

(b) **micro**/scope

(c) **micro**/scopy

(d) **micro**/scop/ist

Note carefully the differences between **-scope**, **-scopy** and **-scopist**.

(e) **micro**/bio/logy

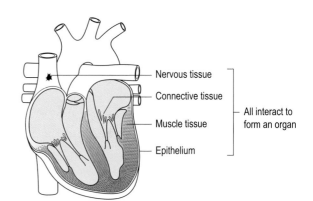

Figure 5 The heart

Organs

Groups of different tissues interact to produce larger structures known as organs; these form the third level of organization. A familiar example is the heart (Fig. 5), which consists of muscle tissue, a covering of epithelium, nerve tissue and connective tissue. All these tissues interact so that the heart pumps blood.

ROOT

Organ
(From a Greek word organon, meaning tool. Here organ/o means body organs.)

Combining form **Organ/o**

WORD EXERCISE 7

Using your Exercise Guide, find the meaning of:

(a) **organ/o**/genesis

(synonymous with organogeny)

(b) **organ/o**/genic

(c) **organ/o**/trophic

Systems

Groups of organs interact to form the fourth level of organization, the system, e.g. the stomach, duodenum, colon, etc. interact to form the digestive system that digests and absorbs food. Units 2–17 introduce medical terms associated with the main body systems.

CASE HISTORY 1

The object of this exercise is to understand words associated with a patient's medical history.

To complete the exercise:

- read through the passage on diagnosis of an AIDs related infection; unfamiliar words are underlined and you can find their meaning using the Word Help

- write the meaning of the medical terms shown in bold print on the lines that follow the Word Help.

Diagnosis of an AIDS related infection

Mr A, a 34-year-old <u>HIV positive</u> patient with symptoms of <u>AIDs</u>, was admitted to the unit following a chest X-ray that revealed a left upper lobe <u>mass</u>.

A <u>CT</u> scan confirmed the presence of a mass within the <u>peripheral aspect</u> of the left upper <u>lobe</u>, and a small left <u>pleural effusion</u>. CT guided fine needle <u>aspiration</u> of the left upper lobe mass was performed and the <u>biopsy</u> material sent to the **histology** laboratory for analysis by the duty **pathologist**.

Cytological examination of direct smears using optical **microscopy** revealed a <u>mucoid</u> background, moderate <u>cellularity</u>, <u>polymorphonuclear</u> **leucocytes** (Am. leukocytes), **lymphocytes** and <u>histiocytes</u>. A significant number of oval yeast-like cells were observed that appeared to be <u>budding</u>. No <u>malignant</u> cells were observed.

A sample of the biopsy material was sent for <u>culture and sensitivity</u> testing to the **microbiology** laboratory. The report was positive for <u>encapsulated</u> fungal yeast forms <u>morphologically</u> compatible with **pathogenic** <u>cryptococcus</u> species (*Cryptococcus neoformans*). Mr A's diagnosis was <u>cryptococcosis</u>, a condition seen mainly in AIDs patients and others with <u>compromised</u> immune systems.

WORD HELP

AIDs acquired immune deficiency syndrome

aspect part of a surface facing a designated direction

aspiration withdrawal by suction of a fluid

biopsy removal and examination of living tissue

budding performing asexual reproduction by producing buds that grow into new cells

cellularity state/condition of being made up of cells

compromised lacking the ability to mount an adequate immune response

cryptococcus a yeast-like fungus that causes disease in humans

cryptococcosis abnormal condition of infection with cryptococcus

CT computed tomography, a technique of using X-rays to image a slice or section through the body

culture & sensitivity testing growing microorganisms in the laboratory and testing them for sensitivity to antibiotics

effusion a fluid discharge into a part/escape of fluid into an enclosed space

encapsulated enclosed on a capsule or sheath

histiocytes the word means a tissue cell (actually a large cell found in connective tissue that helps defend against infection)

HIV-positive presence of antibodies to the human immunodeficiency virus in the blood, it indicates the virus has infected the body

lobe a division of an organ into smaller sections, here a lobe of the lung

malignant dangerous, life threatening

mass lump/collection of cohering cells

morphologically referring to the form and structure of an organism

mucoid resembling mucus

peripheral pertaining to the periphery i.e. the surface of an organ, outermost part, exteriority

pleural pertaining to the pleura/pleural membranes that surround the lungs

polymorphonuclear pertaining to or having nuclei of many shapes

Now write the meaning of the following words from the case history without using your dictionary lists:

(a) histology

(b) pathologist

(c) cytological

(d) microscopy

(e) leucocyte

(Am. leukocyte)

(f) lymphocyte

(g) microbiology

(h) pathogenic

(Answers to the case history exercise are given in the Answers to Word Exercises beginning on page 301)

Quick Reference

Combining forms relating to levels of organization:

Blast/o	immature cell/cell that forms . . .
Chondr/o	cartilage
Cyt/o	cell
Granul/o	granule
Hist/i/o	tissue
Lymph/o	lymph
Melan/o	pigment/melanin
Oo	egg/ovum
Organ/o	organ
Oste/o	bone
Path/o	disease
Spermat/o	sperm

Abbreviations

Some common abbreviations related to cells and tissues are listed below. Note some are not standard and their meaning may vary from one health care setting to another. There is a more extensive list for reference on page 335

Diff	differential blood count (of cell types)
FBC	full blood count (of cells)
GCSF	granulocyte colony stimulating factor
Histo	histology (lab)
HLA	human leucocyte antigen
Lymphos	lymphocytes
NK	natural killer (cells)
Pap	Papanicolaou smear test (of cervical cells)
PCV	packed cell volume
RBC	red blood count/red blood cell
RCC	red cell count
WBC	white blood cell/white blood count

NOW TRY THE WORD CHECK

WORD CHECK

This self-check exercise lists all the word components used in this unit. First write down the meaning of as many word components as you can. Then check your answers using the Exercise Guide and Quick Reference box or the Glossary of Word Components (pp. 347–371.)

Prefixes

micro-

Combining forms of word roots

bio-

blast/o

chem/o

chondr/o

cyt/o

erythr/o

fibr/o

granul/o

hist/i/o

leuc/o

lymph/o

melan/o

oo-

organ/o

oste/o

path/o

spermat/o

tox/o

Suffixes

-blast

-genic

-genesis

-ic

-ical

-ist

-log(ist)

-logy

-lysis

-pathy

-scope

-scop(ist)

-scopy

-tox(ic)

-trophic

NOW TRY THE SELF-ASSESSMENT

SELF-ASSESSMENT

Test 1A

Prefixes, suffixes and combining forms of word roots

Match each word component in Column A with a meaning in Column C by inserting the appropriate number in Column B.

Column A	Column B	Column C
(a) chem/o		1. egg
(b) cyt/o		2. bone
(c) erythr/o		3. white
(d) granul/o		4. study of
(e) hist/i/o		5. pigment (black)
(f) leuc/o		6. sperm cells
(g) -log(ist)		7. chemical
(h) -logy		8. tissue
(i) lymph/o		9. person who studies (specialist)
(j) -lysis		10. small
(k) melan/o		11. specialist who views/examines
(l) micro-		12. breakdown/ disintegration
(m) oo		13. poisonous/ pertaining to poison
(n) oste/o		14. cell
(o) -pathy		15. visual examination
(p) -scope		16. disease
(q) -scop(ist)		17. lymph
(r) -scopy		18. red
(s) spermat/o		19. granule
(t) -tox(ic)		20. viewing instrument

Score

20

Test 1B

Write the meaning of:

(a) chondrolysis

(b) leucocytolysis

(c) histotoxic

(d) osteopathy

(e) lymphoblast

Score

5

Test 1C

This type of test may seem difficult at first but as the terms become familiar you will improve.

Build words that mean:

(a) small cell

(b) person who specializes in the study of disease

(c) person who specializes in the study of disease of cells

(d) scientific study of cartilage

(e) pertaining to disease of cells

Score

5

Check answers to Self-Assessment Tests on page 325.

UNIT 2
THE DIGESTIVE SYSTEM

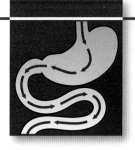

EXERCISE GUIDE

Use this list of word components and their meanings to complete the word exercises in this unit.

Prefixes

a-	without
endo-	inside/within
epi-	upon/above
mega-	large
para-	beside
peri-	around

Suffixes

-aemia	condition of blood
-al	pertaining to
-algia	condition of pain
-clysis	infusion/injection into
-ectomy	removal of
-emia (Am.)	condition of blood
-gram	X-ray/tracing/recording
-graphy	technique of recording/making X-ray
-ia	condition of
-iasis	abnormal condition
-ic	pertaining to
-ist	specialist
-itis	inflammation of
-lith	stone
-lithiasis	abnormal condition of stones
-logist	specialist who studies . . .
-logy	study of
-lysis	breakdown/disintegration
-megaly	enlargement
-oma	tumour/swelling
-pathy	disease of
-scope	instrument used to view/examine
-scopy	technique of viewing/examining
-stomy	formation of an opening into . . .
-tomy	incision into
-toxic	pertaining to poisoning
-uria	condition of the urine

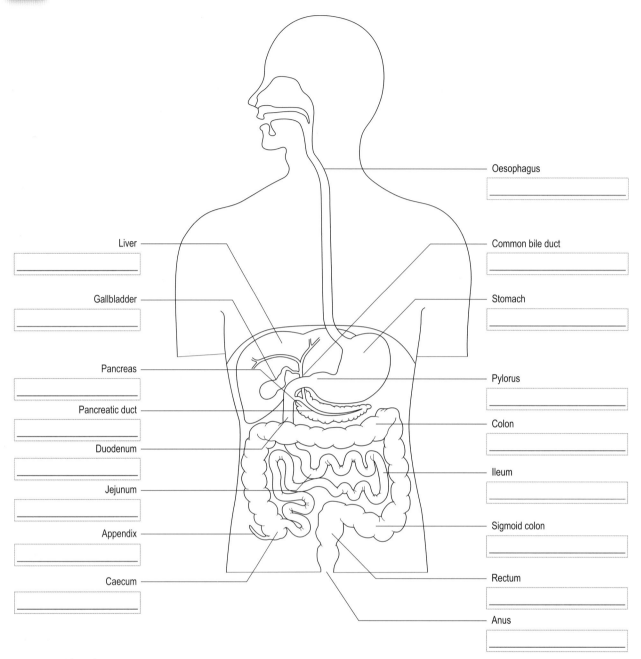

Figure 6   The digestive system

ANATOMY EXERCISE

When you have finished Word Exercises 1–12, look at the word components listed below. Complete Figure 6 by writing the appropriate combining form on each line. (You can check their meanings in the Quick Reference box on page 23)

Appendic/o	Gastr/o	Pancreatic/o
Caec/o, Cec/o (Am.)	Hepat/o	Proct/o
Cholecyst/o	Ile/o	Pylor/o
Choledoch/o	Jejun/o	Rect/o
Col/o	Oesophag/o, Esophag/o (Am.)	Sigmoid/o
Duoden/o	Pancreat/o	

The digestive system

The organs that compose the digestive system digest, absorb and process nutrients taken in as food. Materials not absorbed into the lining of the intestine form the faeces and leave the body through the anus.

Our study of the digestive system begins at the point where food leaves the mouth and enters the gullet or oesophagus.

Use the Exercise Guide at the beginning of this unit to complete Word Exercises 1–12 unless you are asked to work without it.

ROOT

Oesophag
(From a Greek word **oisophagos**, *meaning oesophagus or gullet.)*

Combining forms **Oesophag/o**
　　　　　　　　Esophag/o *(Am.)*

WORD EXERCISE 1

Using your Exercise Guide, find the meaning of:

(a) **oesophag/o**/scope
　　(Am. **esophag/o**/scope)

Remember that, to understand the meaning of these medical terms, we read the components from the suffix towards the beginning of the word.

(b) **oesophag**/ectomy
　　(Am. **esophag**/ectomy)

(c) **oesophag/o**/tomy
　　(Am. **esophag/o**/tomy)

(d) **oesophag**/itis
　　(Am. **esophag**/itis)

Once you have learnt the suffixes in Word Exercise 1, it is easy to work out the meaning of other words with similar endings. Now we will use the same suffixes again with a different word root.

ROOT

Gastr
(From a Greek word **gaster**, *meaning stomach.)*

Combining form **Gastr/o**

WORD EXERCISE 2

Without using your Exercise Guide, write the meaning of:

(a) **gastr/o**/scope

(b) **gastr**/ectomy

(c) **gastr/o**/tomy

(d) **gastr**/itis

Using your Exercise Guide find the meaning of epi-, -ic, -logist, -logy, -pathy and -scopy and then build words that mean:

(e) disease of the stomach

(f) study of the stomach

(g) pertaining to upon or above the stomach

(h) a specialist who studies the stomach

(i) technique of viewing/ examining the stomach

(Remember when building words, the vowel of the combining form is usually dropped if the suffix begins with a vowel.)

Note. A naso **gastr**ic tube (nas/o meaning nose) that passes through the nose to the stomach can be used for suction, irrigation or feeding.

ROOT

Enter
(From a Greek word **enteron**, *meaning intestine or gut.)*

Combining form **Enter/o**

WORD EXERCISE 3

Without using your Exercise Guide, write the meaning of:

(a) **enter**/itis

(b) **enter/o**/pathy

(c) **enter/o**/tomy

Using your Exercise Guide, find the meaning of:

(d) **enter/o**/stomy

Here you need to note the difference between:

-ectomy
A surgical procedure in which a part is removed by cutting. (Synonymous with the words excision and resection.)

-stomy
A surgical procedure in which an opening is made into a cavity or a communication is formed between cavities. The word also refers to the name of the opening or stoma so created e.g. a colostomy is an opening into the colon or the procedure of forming the opening (From the Greek word *stoma* meaning mouth). This word component is also used in anastomosis, an opening or communication formed between two parts (Fig. 7). Note a stoma can be temporary or permanent.

-tomy
A surgical procedure in which an incision is made as at the beginning of an operation.

(e) **enter/o/lith**

Without using your Exercise Guide, build words that mean:

(f) study of the intestine

(g) a person who specialises in the study of the intestines

Now we can put the combining forms of two roots together to make a larger word. Although these words look complicated it is now quite easy to understand their meaning.

Without using your Exercise Guide, write the meaning of:

(h) gastr/o/**enter/o**/logy

(i) gastr/o/**enter/o**/pathy

(j) gastr/o/**enter**/itis

(k) gastr/o/**enter/o**/scopy

Note. When the combining forms of two roots **gastr/o** and **enter/o** are joined, the combining vowel of the first root is retained.

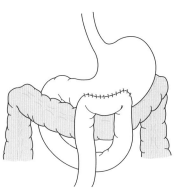

Stomach to intestine (side to side)

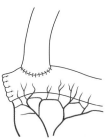

Intestine to intestine (side to end)

Figure 7   Surgical anastomoses

Between the stomach and the small intestine there is an aperture surrounded by a sphincter muscle known as the **pylorus** (see Fig. 6). This acts as a valve that opens periodically to allow digested food to leave the stomach.

ROOT

Pylor
(From a Greek word **pylouros**, *meaning gate-keeper. Here pylor/o means the pylorus, the opening of the stomach into the duodenum encircled by a sphincter muscle.)*

Combining form   **Pylor/o**

WORD EXERCISE 4

Without using your Exercise Guide, write the meaning of:

(a) **pylor/o/gastr/ectomy**

(b) **pylor/o/scopy**

The small intestine

Now we'll examine the small intestine that consists of three parts, the **duodenum, jejunum** and **ileum**. The duodenum is concerned mainly with digestion of food while the jejunum and ileum are specially adapted for the absorption of nutrients. Food is moved along the lumen (internal space) of the intestines and other parts of the alimentary canal by a process called **peristalsis** (from a Greek word *peristellein* meaning to clasp). This is brought about by a wave of contraction of smooth muscle in the wall of the intestine followed by a wave of relaxation.

Note. Although the root **enter** refers generally to intestines, it is often used to mean the small intestine. However, there are special roots that describe the different regions of the intestine; we shall use these in the next three exercises.

ROOT

Duoden
*(From a Latin word **duodeni**, meaning twelve. Here duoden/o means the duodenum, the structure that forms the first 12 inches of the small intestine.)*

Combining form **Duoden/o**

ROOT

Jejun
*(From a Latin word **jejunus**, meaning empty. Here jejun/o means the jejunum, the part of the intestine between the duodenum and ileum approx 2.4 m in length.)*

Combining form **Jejun/o**

ROOT

Ile
*(From a Latin word **ilia**, meaning flanks. Here ile/o means the ileum, the part that forms the lower three-fifths of the small intestine.)*

Combining form **Ile/o**

WORD EXERCISE 5

Without using your Exercise Guide, write the meaning of:

(a) **duoden/o/enter/o/stomy**

(b) **jejun/o/jejun/o/stomy**

Using your Exercise Guide, find the meaning of:

(c) **duoden/o/jejun/al**

Without using your Exercise Guide, build words that mean:

(d) formation of an opening into the ileum

(e) inflammation of the ileum

(Exception to the 'rule' two vowels together)

A permanent opening or **ileostomy** is made when the whole of the large intestine has been removed. This acts as an artificial anus. The ileum opens directly on to the abdominal wall and the liquid discharge from it is collected in a plastic **ileostomy bag** (Fig. 8).

After passing through the small intestine, any remaining material passes into the large intestine. (Note **small bowel** and **large bowel** are used colloquially to mean the small and large intestine.)

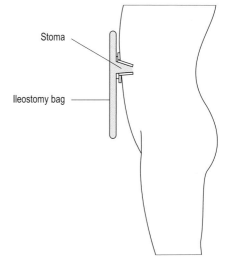

Figure 8 Ileostomy

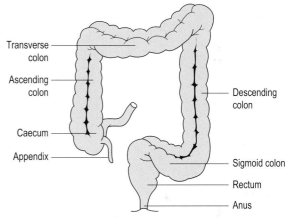

Figure 9 The large intestine

The large intestine

The large intestine has a wider diameter than the small intestine and it is shorter. Its main function is to absorb water from the materials that remain after digestion and eject them from the body as faeces (Am. feces) during defaecation. The large intestine is made up of the **caecum** (Am. cecum), **appendix**, **colon**, **rectum** and **anus** (Fig. 9).

The next six roots refer to the large intestine:

ROOT

Caec
*(From a Latin word **caecus** meaning blind. Here caec/o means the caecum, the blindly ending pouch that is attached to the vermiform appendix and separated from the ileum by the ileocaecal valve.)*

Combining forms **Caec/o**
Cec/o *(Am.)*

ROOT

Append
*(From a Latin word **appendix**, meaning appendage. Here appendic/o means the appendix, a blindly ending sac attached to the caecum.)*

Combining forms   **Appendic/o**
                           Append/o *(Am.)*

ROOT

Col
*(From a Greek word **kolon**, meaning colon, the part of the large intestine (large bowel) extending from the caecum to the rectum.)*

Combining forms   **Col/o, colon/o**

WORD EXERCISE 6

Using your Exercise Guide, find the meaning of:

(a) mega/**colon**

Without using your Exercise Guide, write the meaning of:

(b) **appendic**/itis

(c) **col**/ectomy

(d) **col**/o/stomy
(see Fig. 10)

A colostomy may be temporary or permanent and acts as an opening through which the effluent from the colon is discharged. The effluent is collected in a **colostomy bag** attached to the surface of the abdomen.

Without using your Exercise Guide, build words that mean:

(e) formation of an opening into the caecum (Am. cecum)

(f) removal of the appendix

(g) formation of an opening (anastomosis) between the colon and stomach

ROOT

Sigm
*(From a Greek word **sigma**, meaning the letter S. Here sigmoid/o means the sigmoid colon, the last part of the descending colon that has an S-shape.)*

Combining form   **Sigmoid/o**

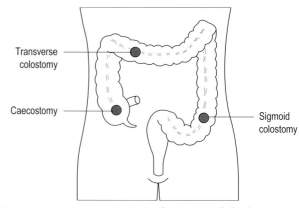

Figure 10   Common sites of stomas of the large intestine (large bowel)

ROOT

Rect
*(From a Latin word **rectus**, meaning straight. Here rect/o means the rectum, the last part of the large intestine which is straight.)*

Combining form   **Rect/o**

ROOT

Proct
*(From a Greek word **proktos**, meaning anus. Here proct/o means the anus or rectum.)*

Combining form   **Proct/o**

WORD EXERCISE 7

Using your Exercise Guide, find the meaning of:

(a) **sigmoid/o**/scopy

(b) para/**rect**/al

(c) peri/**proct**/itis

(d) **proct/o**/clysis

(e) **proct**/algia

Without using your Exercise Guide, build words that mean:

(f) instrument to view anus/ rectum (use proct/o)

(g) formation of an opening between the caecum and anus/rectum (use proct/o)

(h) formation of an opening between the sigmoid colon and caecum (Am. cecum)

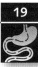

Sometimes the lining of the intestine develops enlarged pouches or sacs. Each is known as a **diverticulum** (pl. **diverticulae**). These can become inflamed as in **diverticulitis** and may have to be removed by **diverticul**ectomy.

The outer layer of the intestines and the lining of the cavity in which they lie consist of serous membrane. This secretes a serum-like fluid called serous fluid that acts as a lubricant. A film of serous fluid allows organs to slide over each other as they move by peristalsis.

ROOT

Peritone
(From Greek words **peri**, *meaning around, and* **teinein**, *meaning to stretch. Here peritone/o means the peritoneum, the serous membrane lining the abdominal and pelvic cavities and covering all abdominal organs.)*

Combining forms **Periton/e/o**

WORD EXERCISE 8

Without using your Exercise Guide, write the meaning of:

(a) **periton**/itis

(b) **peritone**/o/clysis

Accessory organs of the digestive system

The pancreas

This large gland is found beneath the stomach (see Fig. 6). Its function is to produce **pancreatic juice** that is passed to the duodenum where it neutralizes acid and digests food. It can also produce the hormones **insulin** and **glucagon** which are secreted directly into the blood.

ROOT

Pancreat
(From a Greek word **pankreas**, *meaning the pancreas.)*

Combining forms **Pancreat/o**

A combining form **pancreatic/o** *is also derived from this root. It is used to mean the pancreatic duct. This duct transfers pancreatic juice containing digestive enzymes from the pancreas to the duodenum.*

The liver

The liver is the largest abdominal organ and is located just beneath the diaphragm (see Fig. 11). It processes nutrients received from the intestine, stores materials and excretes wastes in the form of **bile** into the intestine.

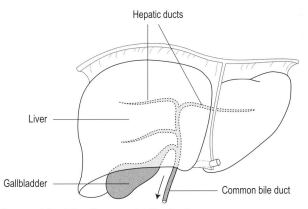

Figure 11   The liver and bile ducts

ROOT

Hepat
(From a Greek word **hepatos**, *meaning the liver.)*

Combining forms **Hepat/o**

A combining form **hepatic/o** *is also derived from this root and is used to mean the hepatic bile duct.*

WORD EXERCISE 9

Using your Exercise Guide, find the meaning of:

(a) **pancreat/o**/lysis

(b) **hepat/o**/megaly

(c) **hepat**/oma

(d) **hepat/o**/toxic

Without using your Exercise Guide, write the meaning of:

(e) **hepatic/o**/gastr/o/stomy

(f) **pancreatic/o**/duoden/al

ROOT

Chol
(From a Greek word **chole**, *meaning bile.)*

Combining form **Chol/e**

Liver cells produce a yellowish-brown waste known as bile. This drains through small canals and hepatic ducts into a sac known as the gallbladder. Bile leaves the gallbladder through the common bile duct and enters the intestine. Although bile is a waste product, the bile salts it contains help to emulsify lipids (fats) in the intestine and neutralize acid entering from the stomach. The structures in which bile is transported are referred to as the **biliary** system (*bili-* meaning bile, *-ary* meaning pertaining to).

WORD EXERCISE 10

Using your Exercise Guide, find the meaning of:

(a) a/**chol**/ia

(b) **chol**/e/lith

(c) **chol**/e/lith/iasis

(d) **chol**/aemia
(Am. chol/emia)

(e) **chol**/uria

A word root commonly combined with **chol/e** is **cyst**, meaning bladder. **Cholecyst/o** literally meaning a bladder of bile is now used to mean the gallbladder.

Without using your Exercise Guide, write the meaning of:

(f) **cholecyst**/o/tomy

(g) **cholecyst**/ectomy

(h) **cholecyst**/o/lith/iasis

A second word root often combined with **chol/e** is **angi** meaning vessel. **Cholangi/o** means bile vessel or bile duct.

Using your Exercise Guide, find the meaning of:

(i) **cholangi**/o/gram

(j) **cholangi**/o/graphy

A third word root often combined with **chol/e** is **doch**, meaning to receive. **Choledoch/o** means the common bile duct, i.e. that which receives the bile.

Without using your Exercise Guide, write the meaning of:

(k) **choledoch**/o/lith/iasis

(l) **choledoch**/o/lith/o/tomy

Here we need to distinguish between three suffixes that often cause some confusion:

-gram
This refers to a tracing. In practice in medicine it usually refers to an X-ray picture, paper recording or to a trace on a screen.

-graphy
This refers to the technique or process of making a recording, e.g. an X-ray or tracing. It can also refer to a written description.

-graph
This means a description or writing but more often it is used in medicine for the name of an instrument that carries out a recording. It is also used to mean a recording or X-ray picture in the term radiograph.

ROOT

Lapar
(From a Greek word **lapara***, meaning loin, the soft part between the ribs and hips. By common usage it has come to mean the abdominal wall.)*

Combining form   **Lapar/o**

WORD EXERCISE 11

Without using your Exercise Guide, write the meaning of:

(a) **lapar**/o/scopy

(b) **lapar**/o/tomy

Laparotomy is an exploratory operation performed when the diagnosis of an abdominal problem is uncertain. With advances in diagnostic procedures such as CT scanning, ultrasonography and laparoscopy, it has become less common.

Laparoscopy is performed using a laparoscope, a device consisting of a thin tube containing a lens system that can be passed through a small hole into the abdominal cavity. The laparoscope allows the internal organs (viscera) to be viewed and manipulated by a surgeon (a procedure commonly called 'keyhole' surgery).

Medical equipment and clinical procedures

The use of medical equipment and clinical procedures enables doctors to make a **diagnosis**, this means naming the patient's disease and distinguishing it from others (from *dia-* meaning through and *-gnosis* meaning knowledge). The information also enables a **prognosis** or forecast of the probable course and termination of a disease to be made (from *pro-* meaning forward).

In this unit we have named several instruments. Let us review their names:

gastroscope	colonoscope
gastroenteroscope	proctoscope
sigmoidoscope	laparoscope

All of these instruments are used to view various parts of the digestive system. Now fibreoptic endoscopes have replaced many of the original viewing instruments. Endoscope means an instrument to view inside (**endo-** within/inside).

Endoscopes utilize flexible/fibreoptic tubes (Fig. 12) that can be inserted into body cavities or into small incisions made in the body wall. Each is provided with illumination and a system of lenses that enables the operator to view the inside of the body. The inclusion of electronic chips at the end of the fibreoptic tube allows the view to be transmitted to a video screen.

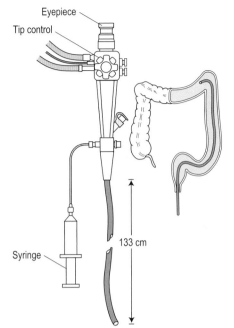

Figure 12   A fibreoptic endoscope used to view the colon

Sometimes the endoscope is used for photography and it is then known as a photoendoscope.

The endoscope can be adapted to view particular areas of the body. In the case of the digestive system, the fibre-optic tube can be passed into the mouth to examine the oesophagus, stomach and intestine. Alternatively it can be passed into the anus to view the rectum and colon. Note that when an endoscope is adapted to examine the stomach it may be referred to as a gastroscope.

Often endoscopes are used to examine the oesophagus, stomach and duodenum at the same examination. This procedure is **pan**endoscopy (**pan-** means all, i.e. all the upper digestive system). Similarly, panendoscopy could be performed on all of the large intestine via the anus.

In addition to viewing cavities, endoscopes can be fitted with a variety of attachments, such as forceps and catheters, and they can then be used for special applications. One such procedure is:

ERCP or **endoscopic, retrograde, cholangiopancreatography**

Let's examine the words separately:

endoscopic	referring to an endoscope
retrograde	going backwards
chol	bile
angio	vessel
pancreato	pancreas
graphy	technique of making a tracing/X-ray recording

Although we cannot deduce the exact meaning from the words we can see why they have been used. Here is the meaning of ERCP:

A technique of making an X-ray (graphy) of the pancreatic and bile vessels (chol/angi/o/pancreat/o) by passing a tube called a catheter backwards (retrograde) into them using an endoscope. Dye is injected through the catheter to outline the vessels on the X-ray.

WORD EXERCISE 12

Match each term in Column A with a description from Column C by placing an appropriate number in Column B.

Column A	Column B	Column C
(a) enteroscope		1. an instrument used to view the rectum or anus
(b) endoscope		2. technique of taking photographs using an endoscope
(c) enteroscopy		3. visual examination of the colon
(d) endoscopy		4. an instrument used to view the intestines
(e) endoscopist		5. visual examination of all cavities, e.g. oesophagus, stomach and duodenum
(f) colonoscopy		6. an instrument used to view body cavities
(g) proctoscope		7. visual examination of the intestine
(h) sigmoidoscopy		8. a person who operates an endoscope
(i) panendoscopy		9. visual examination of body cavities
(j) photoendoscopy		10. visual examination of the sigmoid colon

ANATOMY EXERCISE

Now complete the Anatomy Exercise on page 14.

CASE HISTORY 2

The object of this exercise is to understand words associated with a patient's medical history. To complete the exercise:

• read through the passage on gallstones; unfamiliar words are underlined and you can find their meaning using the Word Help

• write the meaning of the medical terms shown in bold print on the lines that follow the Word Help.

Gallstones (cholelithiasis)

Miss B, a 35-year-old, presented to her general practitioner complaining of pain emanating from the **epigastric** and right hypochondrial regions radiating to the back. The pain lasted for about 3 hours following each meal and was accompanied by nausea and occasional vomiting. Her GP's initial diagnosis was **biliary** colic, and he prescribed the analgesic pethidine. The pain did not resolve and she was admitted to the **gastroenterology** unit.

Initial ultrasound investigations revealed multiple stones in the gallbladder and a dilated common bile duct. A date was set for early elective **laparoscopic cholecystectomy.** Miss B was counselled on her peri-operative drug regimen and was introduced to the concept of patient controlled analgesia (PCA) using a syringe driver. Unfortunately, her elective procedure was delayed by an episode of acute **cholecystitis.**

Once recovered Miss B was admitted again but due to her excessive weight, laparoscopy was deemed inappropriate by the surgeon and she was advised of the associative risks of an alternative procedure.

Vital signs on admission

Pulse 90/minute	Oral temp 37°C	BP 140/70
Height 1.52 m	Weight 85 kg	Smoker 25/day
Moderate drinker	Medication None	

An open cholecystectomy was performed and the inflamed gallbladder found to contain three gallstones each approximately 1.5 cm in diameter. A bile sample was sent for culture and sensitivity testing and a **nasogastric** tube passed. Antibiotic prophylaxis (cefuroxime) was administered prior to her operation and continued for 48 hours. Miss B also received low dose subcutaneous heparin injections as part of her thromboembolic prophylaxis.

The patient tolerated surgery well, PCA controlled her pain and she was apyrexial. In the immediate post-operative period she received an intravenous (i.v.) infusion of dextrose 4%, NaCl 0.18%, KCl 0.05% at a rate of 125 mL/hour.

On day four following her operation, the nasogastric tube and wound drains were removed and i.v. fluid replacement ceased. Miss B left the unit on day six and was provided with diclofenac 50 mg analgesic tablets to be taken up to 3 times daily when required. She agreed to an appointment with the dietician to discuss the desirability of reducing her weight.

WORD HELP

analgesic pain relieving drug

apyrexial absence of fever

culture and sensitivity testing growing microorganisms in the laboratory and testing them for sensitivity to antibiotics

dietician/dietitian specialist who plans and advises on diet with the approval of medical staff

elective voluntary/not an emergency/at a planned date

GP general practitioner (family doctor)

heparin an anticoagulant drug that prevents blood clotting

hypochondrial the region to the side, just below the ribs

intravenous pertaining to within a vein

open refers to surgery via an incision (here into the abdomen)

peri-operative around the time of an operation

post-operative pertaining to after/following an operation

prophylaxis preventative treatment

regimen a regulated scheme (e.g. of taking drugs/medication)

subcutaneous pertaining to under the skin

syringe driver a motorized device that injects medication/drugs into the body

thromboembolic a thrombus or clot moving and blocking another blood vessel

ultrasound using sound waves to produce an image

Now write the meaning of the following words from the case history without using your dictionary lists:

(a) cholelithiasis

(b) epigastric

(c) biliary

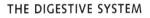
(d) gastroenterology

(e) laparoscopic

(f) cholecystectomy

(g) cholecystitis

(h) nasogastric

(Answers to the case history exercise are given in the Answers to Word Exercises beginning on page 301)

Quick Reference

Combining forms relating to the digestive system:

Appendic/o	appendix
Bil/i	bile
Caec/o	caecum
Cec/o (Am.)	cecum
Chol/e	bile
Cholangi/o	bile vessel/duct
Cholecyst/o	gallbladder
Choledoch/o	common bile duct
Col/o	colon
Colon/o	colon
Diverticul/o	diverticulum
Duoden/o	duodenum
Enter/o	intestine
Esophag/o (Am.)	esophagus
Gastr/o	stomach
Hepat/o	liver
Hepatic/o	hepatic duct
Ile/o	ileum
Jejun/o	jejunum
Lapar/o	flank/abdominal wall
Oesophag/o	oesophagus
Pancreat/o	pancreas
Pancreatic/o	pancreatic duct
Peritone/o	peritoneum
Proct/o	anus/rectum
Pylor/o	pyloric sphincter
Rect/o	rectum
Ser/o	serous/serum
Sigmoid/o	sigmoid colon

Abbreviations

Some common abbreviations related to the digestive system are listed below. Note some are not standard and their meaning may vary from one health care setting to another. There is a more extensive list for reference on page 335

Abdo	abdomen
CD	Crohn's disease
DU	duodenal ulcer

GI	gastrointestinal
GU	gastric ulcer
IUC	idiopathic ulcerative colitis
LLQ	left lower quadrant
pr/PR	per rectum
PU	peptic ulcer
RE	rectal examination
UC	ulcerative colitis
UGI	upper gastrointestinal

Medical Notes

Borborygmi
Rumbling noises caused by movement of gas and fluid in the intestines. From a Greek word *borborizein-* meaning to rumble in the bowels.

Eructation (belching)
The process of expelling of gas from the stomach through the mouth.

Flatus
Gas in the stomach and intestines usually applied to that passed rectally. Flatulence is the presence of large amounts of gas dilating the stomach and intestines. (From a Latin word *flatus* meaning a blowing)

Cancer
Stomach cancer has been linked to excessive alcohol consumption, use of chewing tobacco, and eating smoked or preserved food. Most stomach cancers usually adenocarcinomas, have already metastasized (spread) before they are found because patients treat themselves for the early warning signs of heartburn, belching and nausea. Later warning signs of stomach cancer include chronic indigestion, vomiting, anorexia, stomach pain and blood in the faeces. Surgical removal of the malignant tumours has been the most successful method of treating this condition.

Colorectal cancer is a malignancy, usually adenocarcinoma of the colon and rectum that occurs most frequently after the age of fifty, a low-fibre, high-fat diet and genetic predisposition are known risk factors. Early warning signs of this common type of cancer include changes in bowel habits, faecal (Am. fecal) blood, rectal bleeding, abdominal pain, unexplained anaemia (Am. anemia) or weight loss and fatigue.

Gastro-oesophageal reflux disease (GORD), (Am. Gastro-esophageal reflux disease (GERD))
Backward flow of stomach acid up into the oesophagus (Am. esophagus) causes sensations of burning and pressure behind the breastbone; these symptoms are commonly referred to as heartburn or acid indigestion. In their simplest form GORD symptoms are mild and occur only infrequently. In these cases, avoiding problem foods or beverages, stopping smoking or

losing weight may solve the problem. Additional treatment with over the counter antacids or non-prescription strength acid-blocking medications called H_2-receptor antagonists may also be used. If left untreated, serious pathological (precancerous) lesions may develop in the lining of the oesophagus, these changes are known as Barrett's oesophagus.

Hepatitis

Hepatitis is a general term referring to inflammation of the liver. Hepatitis is characterized by jaundice (a yellowish discoloration of body tissues), liver enlargement, anorexia, abdominal discomfort, grey-white faeces (Am. feces), and dark urine. Various conditions can produce hepatitis, for example, excess alcohol, drugs, toxins and infection with bacteria, viruses or parasites. *Hepatitis A* results from infection by the hepatitis A virus, often acquired from contaminated food. It occurs commonly in young people and ranges in severity from mild to life threatening. Viral *Hepatitis B* is usually more severe, this is also called serum hepatitis because it is transmitted by contaminated blood serum. Hepatitis B causes severe illness that may lead to necrosis of the liver and death. It also predisposes victims to liver cancer. Hepatitis C is transmitted through blood, is common amongst IV drug users and leads to chronic liver disease.

All these conditions may lead to a degenerative condition known as *cirrhosis*. The liver's ability to regenerate damaged tissue is well known, but it has its limits. When the toxic effects of alcohol accumulate faster than the liver can regenerate itself, damaged tissue is replaced with fibrous scar tissue instead of normal tissue. Cirrhosis is the name given to such degeneration.

Inflammatory bowel disease (IBD)
Crohn's disease (regional ileitis)

This is a chronic inflammation of the alimentary tract that usually occurs in young adults. The terminal ileum and rectum are most commonly affected but the disease may be present anywhere from the mouth to the anus. The full thickness of the intestinal wall is inflamed in patches sometimes causing obstruction of the lumen of the intestine. The cause of Crohn's disease is not clear but an immunological abnormality may render the individual susceptible to infection by viruses or other organisms.

Ulcerative colitis

This is a chronic inflammatory disease of the inner lining (mucosa) of the colon and rectum that may ulcerate and become infected. It usually occurs in young adults and begins in the rectum and sigmoid colon. It can spread and involve part or the whole of the colon and the cause is unknown. Surgical removal of the entire colon cures the condition.

Intussusception

A condition in which one part of the intestine telescopes into another, it causes severe colic and intestinal obstruction. The portion that has prolapsed in this way is called an intussusceptum.

Irritable bowel syndrome (IBS)

This is also called spastic colon and is a common chronic non-inflammatory condition that is often caused by stress. Diarrhoea (Am. diarrhea) or constipation with or without pain characterizes irritable bowel syndrome.

Ulcers

An ulcer is an open wound or sore in the area of the digestive system that is acted upon by the gastric juice. The two most common sites for ulcers are the stomach (gastric ulcers) and the upper part of the small intestine or duodenum (duodenal ulcers). Disintegration and death of tissue characterize ulcers as they erode the layers in the wall of the stomach or duodenum. Left-untreated ulcers cause persistent pain and may perforate the digestive tube causing massive haemorrhage (Am. hemorrhage) and widespread inflammation of the abdominal cavity. Most experts now agree that hyperacidity is only partly to blame for most ulcers, the underlying cause is a spiral-shaped bacterium called *Helicobacter pylori*. The presence of this organism in the stomach lining impairs its ability to secrete mucus and opens the way for stomach acid to begin its destruction of the gastric tissue.

Volvulus

Twisting of a section of the intestine so as to occlude its lumen (internal space). Volvulus is a main cause of intestinal obstruction and constitutes a surgical emergency.

NOW TRY THE WORD CHECK

WORD CHECK

This self-check exercise lists all the word components used in this unit. First write down the meaning of as many word components as you can. Then check your answers using the Exercise Guide and Quick Reference box or the Glossary of Word Components (pp. 347–371).

Prefixes

a-

endo-

epi-

mega-

pan-

para-peri-

retro-

Combining forms of word roots

angi/o

appendic/o

bil/i

caec/o
(Am. cec/o)

chol/e

choledoch/o

col/o

colon/o

cyst/o

diverticul/o

duoden/o

enter/o

gastr/o

hepat/o

hepatic/o

ile/o

jejun/o

lapar/o

nas/o

oesophag/o
(Am. esophag/o)

pancreat/o

pancreatic/o

peritone/o

proct/o

pylor/o

rect/o

ser/o

sigmoid/o

tox/o

Suffixes

-aemia
(Am. -emia)

-al

-algia

-ary

-clysis

-ectomy

-grade

-gram

-graph

-graphy

-ia

-iasis

-ic

-ist

-itis

-lith

-lithiasis

-logist

-logy

-lysis

-megaly

-oma

-pathy

-scope

-scopy

-stomy

-tomy

-toxic

-uria

NOW TRY THE SELF-ASSESSMENT

SELF-ASSESSMENT

Test 2A

Below are some combining forms that refer to the anatomy of the digestive system. Indicate which part of the system they refer to by putting a number from the diagram (Fig. 13) next to each word. You can use a number more than once.

(a) pylor/o

(b) gastr/o

(c) proct/o

(d) hepat/o

(e) appendic/o

(f) choledoch/o

(g) col/o

(h) pancreat/o

(i) sigmoid/o

(j) oesophag/o
(Am. esophag/o)

(k) cholecyst/o

(l) ile/o

(m) caec/o
(Am. cec/o)

(n) duoden/o

(o) rect/o

Score [15]

Test 2B

Prefixes and suffixes

Match each prefix or suffix in Column A with a meaning in Column C by inserting the appropriate number in Column B.

Column A	Column B	Column C
(a) a-		1. enlargement
(b) -aemia (Am. -emia)		2. condition of pain
(c) -algia		3. study of
(d) -clysis		4. around
(e) -ectomy		5. injection/infusion
(f) endo-		6. X-ray/tracing
(g) -gram		7. inflammation
(h) -graph		8. condition of urine
(i) -graphy		9. within/inside
(j) -itis		10. beside/near
(k) -lithiasis		11. tumour (Am. tumor)
(l) -logy		12. abnormal condition of stones
(m) mega-		13. all
(n) -megaly		14. without
(o) -oma		15. technique of making an X-ray/tracing/recording
(p) pan-		16. large

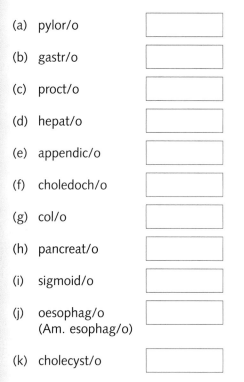

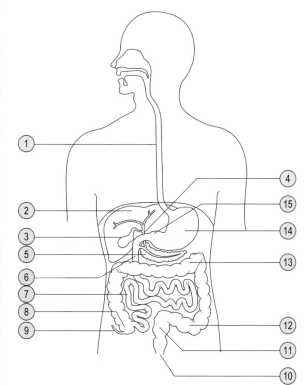

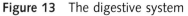

Figure 13 The digestive system

(q) para- [ ]   17. instrument which records

(r) peri- [ ]   18. incision into

(s) -tomy [ ]   19. removal of

(t) -uria [ ]   20. condition of blood

Score [ ]
20

(s) rect/o [ ]   19. liver

(t) sigmoid/o [ ]   20. appendix

Score [ ]
20

Test 2C

Combining forms of word roots

Match each combining form of a word root from Column A with a meaning from Column C by inserting the appropriate number in Column B.

Column A	Column B	Column C
(a) angi/o	[ ]	1. pylorus
(b) appendic/o	[ ]	2. sigmoid colon
(c) caec/o (Am. cec/o)	[ ]	3. peritoneum
(d) chol/e	[ ]	4. jejunum
(e) choledoch/o	[ ]	5. intestine
(f) colon/o	[ ]	6. vessel
(g) cyst/o	[ ]	7. duodenum
(h) duoden/o	[ ]	8. colon
(i) enter/o	[ ]	9. rectum
(j) gastr/o	[ ]	10. rectum/anus
(k) hepat/o	[ ]	11. bladder
(l) jejun/o	[ ]	12. stomach
(m) lapar/o	[ ]	13. oesophagus
(n) oesophag/o (Am. esophag/o)	[ ]	14. bile
(o) pancreat/o	[ ]	15. abdomen/flank
(p) peritone/o	[ ]	16. common bile duct
(q) proct/o	[ ]	17. caecum
(r) pylor/o	[ ]	18. pancreas

Test 2D

Write the meaning of:

(a) gastroenterocolitis [ ]

(b) hepatography [ ]

(c) ileorectal [ ]

(d) proctosigmoidoscope [ ]

(e) pancreatomegaly [ ]

Score [ ]
5

Test 2E

Build words that mean:

(a) inflammation of the duodenum [ ]

(b) condition of pain in the stomach [ ]

(c) incision into the liver [ ]

(d) study of the anus/rectum [ ]

(e) formation of an opening/ anastomosis between the anus and the ileum [ ]

Score [ ]
5

Check answers to Self-Assessment Tests on page 325.

UNIT 3
THE RESPIRATORY SYSTEM

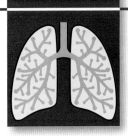

OBJECTIVES

Once you have completed Unit 3 you should be able to:

- understand the meaning of medical words relating to the respiratory system
- build medical words relating to the respiratory system
- associate medical terms with their anatomical position
- understand medical abbreviations relating to the respiratory system.

EXERCISE GUIDE

Use this list of word components and their meanings to complete the word exercises in this unit.

Prefixes

a-	without
dys-	difficult/painful
hyper-	above/excessive
hypo-	below/low
inter-	between
tachy-	fast

Roots/Combining forms

chondr/o	cartilage
esophag/o	esophagus (Am.)
gastr/o	stomach
haem/o	blood
hem/o (Am.)	blood
hepat/o	liver
myc/o	fungus
oesophag/o	oesophagus
radi/o	radiation/X-ray

Suffixes

-al	pertaining to
-algia	condition of pain
-ary	pertaining to
-centesis	surgical puncture to remove fluid
-desis	fixation/bind together by surgery/sticking together
-dynia	condition of pain
-eal	pertaining to
-ectasis	dilatation/stretching
-ectomy	removal of
-genic	pertaining to formation/originating in
-gram	X-ray/tracing/recording
-graphy	technique of recording/making X-ray
-ia	condition of
-ic	pertaining to
-itis	inflammation of
-logy	study of
-meter	measuring instrument
-metry	process of measuring
-osis	abnormal condition/disease of
-pathy	disease of
-plasty	surgical repair/reconstruction
-pexy	surgical fixation/fix in place
-plegia	condition of paralysis
-rrhaphy	stitching /suturing
-rrhea (Am.)	excessive discharge/flow
-rrhoea	excessive discharge/flow
-scope	an instrument to view/examine
-scopy	technique of viewing/examining
-spasm	involuntary contraction
-stenosis	abnormal condition of narrowing
-stomy	formation of an opening into . . .
-tomy	incision into
-us	thing/a structure (indicates an anatomical part)

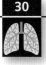

ANATOMY EXERCISE

When you have finished Word Exercises 1–16, look at the word components listed below. Complete Figure 14 by writing the appropriate combining form on each line – more than one component may relate to the same position. (You can check their meanings in the Quick Reference box on p. 37)

Bronch/o	Nasopharyng/o	Pulmon/o
Cost/o	Pharyng/o	Rhin/o
Laryng/o	Phren/o	Steth/o
Lob/o	Pleur/o	Trache/o
Nas/o	Pneumon/o	

enters the blood in exchange for carbon dioxide. During expiration, air containing less oxygen and more carbon dioxide leaves the body. The oxygen obtained through gaseous exchange is required by body cells for cellular respiration, a process that releases energy from food.

Our study of the respiratory system begins at the point where air enters the body, the nose.

Use the Exercise Guide at the beginning of this unit to complete Word Exercises 1–16 unless you are asked to work without it.

The respiratory system

Humans breathe air into paired lungs through the nose and mouth during inspiration. Whilst air is in the lungs gaseous exchange takes place; in this process oxygen

ROOT

Rhin
*(From a Greek word **rhinos**, meaning nose.)*

Combining form **Rhin/o**

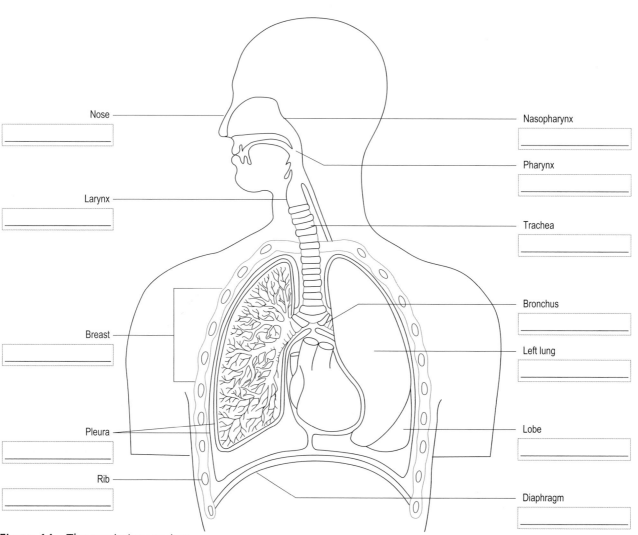

Figure 14 The respiratory system

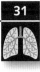

WORD EXERCISE 1

Using your Exercise Guide, find the meaning of:

(a) **rhin/o**/scopy

(b) **rhin/o**/pathy

(c) **rhin**/algia

(d) **rhin**/itis

(e) **rhin/o**/rrhoea
(Am. **rhin/o**/rrhea)

(f) **rhin/o**/plasty

ROOT

Nas
(From a Latin word **nasus**, *meaning nose.)*

Combining form **Nas/o**

WORD EXERCISE 2

Using your Exercise Guide, find the meaning of:

(a) **nas/o**/gastr/ic tube

(b) **nas/o**-oesophag/eal tube
(Am. **nas/o**-esophag/eal)

ROOT

Pharyng
(From a Greek word **pharynx**, *meaning throat. Here pharyng/o means the pharynx, the cone-shaped cavity at the back of the mouth lined with mucous membrane.)*

Combining form **Pharyng/o**

WORD EXERCISE 3

Without using your Exercise Guide, write the meaning of:

(a) **pharyng**/algia

(b) **pharyng/o**/rrhoea
(Am. **pharyng/o**/rrhea)

Without using your Exercise Guide, build words that mean:

(c) surgical repair of the pharynx

(d) inflammation of the nose and pharynx (use rhin/o)

ROOT

Laryng
(From a Greek word **larynx** *meaning the voice box. Here laryng/o means the larynx, the organ that produces the voice.)*

Combining form **Laryng/o**

WORD EXERCISE 4

Using your Exercise Guide, find the meaning of:

(a) **laryng/o**/logy

(b) **laryng/o**/pharyng/ectomy

Without using your Exercise Guide, build words that mean:

(c) technique of viewing the larynx

(d) the study of the nose and larynx (use rhin/o).

When swallowing, food is prevented from falling into the larynx by the **epiglottis**, a thin flap of cartilage lying above the glottis and behind the tongue. When the epiglottis moves, it covers the opening into the larynx and sound-producing glottis. **Epiglott/o** is the combining form derived from epiglottis; inflammation of the epiglottis may produce **epiglott**itis and tumours may be removed by **epiglott**ectomy.

ROOT

Trache
(From Greek **tracheia**, *meaning rough. Here trache/o means the trachea or windpipe, a structure containing rings of cartilage that give it a rough appearance.)*

Combining form **Trache/o**

WORD EXERCISE 5

Using your Exercise Guide, find the meaning of:

(a) **trache/o**/tomy

(b) **trache/o**/stomy

(an operation performed to maintain the airway or the name of the opening so created; see Fig. 15)

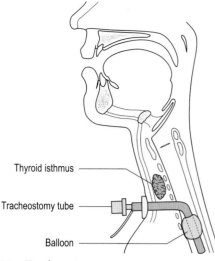

Figure 15   Tracheostomy

ROOT

Bronch

(From a Greek word **bronchos**, *meaning windpipe. Here bronch/o means the bronchi, two large air passages formed by division of the trachea that enter the lungs.)*

Combining forms   Bronch/i/o

WORD EXERCISE 6

Using your Exercise Guide find the meanings of, -gram, -graphy, -rrhoea (Am. -rrhea) and -scope and then build words that mean:

(a) discharge/excessive flow of mucus from bronchi

(b) an X-ray picture of the bronchi

(c) technique of making an X-ray of the bronchi

(d) an instrument for the visual examination of the bronchi

Using your Exercise Guide, find the meaning of:

(e) **bronch**/us (Singular bronchi)

(f) **bronch**/o/plegia

(g) **bronch**/o/rrhaphy

(h) **bronchi**/ectasis

(i) **bronch**/o/myc/osis

(j) **bronch**/o/genic

(k) **bronch**/o/spasm

(l) trache/o/**bronchi**/al

Without using your Exercise Guide, write the meaning of:

(m) laryng/o/trache/o/**bronch**/itis

(n) **bronch**/oesophag/o/stomy (Am. **bronch**/esophag/o/stomy)

> **Note.** The combining form **bronchiol/o** is used when referring to the very small subdivisions of the bronchi known as **bronchioles**, e.g. **bronchiol**itis for inflammation of the bronchioles.

The smallest bronchioles end in microscopic air sacs known as **alveoli** (from Latin *alveus*, meaning hollow cavity). Alveoli form a large surface area of the lungs across which the gases oxygen and carbon dioxide are exchanged and therefore play an essential role in maintaining life. The combining form is **alveol**/o, but few terms are in use, e.g. **alveol**itis.

At the alveolar surface oxygen diffuses into the blood from the cavities of the alveoli, carbon dioxide diffuses in the opposite direction and is lost from the body in expired air. Disorders of the respiratory and cardiovascular systems can affect gaseous exchange and therefore the concentration of these gases in the blood. **Hypoxia** is a condition of deficiency of oxygen in the tissues (*hypo-* meaning below/low, *-oxia* meaning condition of oxygen). **Hypercapnia** is a condition of too much carbon dioxide in the blood (*hyper-* meaning above/ excessive, *-capnia* meaning a condition of carbon dioxide).

Poor oxygenation also results in the presence of large amounts of unoxygenated haemoglobin (Am. hemoglobin) in the blood. This produces **cyanosis**, an abnormal condition in which unoxygenated haemoglobin gives a blue tinge to the skin, lips and nail beds (*cyan/o* meaning blue, *-osis* meaning abnormal condition).

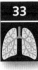

ROOT

Pneumon
(A Greek word, meaning lung.)

Combining form   **Pneumon/o**

WORD EXERCISE 7

Without using your Exercise Guide, write the meaning of:

(a) **pneumon/o**/tomy

(b) **pneumon/o**/rrhaphy

(c) **pneumon**/osis

> **Note.** Pneumonia means a condition of the lungs. It refers to an inflammation of the lungs with exudation caused by infection. (The exudate is a fluid that has escaped from capillaries lining the lungs).

Without using your Exercise Guide, build words that mean:

(d) removal of a lung

(e) disease of a lung

Using your Exercise Guide, find the meaning of:

(f) **pneumon/o**/centesis

(g) **pneumon/o**/pexy

ROOT

Pneum
*(From a Greek word **pneuma**, meaning air. In the following examples pneum/o and pneumat/o means gas or air but they can be used to mean the lungs or breathing.)*

Combining forms   **Pneum/a/o, Pneumat/o**

At this point we need to introduce the word **pneumothorax**. The components of this word refer to air and thorax (chest) but the meaning of the word is not obvious. It means air or gas in the pleural cavity, i.e. the space between the wall of the thorax and the lungs. A pneumothorax is formed by puncture of the chest wall; a stab wound or incision made as part of a surgical procedure can cause this.

WORD EXERCISE 8

Using your Exercise Guide, find the meaning of:

(a) **pneum/o**/haem/o/thorax (Am.
pneum/o/hem/o/thorax; see Fig. 16)

(b) **pneum/o**/radi/o/graphy (This term does not refer specifically to the respiratory system. It is a technique used to enhance the contrast of X-rays of body cavities by injecting air into them.)

A combining form **-pnoea** (Am. **-pnea**), is derived from the Greek word **pnoia** meaning breathing or from **pnein** meaning to breathe.

Using your Exercise Guide, find the meaning of:

(c) a/**pnoea** (Am. a/**pnea**)

(d) dys/**pnoea** (Am. dys/**pnea**)

(e) hyper/**pnoea** (Am. hyper/**pnea**)

(f) hypo/**pnoea** (Am. hypo/**pnea**)

(g) tachy/**pnoea** (Am. tachy/**pnea**)

ROOT

Lob
*(From a Greek word **lobos**, meaning lobe, a rounded section of an organ. In the lungs, lobes are formed by fissures or septa that divide the right lung into three lobes and the left lung into two. Note that other organs in the body are lobar.)*

Combining form   **Lob/o**

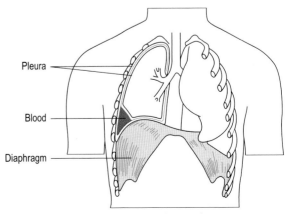

Pleura

Blood

Diaphragm

Figure 16   Haemothorax (Am.hemothorax)

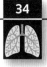

WORD EXERCISE 9

Without using your Exercise Guide, build words that mean:

(a) incision into a lobe

(b) removal of a lobe

ROOT

Pulmon
(From a Latin word **pulmonis**, *meaning lung.)*

Combining form **Pulmon/o**

WORD EXERCISE 10

Using your Exercise Guide, find the meaning of:

(a) **pulmon**/ic

(b) **pulmon**/ary

ROOT

Pleur
(From a Greek word **pleura**, *meaning rib. Here pleur/o means pleura, the shiny membranes covering the lungs and internal surfaces of the thorax. The space in between these membranes is known as the pleural cavity.)*

Combining form **Pleur/o**

WORD EXERCISE 11

Without using your Exercise Guide, write the meaning of:

(a) **pleur**/itis (also called pleurisy)

(b) **pleur/o**/centesis

Without using your Exercise Guide, build a word that means:

(c) technique of making an X-ray/recording of the pleura (pleural cavity)

Using your Exercise Guide, find the meaning of:

(d) **pleur/o**/dynia

(e) **pleur/o**/desis

ROOT

Phren
(A Greek word, meaning midriff. Here phren/o means the diaphragm, the muscular septum separating the thorax and abdomen that acts as the main respiratory muscle.)

Combining form **Phren/o**

WORD EXERCISE 12

Using your Exercise Guide, find the meaning of:

(a) **phren/o**/gastr/ic

(b) **phren/o**/hepat/ic

(c) **phren/o**/pleg/ia

ROOT

Thorac
(From a Greek word **thorax**, *meaning chest.)*

Combining form **Thorac/o, -thorax** *is used as a suffix*

WORD EXERCISE 13

Without using your Exercise Guide, build words that mean:

(a) disease of the thorax

(b) incision into the chest

Without using your Exercise Guide, write the meaning of:

(c) **thorac/o**/centesis

(d) **thorac/o**/scope

Using your Exercise Guide, find the meaning of:

(e) **thorac/o**/stenosis

ROOT

Cost
(From a Latin word **costa**, *meaning rib, one of the twelve pairs of curved bones that form part of the thorax.)*

Combining form **Cost/o**

WORD EXERCISE 14

Using your Exercise Guide, find the meaning of:

(a) inter/**cost**/al

(b) **cost/o**/genic

(c) **cost/o**/chondr/itis

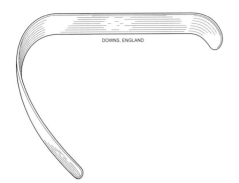

Figure 17 A tongue depressor

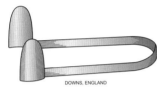

Figure 18 A nasal speculum

Medical equipment and clinical procedures

In this unit we have named several instruments used to examine the respiratory system. Some of those mentioned may be modified fibreoptic endoscopes. Here's a review of their names:

rhinoscope
pharyngoscope
laryngoscope
bronchoscope
thoracoscope

The nose and pharynx can be superficially examined using a source of illumination with a tongue depressor and a nasal speculum (Figs 17 and 18).

> **Note.** The word **speculum** refers to an instrument used to hold the walls of a cavity apart so that its interior can be examined visually.

Other instruments used to investigate the respiratory system include:

Stethoscope

(From a Greek word stethos, meaning breast, and skopein, meaning to examine.) Although this word ends in -scope, which usually refers to an instrument for visual examination, a stethoscope is used to listen to the sounds from the chest.

Spirograph

(From a Latin word spirare, meaning to breathe.) An instrument that records the breathing movements of the lungs.

Spirometer

An instrument that measures the capacity of the lungs. The technique for using this instrument is known as spirometry (synonymous with pneumatometry).

We also need to distinguish between the suffixes:

> **-meter**
> an instrument that measures.
>
> **-metry**
> the technique of measuring, i.e. using a measuring instrument.

Now revise the names and uses of all instruments and clinical procedures mentioned in this unit and then try Exercises 15 and 16.

WORD EXERCISE 15

Match each term in Column A with a description from Column C by placing an appropriate number in Column B.

Column A	Column B	Column C
(a) bronchoscope		1. a person who may use a nasal speculum
(b) laryngoscopy		2. an instrument used to examine the vocal cords
(c) rhinoscope		3. an instrument used to examine the bronchi
(d) pharyngoscope		4. visual examination of the vocal cords
(e) bronchoscopy		5. a device used to allow air through the tracheal wall
(f) rhinologist		6. an instrument used to view the back of the mouth
(g) tracheostomy tube		7. visual examination of the bronchi
(h) laryngoscope		8. an instrument used to view nasal cavities

WORD EXERCISE 16

Match each term in Column A with a description from Column C by placing an appropriate number in Column B.

Column A	Column B	Column C
(a) thoracoscope		1. an instrument used to open the nostrils
(b) stethoscope		2. technique of making an X-ray/ recording of the pleura (pleural cavity)
(c) spirometer		3. technique of recording breathing movements
(d) spirography		4. technique of measuring lung capacity
(e) nasal speculum		5. an instrument used to view the thorax
(f) nasogastric tube		6. an instrument that measures lung capacity
(g) pleurography		7. an instrument used to examine/ listen to the breast
(h) spirometry		8. a tube inserted into the stomach via the nose

ANATOMY EXERCISE

Now complete the Anatomy Exercise on page 30.

CASE HISTORY 3

The object of this exercise is to understand words associated with a patient's medical history.

To complete the exercise:

- read through the passage on chronic obstructive pulmonary disease; unfamiliar words are underlined and you can find their meaning using the Word Help

- write the meaning of the medical terms shown in bold print on the lines that follow the Word Help.

Chronic obstructive pulmonary disease

Mr C is 56 years of age and has a long history of chronic obstructive **pulmonary** disease (COPD). He began smoking at the age of 14 and until 6 years ago smoked approximately 25–30 cigarettes per day but now only smokes 2 or 3 per week. Five years ago he developed a squamous cell carcinoma and had a right upper **lobectomy.**

Mr C has had two acute exacerbations of bronchitis in the past year. His wife says that over the last few days he has become increasingly out of breath and has difficulty in walking, speaking and eating. He was seen in casualty with increasing **dyspnoea (Am. dyspnea)**, **cyanosis** and a productive, purulent sputum.

Vital signs on admission
Pulse 100/min   Oral temp 38°C   BP 150/95

Medication
Home oxygen   salbutamol 5 mg nebulized
therapy   prednisolone 30 mg/day

Blood Gas Analysis

$paCO_2$ 8.90 kPa (4.5–6.1)	Standard bicarbonate 29.2 (22–28)	PEFR 180 L/min
paO_2 4.5 kPa (12–15)	Blood pH 7.05 (7.32–7.42)	

On examination he had a degree of **bronchospasm** and was showing signs of **hypoxia** and **hypercapnia**. His serious condition required his immediate transfer to the intensive therapy unit (ITU) for mechanical ventilatory support. An arterial catheter for blood gas sampling was inserted via the left radial artery, and he was sedated. He was given a muscle relaxant intravenously to enable tracheal intubation and commencement of intermittent positive pressure ventilation (IPPV).

Mr C was initially diagnosed as having basal **pneumonia** in the right lung complicating his COPD. He was administered one intravenous dose of 500 mg of ampicillin followed by 500 mg amoxicillin 8-hourly.

WORD HELP

acute symptoms/signs of short duration

carcinoma a malignant growth of epidermal cells/ a cancer

catheter a tube inserted into the body

chronic lasting/lingering for a long time

exacerbations acute increased severity of symptoms

intravenous pertaining to within a vein

intubation insertion of a tube into a hollow organ in this case the trachea

productive producing e.g. producing mucus/sputum

purulent resembling pus/infected

sedated state of reduced activity usually as a result of medication

sputum material expelled from the respiratory passages by coughing or clearing the throat

squamous pertaining to scale-like/from a squamous epithelium

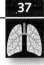

Now write the meaning of the following words from the case history without using your dictionary lists:

(a) pulmonary

(b) lobectomy

(c) dyspnoea (Am. dyspnea)

(d) cyanosis

(e) bronchospasm

(f) hypoxia

(g) hypercapnia

(h) pneumonia

(Answers to the case history exercise are given in the Answers to Word Exercises beginning on page 301)

Quick Reference

Combining forms relating to the respiratory system:

Alveol/o	alveolus
Bronch/o	bronchus
Bronchiol/o	bronchiole
Chondr/o	cartilage
Cost/o	rib
Epiglott/o	epiglottis
Laryng/o	larynx
Lob/o	lobe
Nas/o	nose
Nasopharyng/o	nasopharynx
Pharyng/o	pharynx
Phren/o	diaphragm
Pleur/o	pleura
Pneum/o	gas/air/lung
Pneumon/o	lung/air
-pnoea	breathing
-pnea (Am.)	breathing
Pulmon/o	lung
Rhin/o	nose
Spir/o	to breathe
Steth/o	breast
Thorac/o	thorax
Trache/o	trachea

Abbreviations

Some common abbreviations related to the respiratory system are listed below. Note some are not standard and their meaning may vary from one health care setting to another. There is a more extensive list for reference on page 335.

BRO	bronchoscopy
COPD	chronic obstructive pulmonary disease

CXR	chest X-ray
ET	endotracheal
FVC	forced vital capacity
LLL	left lower lobe
PE	pulmonary embolism
PEFR	peak expiratory flow rate
PFts	pulmonary function tests
RSV	respiratory syncytial virus
SOBE	shortage of breath on exertion
URTI	upper respiratory tract infection

Medical Notes

Asthma
Asthma is an obstructive lung disorder characterized by recurring inflammation of mucous membranes and spasms of smooth muscles in the walls of bronchial air passages. The inflammation and contraction of smooth muscle narrow the airways and make breathing difficult. Initial onset of asthma can occur in children or adults. Stress, heavy exercise, infection or exposure to allergens or other irritants such as dusts, vapours, or fumes can trigger acute episodes of asthma, so called 'asthma attacks'. Many patients with asthma have a family history of allergies. Dyspnoea (Am. dyspnea) is the major symptom but hyperventilation, headaches, numbness and nausea can occur. One way to treat asthma is by using inhaled or systemic bronchodilators that reduce muscle spasms and open the airways. Other types of treatment use anti-inflammatory medications or leukotriene modifiers that reduce the inflammation associated with asthma.

Atelectasis
A condition in which there is collapse of lung tissue with a consequent reduction in gaseous exchange. It may be due to failure of the alveoli to expand in the newborn (congenital atelectasis) or to resorption of air from the alveoli (collapse).

Chronic obstructive pulmonary disease (COPD)
This is a broad term used to describe conditions of progressive, irreversible obstruction of expiratory airflow. Patients with COPD have a productive cough, difficulty in breathing (mainly emptying their lungs), and develop visibly hyperinflated chests. The major disorders observed in people with this condition are bronchitis, emphysema, and asthma.

Cor pulmonale
Failure of the right side of the heart to pump sufficient blood to the lungs, it results from chronic respiratory disease.

Emphysema
In this condition the walls of the alveoli lose their elasticity and remain filled with air on expiration. As emphysema progresses large numbers of alveoli are damaged and they become permanently dilated due to

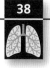

loss of interstitial connective tissue. These changes result in a hyperinflated chest known as a 'barrel chest'. Emphysema is associated with long term exposure to cigarette smoke or air pollution and victims often suffer the effects of hypoxia.

Lung cancer

Lung cancer is a malignancy of pulmonary tissue that not only destroys the vital gas exchange tissues of the lungs but also like other cancers may invade other parts of the body (metastasis). Lung cancer most often develops in damaged or diseased lungs. The most common predisposing condition associated with lung cancer is cigarette smoking (accounting for about 75% of cases). Other factors include exposure to 'second-hand' cigarette smoke, asbestos, chromium, coal products, petroleum products, rust and ionizing radiation (as in radon gas).

Lung cancer may be arrested if detected early in routine chest X-ray films or other diagnostic procedures such as bronchoscopy. Depending on the size, location and exact type of malignancy involved, several strategies are available for treatment. Chemotherapy can cause a cure or remission in selected cases, as can radiation therapy. Photodynamic therapy (PDT) is also used to treat cancer of the lining of the bronchial tubes. Surgery is the most effective treatment known, but less than half of those diagnosed are good candidates for surgery because of extensive metastatic spread.

Pulmonary embolism

A pulmonary embolism is a sudden obstruction of a pulmonary vessel by an embolus. Emboli can form from blood clots, fat, air and infective material. An embolus in a pulmonary vessel obstructs circulation of blood through the lungs.

Pulmonary oedema (Am. edema)

Pulmonary oedema is a condition in which there is an abnormal accumulation of fluid in the intercellular spaces and alveoli of the lungs, it is due to changes in hydrostatic forces in the capillaries or to an increase in capillary permeability. The condition is characterized by severe dyspnoea (Am. dyspnea), it may develop slowly, as in the patient with renal failure or suddenly in the patient with left ventricular failure.

Rale

An abnormal crackling sound heard on inspiration when fluid is present in the bronchi and alveoli.

Restrictive pulmonary disorder

Restrictive pulmonary disorders involve restriction of the alveoli, or reduced compliance, leading to decreased lung inflation. The hallmark of these disorders, regardless of their cause is a decrease in lung volume, inspiratory reserve volume and vital capacity. Factors that restrict breathing can originate within the lung or the environment. Causes of restrictive lung disorders include *alveolar fibrosis* (scarring) secondary to occupa-

tional exposure to asbestos, toxic fumes, coal dust or other contaminants and immunological disease.

Rhonchi

Loud rales (crackling sounds) caused by air passing through bronchi obstructed by secretions. Singular *rhonchus*.

Stridor

A harsh high-pitched sound on inspiration caused by air passing through constricted air passages.

Tuberculosis (TB)

An infectious communicable disease caused by one of two forms of mycobacterium. Humans are the main host for *Mycobacterium tuberculosis* spread either by droplet infection or dust contaminated with infected sputum. *Mycobacterium bovi* (bovine TB) is transmitted from cows to humans via consumption of unpasteurized milk causing initial infection in the alimentary canal. Tuberculosis can affect any organ but in man the main focus is in the lungs and pleurae where it is marked by formation of tubercles and necrotic tissue. Immunization with attenuated BCG (Bacille-Calmette-Guérin) mycobacterium protects susceptible individuals who are identified by skin testing.

NOW TRY THE WORD CHECK

WORD CHECK

This self-check exercise lists all the word components used in this unit. First write down the meaning of as many word components as you can. Then check your answers using the Exercise Guide and Quick Reference box or the Glossary of Word Components (pp. 347–371).

Prefixes

a-

dys-

hyper-

hypo-

inter-

tachy-

Combining forms of word roots

alveol/o

bronch/o

bronchiol/o

chondr/o

cost/o

cyan/o

epiglott/o

gastr/o

haem/o
(Am. hem/o)

hepat/o

laryng/o

lob/o

myc/o

nas/o

oesophag/o
(Am. esophag/o)

pharyng/o

phren/o

pleur/o

pneum/o

pneumon/o

-pnoea (Am. -pnea)

pulmon/o

radi/o

rhin/o

spir/o

sten/o

thorac/o

trache/o

Suffixes

-al

-algia

-ary

-capnia

-centesis

-desis

-dynia

-ectasis

-ectomy

-genic

-gram

-graphy

-ia

-ic

-itis

-logy

-meter

-metry

-osis

-oxia

-pathy

-pexy

-plasty

-plegia

-rrhaphy

-rrhoea
(Am. rrhea)

-scope

-scopy

-spasm

-stomy

-tomy

-us

NOW TRY THE SELF-ASSESSMENT

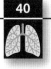

SELF-ASSESSMENT

Test 3A

Below are some combining forms that refer to the anatomy of the respiratory system. Indicate which part of the system they refer to by putting a number from the diagram (Fig. 19) next to each word. The numbers may be used more than once.

(a) bronch/o

(b) nasopharyng/o

(c) phren/o

(d) lob/o

(e) pleur/o

(f) pneum/o

(g) trache/o

(h) laryng/o

(i) pharyng/o

(j) rhin/o

Score

10

Test 3B

Prefixes and Suffixes

Match each prefix and suffix in Column A with a meaning in Column C by inserting the appropriate number in Column B.

Column A	Column B	Column C
(a) -centesis		1. measuring instrument
(b) -desis		2. pertaining to originating in/formation
(c) -dynia		3. opening into/connection between two parts
(d) dys-		4. between
(e) -ectomy		5. abnormal condition/disease of
(f) -genic		6. fixation (by surgery)
(g) hyper-		7. condition of pain
(h) hypo-		8. removal of
(i) inter-		9. excessive flow/discharge
(j) -meter		10. fast
(k) -metry		11. above
(l) -osis		12. difficult/painful
(m) -pexy		13. surgical repair
(n) -plasty		14. puncture
(o) -plegia		15. condition of paralysis
(p) -rrhaphy		16. to bind together
(q) -rrhoea (Am. rrhea)		17. incision into
(r) -stomy		18. below
(s) -tachy		19. technique of measuring
(t) -tomy		20. suturing/stitching

Score

20

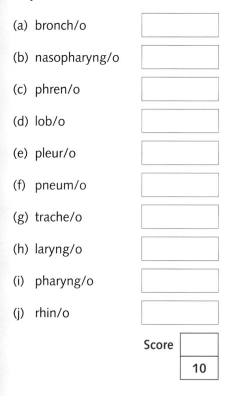

Figure 19 The respiratory system

Test 3C

Combining forms of word roots

Match each combining form in Column A with a meaning in Column C by inserting the appropriate number in Column B.

Column A	Column B	Column C
(a) bronch/o		1. larynx
(b) cost/o		2. diaphragm
(c) enter/o		3. bronchus
(d) epiglott/o		4. thorax
(e) gastr/o		5. intestine
(f) hepat/o		6. pleural membranes
(g) laryng/o		7. stomach
(h) lob/o		8. trachea
(i) myc/o		9. breathing (wind)
(j) nas/o		10. nose (i)
(k) pharyng/o		11. nose (ii)
(l) phren/o		12. fungus
(m) pleur/o		13. lobe
(n) pneum/o		14. pharynx
(o) pneumon/o		15. liver
(p) -pnoea (Am. -pnea)		16. gas/air/wind
(q) rhin/o		17. lung
(r) sten/o		18. epiglottis
(s) thorac/o		19. rib
(t) trache/o		20. narrowing

Score

20

Test 3D

Write the meaning of:

(a) bronchogenic

(b) tracheostenosis

(c) pulmonologist

(d) phrenograph

(e) laryngoplegia

Score

5

Test 3E

Build words that mean:

(a) surgical repair of the bronchus

(b) technique of visually examining bronchi

(c) suturing of the trachea

(d) study of the nose (use rhin/o)

(e) pertaining to the diaphragm and ribs

Score

5

Check answers to Self-Assessment Tests on page 325.

UNIT 4
THE CARDIOVASCULAR SYSTEM

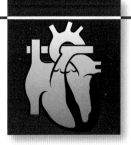

EXERCISE GUIDE

Use this list of word components and their meanings to complete the word exercises in this unit.

Prefixes

a-	without
brady-	slow
dextro-	right
endo-	within/inside
pan-	all
peri-	around
tachy-	fast

Roots/Combining forms

dynam/o	force
ech/o	echo/reflected sound
electr/o	electrical
lith/o	stone
man/o	pressure
my/o	muscle
necr/o	dead, death of
phon/o	sound/voice

Suffixes

-ac	pertaining to
-algia	condition of pain
-ar	pertaining to
-centesis	surgical puncture to remove fluid
-clysis	infusion/injection/irrigation
-ectasis	dilatation/stretching
-ectomy	removal of
-genesis	capable of causing/pertaining to formation

-gram	X-ray/tracing/recording
-graph	usually an instrument that records
-graphy	technique of recording/making X-ray
-ia	condition of
-ic	pertaining to
-itis	inflammation of
-logy	study of
-lysis	breakdown/disintegration
-megaly	enlargement
-meter	measuring instrument
-metry	process of measuring
-oma	tumour/swelling (Am. tumor)
-osis	abnormal condition/disease of
-ous	pertaining to/of the nature of
-pathy	disease of
-plasty	surgical repair/reconstruction
-pexy	surgical fixation/fix in place
-plegia	condition of paralysis
-poiesis	formation
-rrhaphy	stitching/suturing
-sclerosis	abnormal condition of hardening
-scope	an instrument to view/examine
-spasm	involuntary contraction of muscle
-stasis	stopping/controlling/cessation of movement
-stenosis	abnormal condition of narrowing
-tome	cutting instrument
-tomy	incision into
-um	thing/a structure/anatomical part
-us	thing/a structure/anatomical part

ANATOMY EXERCISE

When you have finished Word Exercises 1–16, look at the word components listed below. Complete Figure 20 by writing the appropriate combining form on each line – more than one component may relate to the same position. (You can check their meanings in the Quick Reference box on p. 52)

Aort/o   Pericardi/o   Venacav/o
Arteri/o   Phleb/o   Ven/o
Cardi/o   Valv/o
Myocardi/o   Valvul/o

The cardiovascular system

In order to remain alive, cells within the body need a continuous supply of oxygen and nutrients for their metabolism. Any metabolic wastes excreted by these cells must be transported to the excretory organs where they can be removed from the body. The cardiovascular system provides a transport system for supply and removal of materials to and from the tissue cells; it consists of the heart and blood vessels.

The heart

The heart is a four chambered muscular pump that continuously pushes blood into arteries. The right and left atria (singular – atrium) form the top chambers and the right and left ventricles the lower chambers.

The atria receive blood from veins and push it into the ventricles. The right ventricle then forces blood through the pulmonary arteries to the lungs where it is oxygenated. Simultaneously, the left ventricle forces blood into the systemic circulation through the aorta.

The heart muscle (myocardium) that forms the walls of the chambers, is stimulated to contract rhythmically by a special patch of tissue called the sino-atrial (SA) node or 'pacemaker'. Although the SA node gives the heart the ability to contract by itself, its rate of contraction is determined by nerve impulses from centres in the brain.

The heart muscle receives a supply of fully oxygenated blood from branches of the aorta known as the coronary arteries. If coronary arteries become blocked, the muscle dies triggering a heart attack. Another common cause of death is **heart failure**, defined as the inability of the heart to maintain a flow of blood sufficient to meet the body's needs; the term is most often applied to the heart muscle of either the left or right ventricle. If both ventricles are affected, it is known as **biventricular** heart failure (bi – meaning two).

(The term **atrial** means pertaining to an atrium and **ventricular** means pertaining to a ventricle (-*al* and -*ar* both mean pertaining to.)

Use the Exercise Guide at the beginning of this unit to complete Word Exercises 1–16 unless you are asked to work without it.

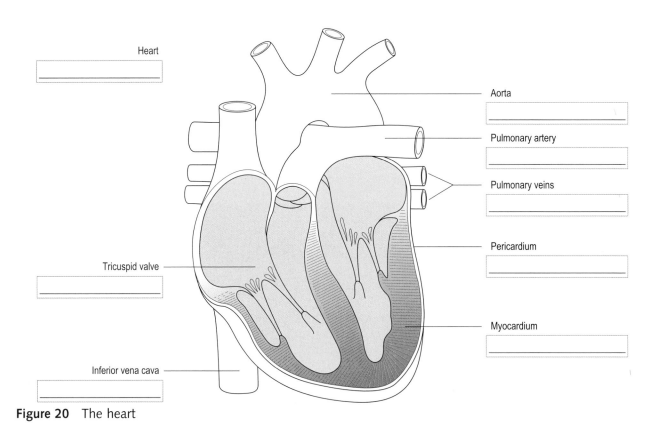

Figure 20 The heart

ROOT

Card
(From a Greek word **kardia***, meaning heart.)*

Combining forms **Card/i/o**

WORD EXERCISE 1

Using your Exercise Guide, find the meaning of:

(a) **cardi**/ac

(b) **cardi**/algia

(c) **cardi**/o/scope

(d) **cardi**/o/graph

(e) **cardi**/o/gram

(f) tachy/**card**/ia

Using your Exercise Guide find the meaning of -logy, -megaly, -pathy, and -plasty and then build words using cardi/o that mean:

(g) enlargement of the heart

(h) surgical repair of the heart

(i) disease of the heart

(j) study of the heart

Using your Exercise Guide, find the meaning of:

(k) my/o/**cardi**/um

(l) **cardi**/o/my/o/pathy

(m) **cardi**/o/rrhaphy

(n) electro/**cardi**/o/graph

(o) endo/**card**/itis

(p) pan/**card**/itis

(q) brady/**card**/ia

(r) dextro/**card**/ia

(s) phon/o/**cardi**/o/graphy

(t) echo/**cardi**/o/graphy

(u) electro/**cardi**/o/gram

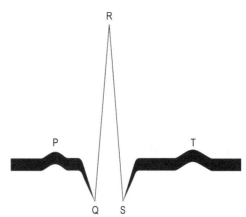
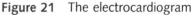

Figure 21 The electrocardiogram

To make an electrocardiogram (ECG; Fig. 21) electrodes are attached to the skin at various sites on the body. The heart muscle generates electrical impulses that can be detected at the surface of the body, amplified and converted into a trace on a screen or paper. The P wave appears when the atria are stimulated, the QRS complex when the impulse passes to the ventricles and the T wave is generated when the ventricles contract. Abnormal electrical activity and changes in heart rate seen in coronary heart disease can be detected from the ECG.

The heart is continuously supplied with blood through coronary arteries. Narrowing of these vessels results in **ischaemia**, a deficient blood supply (*isch-* meaning to check) that produces the chest pain known as **angina pectoris**. If the flow of blood to the heart muscle is interrupted, the muscle dies; this is a **myocardial infarction** or heart attack. Heart muscle deprived of oxygen produces a rapid, uncoordinated, quivering contraction known as **fibrillation**. Applying an electric shock with an instrument known as a defibrillator can sometimes restore normal rhythm.

Around the heart there is a double membranous sac known as the **pericardium** (peri-, prefix meaning around). Between the membranes is the pericardial cavity containing a small amount of fluid. The combining forms of pericardium are **pericard/o** and **pericardi/o**.

WORD EXERCISE 2

Without using your Exercise Guide, build a word that means:

(a) inflammation of the pericardium

Using your Exercise Guide, find the meaning of:

(b) cardi/o/**pericardi**/o/pexy

(c) **pericardi**/o/centesis

(d) **pericardi**/ectomy

ROOT

Valv
*(From Latin **valva**, meaning fold. Here valv/o means a valve, a fold or flap in a tube or passage that permits flow of fluid in one direction only.)*

Combining form   **Valv/o**

Valves control blood flow through the heart. Between the right atrium and the right ventricle there is a **tricuspid valve** (with three flaps or cusps) that allows blood to flow from the right atrium to the right ventricle but not in the opposite direction. Similarly there is a valve on the left side of the heart that allows blood to flow from the left atrium to the left ventricle. This is known as the **bicuspid valve** or the **mitral valve** (with two flaps or cusps).

The **aortic semilunar valve** in the aorta and the **pulmonary semilunar valve** in the pulmonary artery prevent backflow of blood into the ventricles.

WORD EXERCISE 3

Without using your Exercise Guide, build words that mean:

(a) surgical repair of a heart valve

(b) removal of a heart valve

Valvul/o is a New Latin combining form also derived from *valva*; using your Exercise Guide, find the meaning of:

(c) cardio/**valvul**/o/tome

Note. -tome comes from *tomon*, meaning cutter.
Using your Exercise Guide, find the meaning of:

(d) **valvul**/ar

(e) **valv**/o/tomy

The blood vessels

Blood circulates through a closed system of blood vessels throughout the body. It flows away from the heart in arteries that divide into smaller arterioles and then into capillaries. Blood flows back to the heart through venules and then into larger vessels known as veins. The system that supplies blood to the tissues is known as the **arterial system** and that which takes it away the **venous system**. Now we will look at some of the terms concerned with blood vessels.

ROOT

Vas
*(A Latin word, meaning **vessel**. Here vas/o means a blood vessel of any type.)*

Combining forms   **Vas/o**

> **Vascul/o**, *also derived from vas, means a small blood vessel of any type.*

WORD EXERCISE 4

Using your Exercise Guide, find the meaning of:

(a) **vas/o**/spasm

Blood vessels can widen (**vaso**dilatation) and they can narrow (**vaso**constriction) because of the activity of smooth muscle in their walls. If a vessel widens then the blood pressure within it falls. Some drugs are designed to stimulate this action, i.e. reducing blood pressure, and are known as **vasodilators** and antihypertensives.

(b) a/**vascul**/ar

Without using your Exercise Guide, build words using vascul/o that mean:

(c) inflammation of blood vessels

(d) disease of blood vessels

ROOT

Angi
*(From a Greek word **angeion**, meaning vessel. Here angi/o means a blood vessel of any type.)*

Combining form   **Angi/o**

WORD EXERCISE 5

Without using your Exercise Guide, write the meaning of:

(a) **angi/o**/gram

(b) **angi/o**/cardi/o/gram

(c) **angi/o**/cardi/o/graphy

Angiography is the technique of making X-rays or images of blood vessels. Both arteries and veins can be made visible on radiographic film following the injection of a contrast medium. This results in an X-ray film on which the injected vessels cast a shadow showing their size, shape and location.

Digital subtraction angiography (DSA) is very similar, except, instead of having an X-ray film, the X-rays are detected electronically and a computer builds an image of the blood vessels on a monitor.

One problem in visualizing blood vessels is that overlying tissues cast an image on the picture. To eliminate these unwanted images, an X-ray is taken before and after dye is injected. A computer then subtracts the first image from the second, removing the interfering image. The picture produced by DSA is superior to a film-based angiogram.

Without using your Exercise Guide, build words that mean:

(d) study of blood vessels

(e) surgical repair of blood vessels

A common surgical repair is a balloon angioplasty. In this procedure a catheter containing an inflatable balloon is inserted into a narrowed vessel (see Fig. 22). When the balloon is inflated and moved along the lining any fatty plaques are displaced and the flow of blood through the vessel is restored.

Using your Exercise Guide, find the meaning of:

(f) **angi**/oma

(g) **angi**/ectasis

(h) **angi**/o/poiesis

(i) **angi**/o/sclerosis

The above roots refer generally to blood vessels. Now we will look at roots that refer to specific types of vessel.

ROOT

Aort

*(From Greek **aorte**, meaning great vessel. Here aort/o means the aorta, the largest artery in the body. The aorta leaves the left ventricle of the heart and divides into smaller arteries that supply all body systems with oxygenated blood.)*

Combining form **Aort/o**

WORD EXERCISE 6

Without using your Exercise Guide, build words that mean:

(a) disease of the aorta

(b) technique of X-raying the aorta

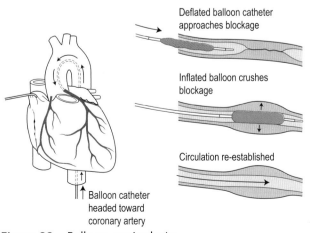

Deflated balloon catheter approaches blockage

Inflated balloon crushes blockage

Circulation re-established

Balloon catheter headed toward coronary artery

Figure 22 Balloon angioplasty

ROOT

Arter

*(From a Greek word **arteria**, meaning artery. The function of arteries is to move blood away from the heart. Arteries divide into smaller arterioles and then into capillaries that exchange materials with the tissue cells.)*

Combining forms **Arter/i/o**

WORD EXERCISE 7

Without using your Exercise Guide, build words using arteri/o that mean:

(a) suturing of an artery

(b) condition of hardening of arteries

Using your Exercise Guide, find the meaning of:

(c) end/**arter**/ectomy

(In this procedure fatty deposits are removed from the lining of the artery.)

(d) **arteri**/o/necr/osis

(e) **arteri**/o/stenosis

ROOT

Vena cav

*(From Latin **vena cavum**, meaning hollow vein. Here venacav/o means the venae cavae, the great veins of the body that drain blood into the heart.)*

Combining form **Venacav/o**

Venae cavae are the great veins of the body; the **superior vena cava** drains blood from the head and upper body the **inferior vena cava** drains blood from the lower parts of the body. They pass their blood into the right atrium of the heart.

WORD EXERCISE 8

Without using your Exercise Guide, write the meaning of:

(a) **venacav**/o/gram

(b) **venacav**/o/graphy

ROOT

Ven

*(From a Latin word **vena**, meaning vein. The function of veins is to transfer blood back to the heart. Capillaries are drained by small vessels called venules, these join and form larger veins. Unlike arteries, veins contain valves that prevent the backflow of blood.)*

Combining form **Ven/o**

WORD EXERCISE 9

Using your Exercise Guide, find the meaning of:

(a) **ven**/ectasis

(b) **ven**/o/clysis

(c) **ven**/ous

Without using your Exercise Guide, build words that mean:

(d) X-ray picture of a vein
(after injection of opaque dye)

(e) technique of making an
X-ray of a vein or the
venous system

ROOT

Phleb
*(From a Greek word **phlebos**, meaning vein.)*

Combining form   **Phleb/o**

WORD EXERCISE 10

Without using your Exercise Guide, write the meaning of:

(a) **phleb**/arteri/ectasis

(b) **phleb**/o/clysis

(c) **phleb**/o/tomy

Using your Exercise Guide, find the meaning of:

(d) **phleb**/o/stasis

(e) **phleb**/o/man/o/meter

(f) **phleb**/o/lith

ROOT

Thromb
*(From a Greek word **thrombos**, meaning a clot. Blood clots are formed mainly of platelets, fibrin and blood cells, they can block blood vessels, restricting or stopping the flow of blood.)*

Combining form   **Thromb/o**

WORD EXERCISE 11

Without using your Exercise Guide, write the meaning of:

(a) **thromb**/o/poiesis

(b) **thromb**/o/phleb/itis

(c) **thromb**/o/end/arter/ectomy

Without using your Exercise Guide, build words that mean:

(d) abnormal condition of
having a clot

(e) removal of a clot

Using your Exercise Guide, find the meaning of:

(f) **thromb**/o/genesis

(g) **thromb**/o/lysis

The sudden blocking of an artery by a clot is referred to as an **embolism**. Thrombi as well as other foreign materials, such as fat, air and infective material can cause emboli. The combining form **embol/o** is used when referring to an **embolus**, e.g. as in **embol**ectomy.

The development of enzymes that can dissolve blood clots in situ has led to the development of **thrombolytic therapies**. For example the drug streptokinase, extracted from bacteria, can be injected into the coronary vessels to lyse a clot and thereby restore blood in the coronary system. The thrombolytic drugs streptokinase, altepase and anistreplase have all been shown to reduce mortality when given by the intravenous route following a heart attack (acute myocardial infarction).

ROOT

Ather
*(From a Greek word **athere**, meaning porridge or meal. Here ather/o means atheroma, a fatty plaque that forms on the inner walls of blood vessels.)*

Combining form   **Ather/o**

The term **ather**oma means a porridge-like tumour and is used to indicate the presence of fatty plaques in the lining of arteries. Atheroma is a common disorder of blood vessels and the presence of such deposits is often related to aspects of one's lifestyle such as smoking, lack of exercise and diets rich in certain types of fat. Atheroma in coronary arteries increases the chance of their becoming blocked, thus predisposing the heart to myocardial infarction.

WORD EXERCISE 12

Without using your Exercise Guide, write the meaning of:

(a) **ather/o**/genesis

(b) **ather/o**/embolus

Atherosclerosis is a common form of arteriosclerosis that results from the presence of atheroma and calcification in vessel walls. Contributing factors to the development of this condition include advanced age, diabetes, high-fat and high-cholesterol diets, hypertension and smoking.

ROOT

Aneurysm
*(From Greek **aneurysma**, meaning a dilatation. Here aneurysm/o means an aneurysm, a dilated vessel, usually an artery. An aneurysm is caused by a localized fault in a vessel wall through a defect, disease or injury; it appears as a pulsating swelling that can rupture.)*

Combining form   Aneurysm/o

WORD EXERCISE 13

Without using your Exercise Guide, write the meaning of:

(a) **aneurysm/o**/plasty

(b) **aneurysm/o**/rrhaphy

ROOT

Sphygm
*(From a Greek word **sphygmos**, meaning pulsation. Here sphygm/o means the pulse, the rhythmical throbbing that can be felt wherever an artery is near to the surface of the body. The pulsation is due to the heart forcing blood into the arterial system at ventricular systole (contraction). Pulse rate is therefore a measure of heart rate.)*

Combining form   Sphygm/o

WORD EXERCISE 14

Using your Exercise Guide, find the meaning of:

(a) **sphygm/o**/dynam/o/meter

(b) **sphygm/o**/man/o/meter

(c) **sphygm/o**/metry

Without using your Exercise Guide, write the meaning of:

(d) **sphygm/o**/graph

(e) **sphygm/o**/gram
(refers to movements created by the arterial pulse)

(f) **sphygm/o**/cardi/o/graph

Note. Man/o comes from Greek *manos*, meaning rare. Manometers were first used for measuring rarefied air, i.e. gases. The combining form **man/o** is now used to mean pressure.

Figure 23 is a drawing of an instrument that uses a manometer to measure blood pressure. Two pressures are measured: the **systolic** pressure when the ventricles of the heart are forcing blood into the circulation, and the **diastolic** pressure which is the pressure within the vessels when the heart is dilating and refilling.

The sphygmomanometer can be used to detect **hypertension**, i.e. a persistently high arterial blood pressure, or **hypotension**, an abnormally low blood pressure. Both of these conditions have a variety of causes.

The **stethoscope** (Fig. 24) is used in conjunction with the sphygmomanometer to listen to the sounds made by blood flowing through the brachial artery when recording the blood pressure.

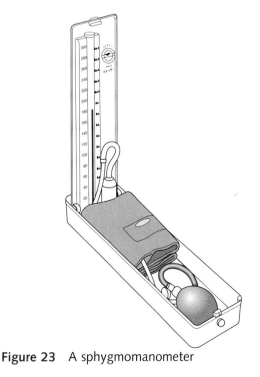

Figure 23   A sphygmomanometer

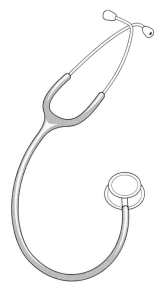

Figure 24   A stethoscope

Note. In medicine the suffix -scope usually refers to an instrument used for visual examination. However, it is used in stethoscope to mean an instrument to examine the breast (from **steth/o** – breast). We can use it in this way because -scope comes from the Greek word *skopein* that means to examine. In practice, a stethoscope is used for listening to body sounds (auscultation).

Medical equipment and clinical procedures

In this unit we have named several instruments that are used to examine the cardiovascular system. The following combining forms have been introduced with them, revise their meanings before completing the next two exercises:

man/o
means pressure. In sphygmo**mano**meter it refers to the pressure of the pulse, i.e. arterial blood pressure.

dynam/o
means power. In sphygmo**dynamo**meter it refers to the force of the pulse (volume and pressure).

Note. Words ending in **-graph** usually refer to a recording instrument and those ending in **-scope** to a viewing instrument. Remember there are exceptions e.g. a radiograph is an X-ray picture and the stethoscope is used for listening to sounds.

Revise the names of all instruments and clinical procedures mentioned in this unit and then complete Exercises 15 and 16.

WORD EXERCISE 15

Match each term in Column A with a description from Column C by placing an appropriate number in Column B.

Column A	Column B	Column C
(a) cardioscope		1. an instrument that measures arterial blood pressure (the pressure of the pulse)
(b) cardiograph		2. an instrument used to cut a heart valve
(c) electro-cardiograph		3. technique of X-raying the heart and blood vessels after injection of radio-opaque dye
(d) cardio-valvotome		4. an instrument that records the heart (beat)
(e) angio-cardiography		5. an instrument that records the electrical activity of the heart
(f) sphygmo-manometer		6. an instrument used to view the heart

WORD EXERCISE 16

Match each term in Column A with a description from Column C by placing an appropriate number in Column B.

Column A	Column B	Column C
(a) echo-cardiography		1. a recording of heart sounds
(b) sphygmo-cardiograph		2. an instrument used to listen to sounds within the chest
(c) stethoscope		3. a tracing or recording of the electrical activity of the heart
(d) phono-cardiogram		4. an instrument that measures the pressure within a vein
(e) electro-cardiogram		5. an instrument that records the pulse and heart beat

| f) | phlebo-manometer | | 6. | technique of recording the heart using reflected ultrasound |

ANATOMY EXERCISE

Now complete the Anatomy Exercise on page 44.

CASE HISTORY 4

The object of this exercise is to understand words associated with a patient's medical history.

To complete the exercise:

- Read through the passage on cardiac failure; unfamiliar words are underlined and you can find their meaning using the Word Help.

- Write the meaning of the medical terms shown in bold print on the lines that follow the Word Help.

Cardiac failure

Mr D, a 65-year-old male builder, was referred by his GP to the **Cardiology** Unit. He had been healthy until 8 months previously but since then he has developed fatigue, exertion dyspnoea (Am. dyspnea) and paroxysmal nocturnal dyspnoea. He also described discomfort in his chest and felt his heart was 'thumping'.

On the morning of admission he had become unwell and was pale, cold and sweating and seemed confused. Initial examination revealed tender, smooth hepatic enlargement and the presence of ascites. His jugular **venous** pulse was raised and pitting oedema (Am. edema) was present in his ankles. Auscultation revealed a left ventricular third sound with **tachycardia** (a gallop rhythm) and crepitations were heard at the lung bases. Mr D was connected to a 12 lead **electrocardiograph** to monitor his heart rate and rhythm. A posteroanterior chest X-ray revealed **cardiomegaly** and pulmonary oedema and he was diagnosed as having acute **biventricular** heart failure.

Mr D was treated with furosemide (frusemide) a diuretic to promote renal excretion of fluid. The loss of fluid provided symptomatic and haemodynamic (Am. hemodynamic) benefits relieving his dyspnoea and reducing ventricular filling pressure. **Cardiac** output was improved by **vasodilator** therapy with ACE inhibitors in combination with positive inotropic agents.

Now write the meaning of the following words from the case history without using your dictionary lists:

(a) cardiology

(b) venous

(c) tachycardia

(d) electrocardiograph

(e) cardiomegaly

(f) biventricular

(g) cardiac

(h) vasodilator

(Answers to the case history exercise are given in the Answers to Word Exercises beginning on page 301)

Quick Reference

Combining forms relating to the cardiovascular system:

Aneurysm/o	aneurysm
Angi/o	vessel
Aort/o	aorta
Arteri/o	artery
Ather/o	atheroma
Atri/o	atrium
Cardi/o	heart
Embol/o	embolism
My/o	muscle
Myocardi/o	myocardium
Pericardi/o	pericardium
Phleb/o	vein
Sphygm/o	pulse
Steth/o	breast
Thromb/o	thrombus/clot
Valv/o	valve
Valvul/o	valve
Vas/o	vessel
Vascul/o	vessel
Venacav/o	vena cava
Ven/o	vein
Ventricul/o	ventricle

Abbreviations

Some common abbreviations related to the cardiovascular system are listed below. Note some are not standard and their meaning may vary from one health care setting to another. There is a more extensive list for reference on page 335.

AAA	abdominal aortic aneurysm
AF	atrial fibrillation
AMI	acute myocardial infarction
CABG	coronary artery bypass grafting
CAD	coronary artery disease
CCU	coronary care unit
CPR	cardiopulmonary resuscitation
CT	coronary thrombosis
ECG	electrocardiogram
iv	intravenous
MI	myocardial infarction
MS	mitral stenosis

Medical Notes

Cardiac tamponade
The compression of the heart caused by an accumulation of fluid in the pericardium.

Claudication
Pain, tension and weakness in a leg upon walking, it is brought on by interference with its blood supply. The pain is relieved by rest and may be caused by a spasm or occlusive arterial disease.

Congestive heart failure (CHF)
CHF is a result of an inadequate pumping action of the heart. Congestion develops when the heart is unable to pump all of the blood it receives and fluid accumulates in the lungs and peripheral tissues. The clinical presentation depends on how quickly heart failure develops and whether it involves the right or left sides of the heart or both.

In patients with *left ventricular failure*, the left ventricle fails to pump blood effectively and as a result blood backs up in the lungs. As a result fluid accumulates in the lungs and patients develop a sensation of breathlessness and have difficulty in breathing, particularly at night (paroxysmal nocturnal dyspnoea (Am. dyspnea)). Often such failure results from coronary artery disease and valve disorders.

In patients with *right ventricular failure*, the right ventricle fails to empty and the right atrium and venae cavae become congested with blood followed by congestion throughout the venous system. The organs first affected are the liver, spleen and kidneys. Oedema (Am. edema) of the limbs and ascites (excess fluid in the peritoneal cavity) usually follow. Symptoms include shortness of breath, pedal (foot) oedema and abdominal pain.

Coronary artery disease (CAD)
Coronary artery disease is one of the leading causes of death. It can result from many causes, all of which reduce the flow of blood to the myocardium (heart muscle). If a coronary artery is occluded, blood cannot reach the heart muscle cells it normally supplies. Deprived of oxygen the cells soon die or are damaged. The death of heart muscle is termed a myocardial infarction (MI) or heart attack. The principal causes are atherosclerosis and the formation of clots in coronary arteries.

Coronary heart disease (CHD)
When symptoms of coronary artery disease appear and begin to affect the patient the term coronary heart disease or CHD is used. Coronary heart disease also called *ischaemic heart disease*, is due to the effects of atheroma causing narrowing or occlusion of one or more branches of the coronary arteries. Narrowing of coronary arteries leads to *angina pectoris* and occlusion to a *myocardial infarction* (heart attack).

Fallot's tetralogy
A congenital defect that results in cardiac function inadequate for a growing child. Four abnormalities are present: stenosis of the pulmonary artery, malposition of the aorta, a ventricular septal defect (a hole between the two ventricles) and right ventricular hypertrophy.

Flutter
An abnormal, rapid and regular rhythm of the atria or ventricles for example, an atrial flutter.

Hypertension
This is a term used to describe a persistently higher than normal blood pressure for a particular age group. Arteriosclerosis contributes to increasing blood pressure with age but it is not the only factor. Hypertension is described as essential, primary or idiopathic when the cause is unknown and as secondary hypertension when it results from other diseases. High blood pressure is of concern because it can damage the heart, brain and kidneys if it remains uncontrolled.

Murmur
An extra heart sound between normal beats for example, a presystolic murmur characteristic of mitral valve stenosis (narrowing).

Myocardial infarction (heart attack)
An infarct is an area of tissue that has died because of lack of a supply of oxygenated blood. The failure of blood supply to cardiac muscle is called a myocardial infarction (MI). The commonest cause is an atheromatous plaque complicated by thrombosis. Myocardial infarction is usually accompanied by severe chest pain which unlike angina pectoris, continues when the individual is at rest. Myocardial infarction is often fatal but recovery is possible if the amount of heart tissue damage is small.

Patent ductus arteriosus
A heart defect in which the ductus arteriosus fails to close at birth. Before birth the duct allows blood to pass between the pulmonary artery and aorta bypassing the pulmonary circulation. Shortly after birth when the pulmonary circulation is established the duct should close completely. Failure to close results in congestion of the lungs and eventual cardiac failure.

Petechia
A small red spot on the skin caused by an effusion of blood (a pinpoint haemorrhage (Am. hemorrhage)). Pleural petechiae.

Rheumatic heart disease
Rheumatic heart disease is an autoimmune disease caused by *Streptococcus pyogenes* (beta-haemolytic group A) that occurs most often in children. The antibodies developed to combat the infection damage the heart. A few weeks after an improperly treated streptococcal infection, the cardiac valves and other tissues in the body may become inflamed, a condition called *rheumatic fever*. If severe, the inflammation can result in stenosis (narrowing) and other deformities of the valves, and damage to the chordae tendinae or myocardium.

Varicose veins
Varicose veins are enlarged veins in which blood tends to pool rather than continue on toward the heart. The condition commonly occurs in superficial veins in areas seen externally as varicosities. The great saphenous vein, the largest superficial vein in the leg often becomes varicose in people who stand for long periods. The force of gravity slows the return of venous blood to the heart in such cases, causing blood engorged-veins to dilate. As the veins dilate, the distance between the flaps of venous valves widens eventually making them incompetent (leaky). Incompetence of valves causes even more pooling in affected veins, a positive feedback mechanism. Haemorrhoids (Am. hemorrhoids) also called *piles*, are varicose veins in the anal canal.

NOW TRY THE WORD CHECK

WORD CHECK

This self-check exercise lists all word components used in this unit. First write down the meaning of as many word components as you can. Then check your answers using the Exercise Guide and Quick Reference box or the Glossary of Word Components (pp. 347–371).

Prefixes

a-

bi-

brady-

dextro-

endo-

hyper-

hypo-

pan-

peri-

tachy-

Combining forms of word roots

aneurysm/o

angi/o

aort/o

arteri/o

ather/o

atri/o

cardi/o

ech/o

electr/o

embol/o

dynam/o

isch/o

man/o

my/o

necr/o

pericardi/o

phleb/o

phon/o

sphygm/o

sten/o

steth/o

thromb/o

valv/o

valvul/o

vas/o

vascul/o

venacav/o

ven/o

ventricul/o

Suffixes

-algia

-ar

-centesis

-clysis

-ectasis

-ectomy

-genesis

-gram

-graph

-graphy

-ia

-ic

-itis

-ium

-lith

-logy

-lysis

-megaly

-meter

-metry

-oma

-osis

-ous

-pathy

-pexy

-plasty

-poiesis

-rrhage

-rrhaphy

-sclerosis

-scope

-stasis

-tome

-tomy

-um

NOW TRY THE SELF-ASSESSMENT

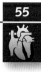

SELF-ASSESSMENT

Test 4A

Below are some combining forms that refer to the anatomy of the cardiovascular system. Indicate which part of the system they refer to by putting a number from the diagram (Fig. 25) next to each word.

(a) aort/o

(b) venacav/o

(c) endocardi/o

(d) valv/o

(e) pericardi/o

(f) myocardi/o

Score

6

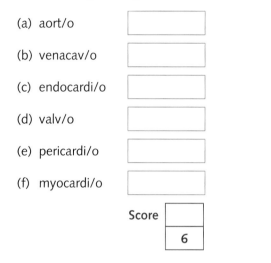

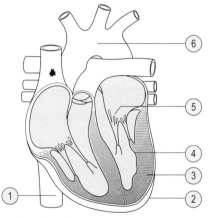

Figure 25   The heart

Test 4B

Prefixes and suffixes

Match each prefix or suffix in Column A with a meaning in Column C by inserting the appropriate number in Column B.

Column A	Column B	Column C
(a) a-		1. formation (i)
(b) -ac		2. formation (ii)
(c) bi-		3. infusion/injection
(d) brady-		4. two
(e) -clysis		5. fast

Column A	Column B	Column C
(f) dextro-		6. pertaining to
(g) -ectasis		7. without
(h) endo-		8. dilatation
(i) -genesis		9. fixation
(j) -megaly		10. right
(k) pan-		11. around
(l) peri-		12. stopping/cessation
(m) -pexy		13. abnormal condition of narrowing
(n) -poiesis		14. condition of hardening
(o) -rrhaphy		15. slow
(p) -sclerosis		16. thing/structure/ anatomical part
(q) -stasis		17. stitching/suturing
(r) -stenosis		18. all
(s) tachy-		19. enlargement
(t) -um		20. inside

Score

20

Test 4C

Combining forms of word roots

Match each combining form in Column A with a meaning in Column C by inserting the appropriate number in Column B.

Column A	Column B	Column C
(a) aneurysm/o		1. echo/reflected sound
(b) angi/o		2. artery
(c) aort/o		3. death/corpse
(d) arteri/o		4. sound
(e) ather/o		5. valve
(f) cardi/o		6. aorta

Column A	Column B	Column C
(g) dynam/o		7. porridge (yellow plaque on wall of blood vessel)
(h) ech/o		8. heart
(i) man/o		9. vessel (i)
(j) my/o		10. vessel (ii)
(k) necr/o		11. force
(l) phleb/o		12. aneurysm (swelling)
(m) phon/o		13. pressure/rare
(n) sphygm/o		14. muscle
(o) sten/o		15. vein (i)
(p) steth/o		16. vein (ii)
(q) thromb/o		17. clot
(r) valv/o		18. narrowing
(s) vas/o		19. pulse
(t) ven/o		20. breast

Score [20]

Test 4D

Write the meaning of:

(a) cardiovalvulitis

(b) aortorrhaphy

(c) angioscope

(d) phlebostenosis

(e) thromboendarteritis

Score [5]

Test 4E

Build words that mean:

(a) inflammation of an artery associated with a thrombosis

(b) puncture of the heart

(c) disease of an artery

(d) removal of a vein

(e) study of the heart and blood vessels (use angi/o)

Score [5]

Check answers to Self-Assessment Tests on page 325.

UNIT 5
THE BLOOD

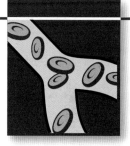

EXERCISE GUIDE

Use this list of word components and their meanings to complete the word exercises in this unit.

Prefixes

a-	without
an-	without/not
ellipto-	shaped like an ellipse
hyper-	above/abnormal increase
hypo-	below/abnormal decrease
iso-	equal/same
macro-	large
micro-	small
normo-	normal/rule
peri-	around
poikil/o	varied/irregular
poly-	many

Roots/Combining forms

cyt/e/o	cell
dynam/o	force/movement
fibr/o	fibre
path/o	disease
pericardi/o	pericardium
septic/o	sepsis/infection/putrefaction

Suffixes

-aemia	condition of blood
-apheresis	removal
-blast	germ cell/cell, cell that forms
-chromia	condition of colour/haemoglobin
-crit	separate/device for measuring cells
-cytosis	abnormal condition of cells (too many)
-emia (Am.)	condition of blood
-genesis	capable of causing/pertaining to formation of
-globin	protein
-ia	condition of
-ic	pertaining to
-ium	structure/anatomical part
-logy	study of
-lysis	breakdown/disintegration
-meter	measuring instrument
-oma	tumour/swelling (Am. tumor)
-osis	abnormal condition/disease of
-penia	condition of lack of/deficiency
-poiesis	formation
-ptysis	spitting up
-rrhage	bursting forth (of blood/bleeding)
-stasis	stopping/controlling/cessation of movement
-toxic	pertaining to poisoning
-um	thing/structure/anatomical part
-uria	condition of urine

ANATOMY EXERCISE

When you have finished Word Exercises 1–7, look at the word components listed below. Complete Figure 26 by writing the appropriate combining form on each line – more than one component may to the same position. (You can check their meanings in the Quick Reference box on p. 63)

Bas/o   Leucocyt/o   Plasma-
Eosin/o   (Am. leukocyt/o)   Thrombocyt/o
Erythrocyt/o   Lymphocyt/o
Haem/o   Monocyt/o
(Am. hem/o)   Neutr/o

The blood

Blood is a complex fluid classified as a connective tissue because it contains cells, plus an intercellular matrix known as plasma. Here we can see the main components of whole blood:

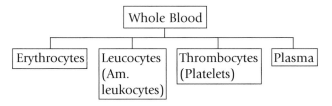

The blood cells carry out a variety of functions: erythrocytes (red blood cells) transport gases whilst leucocytes (white blood cells) defend the body against invasion by microorganisms and foreign antigens. Thrombocytes, or platelets, are actually fragments of larger cells concerned with the formation of blood clots following injury.

The plasma carries nutrients, wastes, hormones, antibodies and blood-clotting proteins. The study of blood is very important in medicine for the diagnosis of disease.

Use the Exercise Guide at the beginning of the unit to complete Word Exercises 1–7 unless you are asked to work without it.

ROOT

Haem
*(From a Greek word **haima**, meaning blood.)*

Combining forms   **Haem/o, haemat/o, -aem-** (Am. **Hem/o, hemat/o, -em-**)

WORD EXERCISE 1

Using your Exercise Guide, find the meaning of:

(a) **haemat/o**/logy
(Am. **hemat/o**/logy)

(b) **haem/o**/path/o/logy
(Am. **hem/o**/path/o/logy)

(c) **haem/o**/dynam/ics
(Am. **hem/o**/dynam/ics)

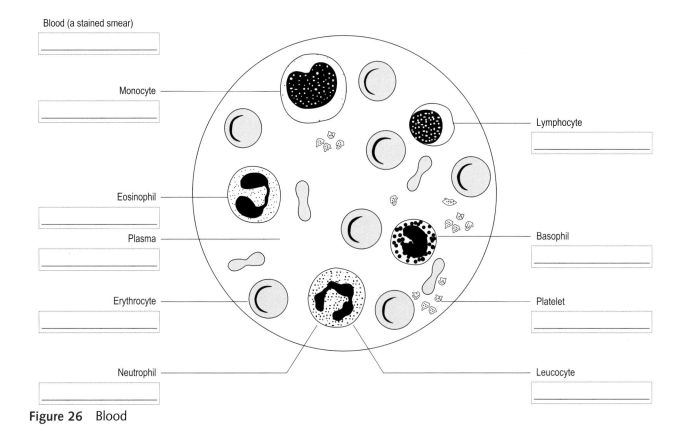

Figure 26   Blood

(d) **haem/o**/poiesis
   (Am. **hem/o**/poiesis)

(e) **haem/o**/stasis
   (Am. **hem/o**/stasis)

(f) **haem/o**/pericardi/um
   (Fig. 27)
   (Am. **hem/o**/pericardi/um)

(g) **haem/o**/ptysis
   (Am. **hem/o**/ptysis)

Using your Exercise Guide look up the meaning of -lysis, -oma, -rrhage and -uria, then build words that mean:

(h) Swelling containing blood
   (use haemat/o, Am. hemat/o)

(i) Breakdown/disintegration of blood

(j) Condition of blood in the urine
   (use haemat/o, Am. hemat/o)

(k) Bursting forth of blood

Using your Exercise Guide, find the meaning of:

(l) poly/cyt/**haem**/ia
   (Am. poly/cyt/**hem**/ia)

(m) an/**aem**/ia
   (Am. an/**em**/ia)

(n) septic/**aem**/ia
   (Am. septic/**em**/ia)

Haemoglobin is a red pigment (globular protein) found inside red blood cells, it functions to transport oxygen and carbon dioxide. The haemoglobin present in the blood is of great importance to the efficiency of gaseous transport and several types of investigation are performed to estimate its concentration.

The three medical terms that follow use the combining form **haemoglobin/o** meaning haemoglobin.

Using your Exercise Guide, find the meaning of:

(o) **haemoglobin/o**/meter
   (Am. **hemoglobin/o**/meter)

Without using your Exercise Guide, write the meaning of:

(p) **haem/o**/globin
   (Am. **hem/o**/globin)

(q) **haemoglobin**/uria
   (Am. **hemoglobin**/uria)

The amount of haemoglobin within red blood cells can be estimated and abnormal levels are found in some patients. Terms describing these conditions have been formed from the suffix **-chromia** (from Greek *chroma*, meaning colour). Here the colour refers to the red pigment haemoglobin.

Using your Exercise Guide, find the meaning of:

(r) hypo/**chrom**/ia

(s) hyper/**chrom**/ia

(t) normo/**chrom**/ic

Another common term relating to the colour of haemoglobin is **cyanosis**. **Cyan/o** means blue. In the absence of oxygen, haemoglobin develops a bluish tinge. Nailbeds, lips and skin show signs of cyanosis (i.e. look blue) when oxygenation of the blood is deficient. Tissues deprived of oxygen can also be described as **anoxic**.

Now we will examine word roots that refer to the different types of blood cells. All of these cells are suspended in the liquid matrix of the blood known as plasma.

ROOT

Erythr
*(From a Greek word **erythros**, meaning red. Here erythr/o means red blood cell or erythrocyte.)*

Combining form   **Erythr/o**

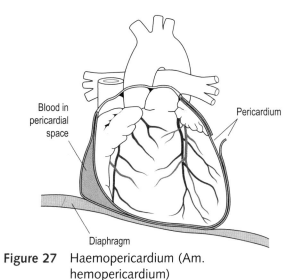

Blood in pericardial space

Pericardium

Diaphragm

Figure 27   Haemopericardium (Am. hemopericardium)

WORD EXERCISE 2

Using your Exercise Guide, find the meaning of:

(a) **erythr/o**/penia

(b) **erythr/o**/genesis

(c) **erythr/o**/blast

(This refers to the cell which eventually forms the mature erythrocyte.)

Without using your Exercise Guide, write the meaning of:

(d) **erythr/o**/poiesis

(e) **erythr/o**/cyt/o/lysis

(f) **erythr/o**/cyt/haem/ia
(Am. **erythr/o**/cyt/hem/ia)

This last condition is synonymous with **erythrocytosis** meaning an abnormal condition of red cells, i.e. too many red cells. This condition is usually a physiological response to low levels of oxygen circulating in the blood. Besides changes in number, individual erythrocytes can suffer from various abnormalities, some of which are listed below.

Using your Exercise Guide, find the meaning of:

(g) micro/**cytosis**

(NB: Cytosis is used in (g) to (k) to mean too many red blood cells.)

(h) macro/**cytosis**

(i) ellipto/**cytosis**

(j) an/iso/**cytosis**

(k) poikilo/**cytosis**

(l) normo/**cyt**/ic

ROOT

Reticul
(From a Latin word **reticulum**, *meaning a small net. Here reticul/o means reticulocyte, a very young erythrocyte lacking a nucleus; its cytoplasm gives it a net-like appearance when stained with basic dyes.)*

Combining form **Reticul/o**

WORD EXERCISE 3

Without using your Exercise Guide, build words that mean:

(a) an immature reticulocyte

(b) condition of too many reticulocytes

(c) condition of deficiency of reticulocytes

ROOT

Leuc
(From a Greek word **leukos**, *meaning white. Here leuc/o means white blood cell or leucocyte.)*

Combining forms **Leuc/o, leuk/o**
*(**Leuc/o** is more commonly used in the UK, **leuk/o** in America.)*

WORD EXERCISE 4

Without using your Exercise Guide, build words that mean:

(a) condition of deficiency of white cells

(b) the formation of white blood cells

Without using your Exercise Guide, write the meaning of:

(c) **leuc/o**/cyto/genesis
(Am. **leuk/o**/cyto/genesis)

(d) **leuk**/aem/ia
(Am. **leuk**/em/ia. This is a malignant condition, i.e. a type of cancer.)

(e) **leuc/o**/cytosis
(Am. **leuk/o**/cytosis. This refers to an excess of white cells as seen during infection.)

(f) **leuc/o**/cyt/oma
(Am. **leuk/o**/cyt/oma)

(g) **leuc/o**/blast
(Am. **leuk/o**/blast)

(h) **leuc/o**/blast/osis
(Am. **leuk/o**/blast/osis)

THE BLOOD

Using your Exercise Guide, find the meaning of:

(i) **leuc/o**/toxic
(Am. **leuk/o**/toxic)

Leucocyte is a general term meaning white cell but there are many types of white cell. Some leucocytes contain granules and are known as **granulocytes**, those without granules are called **agranulocytes** (*a*- meaning without, *granul/o*- granule and *-cyte* cell).

Among the commonest granulocytes are polymorphonuclear granulocytes or polymorphs. These all have nuclei which show many shapes (*poly* – many, *morph/o* – shape). There are three types of polymorph:

Neutrophils
From *neuter*, meaning neither, and *philein*, meaning to love. These cells stain well with (love) **neutral** dyes. Neutrophils engulf microorganisms that have entered the blood and destroy them. These cells are sometimes referred to as phagocytes (*phag/o* means to eat, i.e. cells that eat). The process of engulfing particles is known as phagocytosis.

Basophils
These cells stain well with basic (alkaline) dyes.

Eosinophils
These cells stain well with acid dyes like eosin, a red dye.

Among the agranular leucocytes are lymphocytes and large monocytes (mono means single). The latter can leave the blood and wander to sites of infection. Lymphocytes will be studied in Unit 6.

Note. The condition **pancytopenia** refers to an abnormal depression of all the cellular components of the blood (*pan*- meaning all, *cyt/o*- cell and *-penia* condition of deficiency).

ROOT

Myel
(*From a Greek word* **myelos**, *meaning marrow. Here myel/o means bone marrow, the substance that fills the medullary cavity and spaces of bone; it contains the blood forming tissue that produces blood cells. Myel/o also means myelocyte, a precursor cell of the polymorphonuclear series of granulocytes found in the bone marrow.*)

Combining form   Myel/o

WORD EXERCISE 5

Without using your Exercise Guide, write the meaning of:

(a) **myel/o**/cyte

(b) **myel/o**/fibr/osis

Without using your Exercise Guide, build words that mean:

(c) a germ cell of the marrow

(d) a tumour (Am. tumor) of myeloid tissue

WORD EXERCISE 6

We have already used the combining form **thromb/o** meaning clot; here it is combined with **-cyte** to make **thrombocyte**. Thrombocytes or **platelets** are fragments of cells that circulate in the blood. They play a major role in the clotting of blood.

Without using your Exercise Guide, write the meaning of:

(a) **thrombocyt/o**/penia

(b) **thrombocyt/o**/poiesis

(c) **thrombocyt/o**/lysis

(d) **thrombocyt/o**/pathy

The numbers and proportions of blood cells found in whole blood are important in the diagnosis of disease. The percentage volume of erythrocytes is known as the **haematocrit** (Am. hematocrit) (from Greek *krinein*, meaning to separate/judge/discern). The word haematocrit is also used for the apparatus that measures the volume of erythrocytes in a blood sample.

Now write down what is meant by:

(e) **thrombocyt/o**/crit

The number of blood cells can be counted using a device known as a **haemocytometer**. The simplest type of counter consists of a specially designed microscope slide that holds a precise volume of blood and a grid for the manual counting of cells. Today, the process of counting cells is performed automatically in a Coulter counter. A doctor may request particular types of cell count to aid diagnosis, for example:

Blood count

A count of the number of red cells and/or white cells in a sample of blood. Reference intervals for the number of cells in a sample from a healthy person are:

Red blood cells (erythrocytes) $4.5–6.5 \times 10^{12}/L$ in men, $3.8–5.3 \times 10^{12}/L$ in women

White cells (leucocytes) $4.0–11.0 \times 10^{9}/L$.

Differential count

A count of the proportions of different types of cells in stained smears. Examples of reference intervals for the number of cells in a sample from a healthy person are:

Neutrophils (30–75%) $2.5–7.5 \times 10^{9}/L$

Basophils (<1%) $<0.1 \times 10^{9}/L$

Eosinophils (1–6%) $0.04–0.4 \times 10^{9}/L$

Platelet count

A count of the number of platelets in a sample of blood. The reference interval for the number of platelets in a sample from a healthy person is: $150–400 \times 10^{9}/L$.

Techniques have been developed to take blood from a donor, remove wanted or unwanted components from it and return the cells in fresh or frozen plasma back into the body. When plasma is removed the technique is known as **plasmapheresis**. Plasma refers to the liquid matrix of the blood in which cells are suspended and nutrients and wastes dissolved. Apheresis is from the Greek *aphairesis*, meaning a taking away.

Without using your Exercise Guide, write the meaning of:

(f) erythrocyt/**apheresis**

(g) thrombocyt/**apheresis**

(h) leuc/**apheresis**

Column A	Column B	Column C
(a) plasmapheresis		1. a count of numbers of blood cells/Litre of blood
(b) differential count		2. an instrument that estimates the percentage volume of red cells in blood or the actual value (as a percentage of the volume) of red cells in blood
(c) haematocrit		3. an estimate of proportions/ numbers of white cells in a stained smear
(d) haemoglobi-nometer		4. continuous removal of plasma from blood and retransfusion of cells
(e) blood count		5. an instrument that measures amount of haemoglobin in a sample

ANATOMY EXERCISE

Now complete the Anatomy Exercise on page 58.

Medical equipment and clinical procedures

Revise the names of all instruments and clinical procedures mentioned in this unit and then complete Exercise 7.

WORD EXERCISE 7

Match each term in Column A with a description from Column C by placing an appropriate number in Column B.

CASE HISTORY 5

The object of this exercise is to understand words associated with a patient's medical history.

To complete the exercise:

- read through the passage on aplastic anaemia (Am. anemia); unfamiliar words are underlined and you can find their meaning using the Word Help

- write the meaning of the medical terms shown in bold print on the lines that follow the Word Help.

Aplastic anaemia (Am. aplastic anemia)

Mr E, a 44-year-old chemistry teacher and former industrial chemist, had been unwell for many weeks before seeking advice from his <u>GP</u>. He complained of headache, breathlessness, fatigue and <u>palpitation</u>; the previous day he had become concerned about his condition following a severe <u>epistaxis</u> and **haemoptysis** (Am. hemoptysis). On examination he appeared to have a lower respiratory tract infection and <u>oral thrush</u>. Initial blood investigation revealed a **pancytopenia,** and he was referred to the Haematology (Am. Hematology) Department.

Mr E looked pale and was troubled by <u>ulcerative lesions</u> in his mouth and pharynx. There was no <u>lymphadenopathy</u> or <u>hepatosplenomegaly</u>. A bone marrow <u>trephine biopsy</u> and <u>smear</u> confirmed a <u>hypocellularity</u> with the virtual absence of <u>reticulocytes</u>; no **leukaemic** or <u>neoplastic</u> cells were observed. Detailed <u>haematological</u> (Am. hematological) examination revealed a **normochromic**, **normocytic** anaemia with **granulocytopenia** and **thrombocytopenia.**

Mr E was diagnosed with a severe, <u>secondary</u> **aplastic** anaemia (Am. anemia) and was advised of its serious <u>prognosis</u>. He resigned from his post as a teacher and a programme of supportive care aimed at treating his respiratory tract infection was established. He is currently being assessed for bone marrow transplantation by his <u>HLA identical</u> brother.

WORD HELP

aplastic pertaining to without growth/unable to form new cells

epistaxis a nose bleed

GP general practitioner (family doctor)

haematological pertaining to study of blood (Am. hematological)

hepatosplenomegaly enlargement of the spleen and liver

HLA identical human leucocyte (Am. leukocyte) antigen, important for cross-matching of donor and recipient

hypocellularity condition of below normal number of cells

lesion pathological change in a tissue

lymphadenopathy disease of lymph nodes

neoplastic pertaining to new, abnormal growth of cells (cancer cells)

oral thrush fungal infection in the mouth (with *Candida albicans*)

palpitation unusual awareness of one's heartbeat

prognosis a forecast of the probable course and outcome of a disease

reticulocyte an immature erythrocyte

secondary here refers to a second type of aplastic anaemia caused by direct damage of the bone marrow by chemicals, radiation or infection

smear spreading material across a slide for microscopic examination

trephine biopsy using a trephine (device that removes a circular disc of bone) to take a sample of bone marrow

ulcerative having the form of an ulcer

Now write the meaning of the following words from the case history without using your dictionary lists:

(a) haemoptysis (Am. hemoptysis)

(b) pancytopenia

(c) leukaemic (Am. leukemic)

(d) normochromic

(e) normocytic

(f) granulocytopenia

(g) thrombocytopenia

(h) anaemia (Am. anemia)

(Answers to the case history exercise are given in the Answers to Word Exercises beginning on page 301)

Quick Reference

Combining forms relating to the blood:

Cyt/o,-cyte	cell
Erythr/o	red
Erythrocyt/o	erythrocyte/red cell
Fibr/o	fibre
Globin/o	protein
Granul/o	granule
Haem/o	blood

Hem/o (Am.)	blood
Leuc/o	white
Leucocyt/o	leucocyte/white cell
Leuk/o (Am.)	white
Leukocyt/o (Am.)	leukocyte/white cell
Lymphocyt/o	lymph cell
Monocyt/o	monocyte
Morph/o	shape/form
Myel/o	bone marrow/myelocyte
Phag/o	eating/consuming
Reticul/o	immature erythrocyte
Thromb/o	clot
Thrombocyt/o	thrombocyte/platelet

Abbreviations

Some common abbreviations related to the blood are listed below. Note some are not standard and their meaning may vary from one health care setting to another. There is a more extensive list for reference on page 335.

ALL	acute lymphocytic leukaemia (Am. leukemia)
AML	acute myeloid leukaemia (Am. leukemia)
Diff	differential blood count (of cell types)
ESR	erythrocyte sedimentation rate
FBC	full blood count
Hb	haemoglobin (Am. hemoglobin)
Hct	haematocrit (Am. hematocrit)
MCH	mean corpuscular haemoglobin (Am. hemoglobin)
MCHC	mean corpuscular haemoglobin (Am. hemoglobin) concentration
PCV	peaked cell volume
RBC	red blood cell/count
WBC	white blood cell/count

Medical Notes

Anaemia (Am. anemia)

The term anaemia is used to describe different disease conditions caused by an inability of the blood to carry sufficient oxygen to the body cells. The condition can result from inadequate numbers of red blood cells or a deficiency of haemoglobin (Am. hemoglobin) within them. Signs and symptoms are related to the inability of the blood to supply body cell with sufficient oxygen. All types of anaemia lead to a feeling of fatigue and intolerance to cold conditions. There are many types, for example:

Acute blood loss anaemia is a loss of red blood cells due to haemorrhage (Am. hemorrhage) often associated with trauma, extensive surgery or other situation involving a sudden loss of blood.

Aplastic anaemia is characterized by an abnormally low number of red blood cells. Although idiopathic forms of this disease occur, most cases result from destruction of bone marrow by drugs, toxic chemicals or radiation. As many different cells in the bone marrow are affected, aplastic anaemia is usually accompanied by a decreased number of white blood cells and platelets. Bone marrow transplants have been successful in treating some cases.

Folate deficiency anaemia is similar to pernicious anaemia because it also causes a decrease in the red blood cell count resulting from a vitamin deficiency. In this condition it is folic acid (Vitamin B_9) that is deficient. Folic acid deficiencies are common among alcoholics and other malnourished individuals.

Iron deficiency anaemia is the most common type of anaemia. It is caused by inadequate absorption of dietary iron or excessive loss from the body. Iron (Fe) is a critical component of the haemoglobin molecule and without it the body cannot manufacture enough haemoglobin. Red blood cells seen in this type of anaemia are classed as hypochromic meaning they have an abnormally low haemoglobin content.

Pernicious anaemia is characterized by insufficient production of red blood cells due to a lack of vitamin B_{12}. Vitamin B_{12} is absorbed from the diet and used in the formation of new red blood cells in the bone marrow. In many cases, the condition results from the failure of the stomach lining to produce intrinsic factor, a substance that allows vitamin B_{12} to be absorbed. Pernicious anaemia can be fatal if not successfully treated; one method of treatment involves intramuscular injections of vitamin B_{12}.

Sickle-cell anaemia is characterized by the manufacture of an abnormal haemoglobin (Hb^S) that causes red blood cells to assume a sickle shape when deoxygenated. The sickle cells easily rupture, increase the viscosity of blood and stick to the walls of small blood vessels restricting blood supply to tissues. The condition originated in Africa and is more common in black people.

Granulocytopenia (neutropenia)

Granulocytopenia is a general term used to indicate an abnormal reduction in the number of circulating granulocytes (polymorphonuclear leucocytes (Am. leukocytes)) and is commonly called neutropenia because forty to seventy-five percent of granulocytes are neutrophils. A reduction in the number of circulating granulocytes occurs when production does not keep pace with the normal removal of cells or when the life span of the cells is reduced. Extreme shortage or absence of granulocytes is called agranulocytosis. Cytotoxic drugs, irradiation damage, disease of bone marrow and severe microbial infections may cause inadequate formation of granulocytes.

Haemophilia (Am. hemophilia)

Haemophilia is an inherited disorder caused by a gene linked to the X-chromosome, it affects one in every ten thousand males worldwide. The condition results from a failure to produce one or more plasma proteins responsible for blood clotting and is characterized by a relative inability to form blood clots. Sufferers experience severe episodes of prolonged bleeding often without signs of trauma. Minor blood vessel injuries common in ordinary life can be life threatening as they result in excessive loss of blood. There is also recurrent bleeding into joints causing pain and damage to articular cartilage. The most common form is called haemophilia A caused by absence of Factor VIII protein; this affects more than three hundred thousand people around the world.

Leukaemia (Am. leukemia)

The term leukaemia applies to a group of malignant diseases characterized by proliferation of white blood cell precursors in the bone marrow. The leukaemic cells may eventually leave the bone marrow and infiltrate the lymph nodes, liver, spleen, central nervous system and other parts of the body. Approximately five percent of all deaths are due to leukaemia. Continuous production and accumulation of immature leucocytes (Am. leukocytes) characterize acute leukaemia. Overproduction of these cells leads to crowding out of normal bone marrow cells and platelets, and results in bleeding problems. In chronic leukaemia there is an accumulation of mature leucocytes in the blood that do not die at the end of their normal span.

There are many different types of leukaemia, including acute lymphocytic leukaemia (ALL), acute myelogenous leukaemia (AML), and chronic myelogenous leukaemia (CML).

Polycythaemia (Am. polycythemia)

In this condition there are an abnormally large number of erythrocytes in the blood. This increases blood viscosity, slows the rate of flow and increases the risk of intravascular clotting, ischaemia (Am. ischemia) and infarction. *Polycythaemia rubra vera* is a primary condition of unknown cause in which there is an abnormal excessive production of erythrocyte precursors.

Purpura

A condition in which multiple pinpoint haemorrhages (Am. hemorrhages) accumulate under the skin and mucous membranes. The lesions appear as purple spots and are due to bleeding caused by a reduction in the number of platelets (thrombocytopenia).

Thalassaemia (Am. thalassemia)

An inherited condition caused by the presence of autosomal recessive genes seen most commonly in populations living around the Mediterranean Sea and South East Asia. Reduced or absent synthesis of globin chains of haemoglobin (Am. hemoglobin) characterizes the condition. How an individual is affected depends on the genes they have inherited, they can be asymptomatic or have mild to severe anaemia (Am. anemia).

Thrombocytopenia

A condition characterized by bleeding from many small blood vessels throughout the body, most visibly in the skin and mucous membranes. If the number of thrombocytes falls to 20 000/mm^3 or less (normal range is 150 000–400 000/mm^3) catastrophic bleeding may occur. Although a number of different mechanisms can result in thrombocytopenia, the usual cause is bone marrow destruction by drugs, immune system disease, chemicals, radiation or cancer.

NOW TRY THE WORD CHECK

WORD CHECK

This self-check exercise lists all the word components used in this unit. First write down the meaning of as many word components as you can. Then check your answers using the Exercise Guide and Quick Reference box or the Glossary of Word Components (pp. 347–371).

Prefixes

a-

an-

basi-

ellipto-

eosino-

hyper-

hypo-

iso-

macro-

micro-

neutro-

normo-

pan-

peri-

poikil/o

poly-

Combining forms of word roots

cardi/o

cyan/o

cyt/o

dynam/o

erythr/o

fibr/o

globin/o

granul/o

haem/o
(Am. hem/o)

leuc/o
(Am. leuk/o)

monocyt/o

morph/o

myel/o

norm/o

ox/y

path/o

phag/o

reticul/o

sept/i

thromb/o

thrombocyt/o

Suffixes

-aemia
(Am. -emia)

-apheresis

-blast

-chromia

-crit

-cytosis

-genesis

-ic

-ium

-logy

-lysis

-meter

-oma

-osis

-penia

-phil

-poiesis

-rrhage

-stasis

-toxic

-um

-uria

NOW TRY THE SELF-ASSESSMENT

SELF-ASSESSMENT

Test 5A

Below are some combining forms that relate to the components of blood. Indicate which part of the blood they refer to by putting a number from the diagram (Fig. 28) next to each word. You may use a number more than once.

(a) plasma

(b) erythr/o

(c) haemoglobin/o
(Am. hemoglobin/o)

(d) leucocyt/o
(Am. leukocyt/o)

(e) thrombocyt/o

Score

5

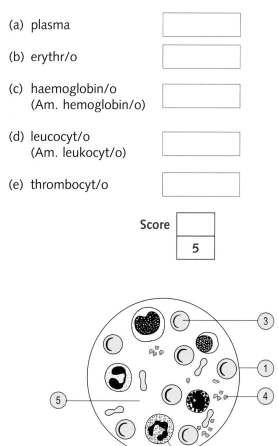

Figure 28 Blood

Test 5B

Prefixes, suffixes and combining forms of word roots

Match each word component in Column A with a meaning in Column C by inserting the appropriate number in Column B.

Column A	Column B	Column C
(a) -aemia (Am. -emia)		1. condition of urine
(b) an-		2. disintegration/ breakdown

Column A	Column B	Column C
(c) iso-		3. red
(d) baso-		4. measuring instrument
(e) -blast		5. abnormal condition/ disease of
(f) -chromia		6. basic/alkaline
(g) ellipt/o		7. white
(h) eosin/o		8. clot
(i) erythr/o		9. equal/same
(j) granul/o		10. condition of blood
(k) leuc/o (Am. leuk/o)		11. disease
(l) -lysis		12. granule
(m) macro-		13. germ cell
(n) -meter		14. cessation of flow
(o) micro-		15. affinity for/loving
(p) neutr/o		16. condition of deficiency/lack of
(q) -osis		17. not/without
(r) -pathy		18. small
(s) -penia		19. -condition of colour/haemoglobin
(t) -phil		20. oval/elliptoid
(u) sept/i		21. large
(v) -stasis		22. eosin (acid dye)
(w) thromb/o		23. neutral
(x) -uria		24. decay/sepsis/ infection

Score

24

Test 5C

Write the meaning of:

(a) leucocyturia
    (Am. leukocyturia)

(b) myelocytosis

(c) erythrocyturia

(d) thrombocythaemia
    (Am. thrombocythemia)

(e) phagocytolysis

Score

5

Test 5D

Build words that mean:

(a) any disease of blood
    (use haem/o, Am. hem/o)

(b) condition of deficiency in
    the number of red cells

(c) a physician who specializes
    in the study of blood
    (use haemat/o, Am. hemat/o)

(d) pertaining to the poisoning
    of blood

(e) condition of deficiency in the
    number of neutrophils

Score

5

Check answers to Self-Assessment Tests on page 325.

Test your recall of the meanings of word components in Units 1–5 by completing the appropriate self-assessment tests in Unit 22 on page 289.

UNIT 6
THE LYMPHATIC SYSTEM AND IMMUNOLOGY

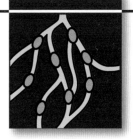

OBJECTIVES

Once you have completed Unit 6 you should be able to:

- understand the meaning of medical words relating to the lymphatic system and immunology

- build medical words relating to the lymphatic system and immunology

- associate medical terms with their anatomical position

- understand medical abbreviations relating to the lymphatic system and immunology.

EXERCISE GUIDE

Use this list of word components and their meanings to complete the word exercises in this unit.

Prefixes

auto-	self

Roots/Combining forms

aden/o	gland
angi/o	vessel
cyt/e/o, -cyte	cell
helc/o	ulcer
hepat/o	liver
path/o	disease
pharyng/o	pharynx
port/o	portal vein

Suffixes

-aemia	condition of blood
-cele	swelling/protrusion/hernia
-cytosis	abnormal increase in cells
-eal	pertaining to
-ectasis	dilatation/stretching
-ectomy	removal of
-emia (Am.)	condition of blood

-genesis	pertaining to formation
-genic	pertaining to formation/originating in
-globulin	protein
-gram	X-ray/tracing/recording
-graphy	technique of recording/making X-ray
-ic	pertaining to
-itis	inflammation of
-ity	state/condition
-logy	study of
-lysis	breakdown/disintegration
-malacia	condition of softening
-megaly	enlargement
-oma	tumour (Am.tumor)/swelling
-osis	abnormal condition/disease of
-pathy	disease of
-pexy	surgical fixation/fix in place
-poiesis	formation
-rrhagia	condition of bursting forth
-rrhea (Am.)	excessive discharge/flow
-rrhoea	excessive discharge/flow
-tic	pertaining to
-tome	cutting instrument

ANATOMY EXERCISE

When you have finished Word Exercises 1–8, look at the word components listed below. Complete Figure 29 by placing the appropriate combining form on each line. (You can check their meanings in the Quick Reference box on p. 75.)

Lymphaden/o   Splen/o   Tonsill/o
Lymphangi/o   Thym/o

The lymphatic system

The lymphatic system consists of capillaries, vessels, ducts and nodes that transport a fluid known as lymph. Lymph is formed from the tissue fluid that surrounds all tissue cells. The system performs three important functions: (i) transportation of lymphocytes that defend the body against infection and foreign antigens, (ii) transportation of lipids and (iii) the drainage of excess fluid from the tissues.

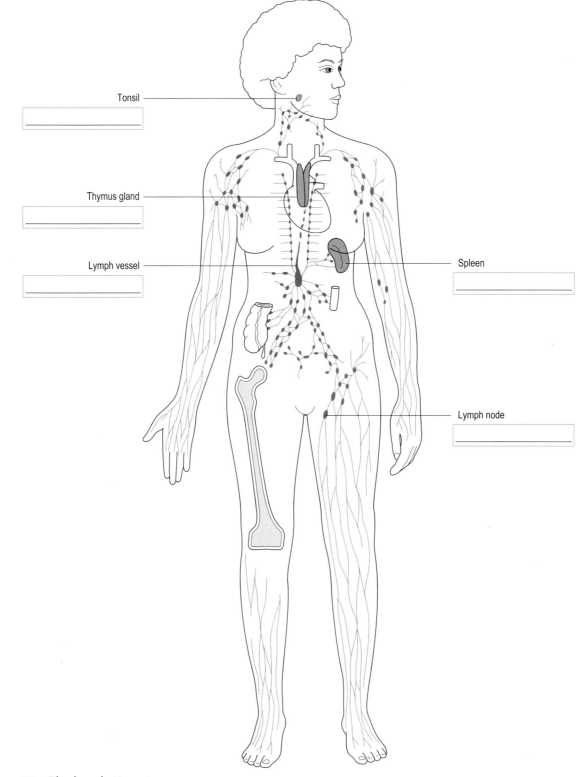

Tonsil

Thymus gland

Lymph vessel

Spleen

Lymph node

Figure 29 The lymphatic system

We'll begin by examining the terms associated with the cells and components of the system. Use the Exercise Guide at the beginning of this unit to complete Word Exercises 1–8 unless you are asked to work without it.

ROOT

Lymph
(From Latin **lympha**, *meaning water. Here lymph/o means lymph or lymphatic tissue.)*

Combining forms **Lymph/a/o**

WORD EXERCISE 1

Using your Exercise Guide, find the meaning of:

(a) **lymph**/o/cyt/osis

(b) **lymph**/o/rrhagia

(c) **lymph**/angi/o/graphy

(d) **lymph**/angi/o/gram

(e) **lymph**/angi/ectasis

Note. The next four words use the combining form lymphaden/o meaning lymph gland. The structures referred to by this combining form are no longer called glands because unlike true glands, they do not produce secretions. Lymphaden/o is now used to mean lymph node. A node is a mass of lymphoid tissue containing cells that defend the body against noxious agents such as microorganisms and toxins.

(f) **lymphaden**/oma

(g) **lymphaden**/ectomy

(h) **lymphaden**/o/pathy

(i) **lymphaden**/itis

Lymph nodes consist of lymphatic channels held in place by fibrous connective tissue that forms a capsule. The nodes contain **lymphocytes** (lymph cells, *-cyte* meaning cell), and special cells called **macrophages** (large-eaters) which, like neutrophils, can engulf foreign substances and microorganisms by phagocytosis. Lymph nodes often trap and destroy malignant cells as well as microorganisms. During infection lymphocytes and macrophages multiply rapidly, causing the nodes to swell; they may become inflamed and sore. Lymphocytes and macrophages leave the nodes in lymph (a clear fluid) that eventually drains through ducts into blood vessels near the heart. These cells then circulate in the blood and form a proportion of the white blood cell population.

If disease in the lymphatic system is suspected, a **nodal biopsy** (*nod-* meaning node and *-al* meaning pertaining

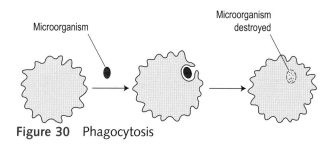

Microorganism / Microorganism destroyed

Figure 30 Phagocytosis

to) may be performed; in this procedure a node is removed for examination by a histopathologist (*hist/o* meaning tissue, *path/o* disease and *-logist* a specialist who studies).

The macrophages that line the lymph organs are part of a large system of cells known as the **reticuloendothelial system** or macrophage system. Cells that form this network have a common ancestry and carry out phagocytosis (Fig. 30) in the liver, bone marrow, lymph nodes, spleen, nervous system, blood and connective tissues. Macrophages found in connective tissues are known as **histiocytes** (i.e. tissue cells). If there is an increase in the number of histiocytes without infection this is known as a **histiocytosis**.

Distinct patches of lymphatic tissue have been given specific names; the familiar ones mentioned here include the spleen, tonsils, adenoids and thymus.

ROOT

Splen
(A Greek word, meaning spleen. The spleen has four main functions: destruction of old blood cells, blood storage, blood filtration and participation in the immune response.)

Combining form **Splen/o**

WORD EXERCISE 2

Using your Exercise Guide, find the meaning of:

(a) **splen**/o/megaly

(b) **splen**/o/hepat/o/megaly

(c) **splen**/o/pexy

(d) **splen**/o/cele

(e) **splen**/o/malacia

(f) **splen**/o/lysis

Without using your Exercise Guide, write the meaning of:

(g) **splen**/o/gram

(h) **splen**/o/port/o/gram

(**Port/o** refers to the portal vein that drains blood from the intestines, stomach, pancreas and spleen into the liver.)

ROOT

Tonsill
*(From Latin **tonsillae**, meaning tonsils. These form a ring of lymphoid tissue at the back of the mouth and nasopharynx. They are important in the formation of antibodies and lymphocytes.)*

Combining form **Tonsill/o**

WORD EXERCISE 3

Without using your Exercise Guide, build words that mean:

(a) inflammation of the tonsils

(b) removal of the tonsils

Using your Exercise Guide, find the meaning of:

(c) **tonsill/o/pharyng/eal**

(d) **tonsill/o/tome**

Note. The enlarged, single nasopharyngeal tonsil is known as the **adenoids**. Sometimes this obstructs the passage of air or interferes with hearing when it blocks the entrance to the auditory tube. Removal of the adenoids is known as an **adenoid**ectomy.

ROOT

Thym
*(From a Greek word **thymos**, meaning soul or emotion. Here, thym/o means the thymus gland that lies high in the chest above the aorta. It controls the development of the immune system in early life.)*

Combining forms **Thym/o, thymic/o**

WORD EXERCISE 4

Without using your Exercise Guide, build words using thym/o that mean:

(a) a cell of the thymus

(b) disease of the thymus

(c) protrusion/swelling of the thymus

Using your Exercise Guide, find the meaning of:

(d) **thym/elc/osis**
(Look up helc.)

(e) **thymic/o/lympha/tic**

Immunology

Immunology is the scientific study of immunity and related disciplines such as immunotherapy and immunochemistry. Immunological research has intensified recently because of the spread of the immunodeficiency virus (HIV) that causes AIDS. Many pharmaceutical companies are actively engaged in the search for vaccines and new treatments based on our increased knowledge of the immune process.

Immunity is the condition of being immune to infectious disease and antigenic substances that might damage the body. It is brought about by the production of antibodies and cells that destroy invading pathogens before they can do us harm. During our lifetime we naturally acquire immunity to common disease-producing organisms, such as viruses that cause colds and influenza. We can also artificially acquire immunity to more serious diseases by vaccination.

Understanding the meaning of the following terms will help you understand the basis of the immune process.

Antigen
An antigen is any foreign substance that enters the body and stimulates antibody production or a response associated with sensitized T-cells. Note, antigens will be present on the surface of any foreign cell that enters the body and these will provoke a response from the immune system.

Antibody
An antibody is a chemical that circulates in the blood destroying or precipitating specific foreign substances (antigens) that have entered the body. (*Anti-* means against, *-body* is an Anglo-Saxon word, in this case referring to a foreign body.)

ROOT

Immun
*(From Latin **immunis**, meaning exempt from public burden. Here, immun/o means immunity i.e. exemption from disease.)*

Combining form **Immun/o**

WORD EXERCISE 5

Using your Exercise Guide, look up the meaning of -logy and path/o, and then build words that mean:

(a) the study of immunity

(b) branch of medicine concerned with the study of immune reactions associated with disease

Using your Exercise Guide, find the meaning of:

(c) **immun/o**/genesis

(d) auto/**immun**/ity

(e) **immun/o**/globulin

Two basic types of cell bring about immunity:

T-cells (thymic cells)

T-cells are types of lymphocyte formed in the bone marrow of the embryo that move to the thymus to be processed into T-cells (hence the name T-cell). The T-cells then move to other parts of the lymphatic system where they are responsible for the **cell-mediated response**. Once sensitized to a specific antigen, these cells multiply rapidly, producing various cell types all of which play a role in the immune response. One type of cell that forms is the cytotoxic (killer) T-cell, this attacks and kills infectious microorganisms containing the specific antigen. These cells are particularly effective against slowly growing bacteria and fungi, cancer cells and skin grafts.

B-cells

B-cells are types of lymphocyte named for historical reasons after the site where they were first seen in birds, the Bursa of Fabricius. In humans, B-cells first differentiate in the fetal liver and transform into large **plasma cells** when confronted with specific antigens. Once sensitized by an antigen, the plasma cell multiplies to form a large clone of similar cells (**plasmacytosis**). Each cell in the clone secretes the same antibody to the sensitizing antigen; this is known as the **humoral response**. Some antibodies activate a protein in the blood known as **complement**, which aids the antibody in destroying antigen. (Note, plasmacytosis means an excess of plasma cells in the blood).

ROOT

Ser
*(From a Latin word **serum**, meaning whey. Here, ser/o means serum, the clear portion of any liquid separated from its more solid elements. Blood serum is the supernatant liquid formed when blood clots; it can be used as a source of antibodies.)*

Combining form **Ser/o**

WORD EXERCISE 6

Without using your Exercise Guide, build a word that means:

(a) the scientific study of sera

Serum investigations can lead to a patient being seronegative or seropositive for the presence of a particular antibody. For example a person assessed as HIV positive has antibodies in their blood to the human immunodeficiency virus. This means that the virus has entered their body and stimulated their immune system to make antibodies. If the virus is not destroyed by the immune system or inhibited by drug therapy it will continue to replicate and lead to the development of AIDS.

> Seronegative
> means showing a lack of antibody.
>
> Seropositive
> means showing the presence of a high level of antibody.

ROOT

Py
*(From a Greek word **pyon**, meaning pus.)*

Combining form **Py/o**

Pus is a yellow, protein-rich liquid, composed of tissue fluids containing bacteria and leucocytes. When a wound is forming or discharging pus it is said to be **suppurating**. Pus is formed in response to certain types of infection.

WORD EXERCISE 7

Using your Exercise Guide, find the meaning of:

(a) **py**/aemia
   (Am. **py**/emia)

(b) **py/o**/genic

(c) **py/o**/rrhoea
   (Am. **py/o**/rrhea)

(d) **py/o**/poiesis

The immune response of the lymphatic system not only resists invasion by infective organisms but also functions to identify and destroy everything described as 'non-self', i.e. foreign antigens that have entered the body, such as transplanted organs or body cells that have become malignant.

Patients infected with microorganisms, for example those who present with tonsillitis, experience swollen lymph nodes and their blood counts indicate an increase in circulating white blood cells. The nodes swell because they contain plasma cells and T-cells forming clones of cells to 'fight' the infection. Once the foreign cells have been destroyed, the nodes return to their normal size. The response of the body to the initial sensitization with the antigen is called the *primary response*.

An important feature of the immune response is that some activated B-cells develop into **memory B-cells** rather than plasma cells. These remain in the nodes and other lymphoid tissue ready to respond should the same antigen enter the body again. If the same antigen is contacted the memory B-cells divide rapidly to produce plasma cells. These release large amounts of antibody, destroying the antigen before symptoms appear.

In a similar way some **memory T-cells** remain in the lymphoid tissue, and can be rapidly activated in response to another contact with the same antigen. The accelerated and increased response of the memory cells is called the *secondary response*, and it endows us with immunity.

Medical equipment and clinical procedures

Revise the names of all instruments and clinical procedures mentioned in this unit and then try Exercise 8. Make sure you know the meaning of the suffixes -**gram** and -**graphy**.

WORD EXERCISE 8

Match each term in Column A with a description from Column C by placing an appropriate number in Column B.

Column A	Column B	Column C
(a) tonsillotome		1. X-ray picture of the portal veins and spleen
(b) lymphangio-graphy		2. X-ray picture of the lymphatic system
(c) lymphadeno-graphy		3. an instrument used for cutting tonsils
(d) lymphogram		4. technique of making an X-ray of lymph vessels
(e) spleno-portogram		5. technique of making an X-ray of the lymphatic system
(f) lymphography		6. technique of making an X-ray of lymph nodes

ANATOMY EXERCISE

Now complete the Anatomy Exercise on page 70.

Now complete the Anatomy Exercise on page 70.

CASE HISTORY 6

The object of this exercise is to understand words associated with a patient's medical history.

To complete the exercise:

- read through the passage on non-Hodgkin's lymphoma; unfamiliar words are underlined and you can find their meaning using the Word Help

- write the meaning of the medical terms shown in bold print on the lines that follow the Word Help.

Non-Hodgkin's lymphoma

Mr F, a 48-year-old male, presented to his <u>GP</u> with a painless swelling in the right <u>axilla</u>. The lump had been present for at least two months before his consultation and he had not been unduly concerned until he noticed a similar lump in his left axilla that appeared to be increasing in size. The patient indicated he had a good appetite and denied weight loss. There had been no change to his bowel and bladder habits and apart from a recent cold and **tonsillitis** he had not suffered any infection. He had smoked for 32 years and admitted moderate drinking. The only problem he mentioned was difficulty in sleeping; sometimes he would wake sweating copiously.

Examination revealed prominent lymph node enlargement in the right and left axillae and <u>inguinal</u> areas. The largest node was located in the right axilla, approximately 2 cm across. Examination of the head and neck also revealed enlarged <u>cervical</u> nodes, the largest approximately 1.5 cm across. The nodes were firm, tender and rubbery on <u>palpation</u>.

Cardiovascular and pulmonary examination was normal. He had **splenomegaly** that was palpable 3 cm below the left <u>costal</u> margin. His tonsils appeared swollen. It was evident from initial examination that Mr F was suffering from a generalized **lymphadenopathy** that did not appear to be associated with infection.

Mr F underwent axillary **nodal** <u>biopsy</u> and his specimen was sent to **histopathology**. Examination of the tissue revealed a <u>follicular</u>, small, <u>cleaved</u> cell <u>non-Hodgkin's</u> **lymphoma** (NHL). This was followed by a <u>bilateral</u> bone marrow <u>trephine</u> biopsy that demonstrated cells suspicious for lymphoma similar to those found in the nodes. The **lymphocytes** forming the tumour (Am. tumor) were classified as being of **B-cell** origin. Computerized <u>tomography</u> (CT) was used to assess nodal enlargement and he was referred to the <u>oncology</u> department for <u>staging</u>.

Mr F underwent four cycles of <u>chemotherapy</u> (<u>CHOPS</u>) and since then no disease is evident in his bone marrow and his lymphadenopathy has <u>regressed</u>.

WORD HELP

axilla the armpit (Pl. axillae)

bilateral pertaining to two sides

biopsy removal and examination of living tissue

cervical pertaining to the neck

chemotherapy treatment with chemicals, i.e. cytotoxic drugs that kill cancer cells

CHOPS type of chemotherapy regimen (using **c**yclophosphamide, **h**ydroxydaunorubicin, **o**ncovin and **p**rednisolone)

cleaved cut/separated (here refers to indentations in the nucleus of a lymph cell)

costal pertaining to the ribs

follicular pertaining to a follicle (here a well-defined collection of multiplying lymph cells)

GP general practitioner (family doctor)

inguinal pertaining to the groin

non-Hodgkin's not Hodgkin's disease, a type of lymphoma named after Thomas Hodgkin (b.1798 London physician)

oncology study of tumours (Am. tumors)/cancers

palpation act of feeling with the fingers using light pressure

regressed reverted (towards former condition)

staging a system of classifying malignant disease that will influence its treatment

tomography technique of using X-rays to image a section through the body

trephine an instrument with a circular cutting edge that removes a disc of tissue

Quick Reference

Combining forms relating to the lymphatic system and immunology:

Aden/o	gland
Adenoid-	adenoids
Cyt/o, -cyte	cell
-globulin	protein
Hist/i/o	tissue
Immun/o	immune
Lymph/o	lymph
Lymphaden/o	lymph node
Lymphangi/o	lymph vessel
Phag/o	eating/consuming
Plasma-	plasma cell
Py/o	pus
Ser/o	serum
Splen/o	spleen
Thym/o	thymus gland
Thymic/o	thymus gland
Tonsill/o	tonsil

Abbreviations

Some common abbreviations related to the lymphatic system are listed below. Note some are not standard and their meaning may vary from one health care setting to another. There is a more extensive list for reference on page 335.

AIDS	acquired immune deficiency syndrome
ALL	acute lymphocytic leukaemia (Am. leukemia)
BM (T)	bone marrow (trephine)
CLL	chronic lymphocytic leukaemia (Am. leukemia)
HLA	human leucocyte antigen (Am. leukocyte)
Ig	immunoglobulin
LAS	lymphadenopathy syndrome
Lymphos	lymphocytes
T & A	tonsils and adenoids
TD	thymus-dependent cells
TI	thymus-independent cells
TLD	thoracic lymph duct

Now write the meaning of the following words from the case history without using your dictionary lists:

(a) tonsillitis

(b) splenomegaly

(c) lymphadenopathy

(d) nodal

(e) histopathology

(f) lymphoma

(g) lymphocyte

(h) B-cell

(Answers to the case history exercise are given in the Answers to Word Exercises beginning on page 301.)

Medical Notes

Acquired immune deficiency syndrome

Acquired immune deficiency syndrome (AIDS) was first recognized in 1981. The condition is caused by the human immunodeficiency virus (HIV). HIV is a retrovirus containing RNA that once transcribed into DNA in the host cell directs it to produce new viruses. When the CD4 subset of T-lymphocytes are infected, they are destroyed and immunity is seriously impaired. When each T-lymphocyte dies, it releases new retroviruses that can spread the infection. As the HIV infection progresses, more and more CD4 lymphocytes are lost; this change is one of the principle clinical methods for monitoring AIDS. When T-lymphocyte and helper T-cell function is impaired, infectious organisms and cancer cells can grow and spread much more easily than normal. Infections and tumours that rarely occur in healthy people such as *Pneumocystis carinii* pneumonia (a protozoal infection) and Karposi's sarcoma (a type of skin cancer) are frequently seen in AIDS patients. As their immune system is deficient, AIDS patients usually die from one of these infections or cancers.

HIV is spread by direct contact of body fluids usually through sexual contact, blood transfusions, intravenous use of contaminated needles and breast-feeding by infectious mothers.

Allergy
The term allergy is used to describe hypersensitivity of the immune system to relatively harmless environmental antigens. Antigens that trigger an allergic response are called allergens. Almost any substance can be an allergen for some individuals. Before such a sensitization reaction occurs, a susceptible person must be exposed repeatedly to an allergen triggering the production of antibodies. Exposure to the allergen causes antigen-antibody reactions that trigger the release of histamine, kinins and other inflammatory substances. In some cases these substances may cause constriction of the airways, relaxation of blood vessels and irregular heart rhythms that can progress to a life-threatening condition called anaphylactic shock. However, more typical allergy symptoms include a runny nose, conjunctivitis and urticaria (hives). Drugs called antihistamines are often used to relieve the symptoms of this type of allergy.

Anaphylaxis
A life-threatening condition resulting from an extreme hypersensitivity reaction to a previously encountered allergen such as a wasp-sting.

Atopy
A familial (inherited) condition in which individuals have an increased tendency to develop an allergy such as eczema, asthma or rhinitis.

Autoimmunity
Autoimmunity is an inappropriate and excessive response to self-antigens. Disorders that result from autoimmune responses are called autoimmune diseases. Self-antigens are molecules that are native to a person's body and that are used by the immune system to identify the components of 'self'. In autoimmunity the immune system inappropriately attacks these antigens. A common autoimmune disease is rheumatoid arthritis in which inflammatory changes affect joints, the heart, blood vessels and skin.

Human leucocyte antigens (HLAs)
These are chemicals (glycoproteins) found on the surface of nucleated cells that were first discovered on leucocytes (Am. leukocytes). They act as antigens that are important when donors and recipients are cross-matched for organ transplantation. Rejection occurs when donor and recipient HLAs do not match.

Isoimmunity
Isoimmunity is a normal but often undesirable reaction of the immune system to antigens from a different individual of the same species. Isoimmunity is important in two situations, pregnancy and tissue transplants. During pregnancy antigens from a fetus may enter the mother's blood and sensitize her immune system. Antibodies that are formed as a result of this sensitization may then enter the fetal circulation and cause an inappropriate reaction. An example is erythroblastosis fetalis in which a Rhesus −ve mother makes antibodies to her Rhesus +ve fetus causing haemolysis (Am. hemolysis) and phagocytosis of her baby's red blood cells.

Isoimmunity is also of great importance in tissue or organ transplants. The immune system sometimes reacts against foreign antigens in grafted tissue causing a rejection syndrome.

Lymphoedema (Am. lymphedema)
Lymphoedema is an abnormal condition in which swelling of the tissues in the extremities occurs because of an obstruction of the lymphatics and accumulation of lymph. The most common causes are tumours and surgery.

Congenital lymphoedema (Milroy's disease) due to deficient development of lymph vessels is more often seen in women between the ages of 15 and 25 years of age. The obstruction can be in the lymphatic vessels or in the lymph nodes themselves.

Lymphoma
Lymphoma is a term that refers to a tumour (Am. tumor) of the cells of lymphoid tissue. Lymphomas are often malignant but in rare cases can be benign. They usually originate in isolated lymph nodes but can involve lymphoid tissue in the liver, spleen and gastrointestinal tract. Widespread involvement is common because the disease spreads from node to node through the lymphatic vessels. The exact cause of these neoplasms is unknown. The two principle categories of lymphoma are Hodgkin's disease and non-Hodgkin's lymphoma.

> **Hodgkin's disease** is a malignancy with an uncertain cause, some pathologists believe it originates as a viral-induced tumour of T-cells. The condition usually begins as painless, non-tender enlarged lymph nodes in the neck or axilla. Soon, lymph nodes in other regions enlarge in the same manner. If those near the trachea or oesophagus swell, the increased pressure results in difficulty in breathing or swallowing. Lymphoedema (Am. lymphedema), anaemia (Am. anemia), leucocytosis (Am. leukocytosis), fever and weight-loss occur as the condition progresses. Hodgkin's disease is potentially curable with radiation therapy provided it has not spread

beyond the lymphatic system. Chemotherapy is used in addition to radiation therapy in more advanced cases.

Non-Hodgkin's lymphoma is the name given to a malignancy of lymphoid tissue other than Hodgkin's disease; examples include multiple myeloma and Burkitt's lymphoma. The cause is uncertain but has been hypothesized to be a virus. Manifestations are similar to Hodgkin's disease but there is usually a more generalized involvement of lymph nodes and the central nervous system is often involved. Radiation and chemotherapy are treatments of choice.

NOW TRY THE WORD CHECK

WORD CHECK

This self-check exercise lists all the word components used in this unit. First write down the meaning of as many word components as you can. Then check your answers using the Exercise Guide and Quick Reference box or the Glossary of Word Components (pp. 347–371).

Prefixes

anti-

auto-

macro-

Combining forms of word roots

aden/o

angi/o

cyt/o

-globulin

helc/o

hepat/o

hist/i/o

immun/o

lymph/o

lymphaden/o

lymphangi/o

phag/o

pharyng/o

plasm/a

port/o

py/o

reticul/o

ser/o

splen/o

thym/o

tonsill/o

Suffixes

-aemia (Am. -emia)

-al

-cele

-eal

-ectasis

-ectomy

-genesis

-genic

-gram

-graphy

-ia

-ic

-itis

-ity

-logy

-lysis

-malacia

-megaly

-oma

-osis

-pathy

-pexy

-poiesis

-rrhagia

-rrhoea (Am. -rrhea)

-tic

-tome

NOW TRY THE SELF-ASSESSMENT

SELF-ASSESSMENT

Test 6A

Below are some medical terms that refer to the anatomy of the lymphatic system. Indicate which part of the system they refer to by putting a number from the diagram (Fig. 31) next to each word.

(a) lymphaden/o

(b) splen/o

(c) thym/o

(d) tonsill/o

(e) lymphangi/o

Score

5

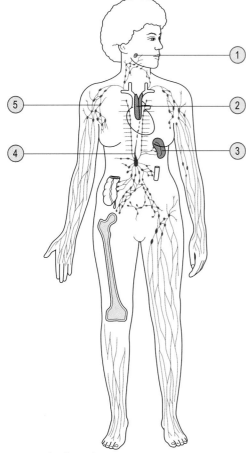

Figure 31 The lymphatic system

Test 6B

Prefixes, suffixes and combining forms of word roots

Match each word component in Column A with a meaning in Column C by inserting the appropriate number in Column B.

Column A	Column B	Column C
(a) aden/o		1. protein/ball
(b) angi/o		2. swelling/hernia/ protrusion
(c) anti-		3. immune
(d) auto-		4. self
(e) -cele		5. vessel
(f) -globin		6. pus
(g) -gram		7. cutting instrument
(h) helc/o		8. against
(i) immun/o		9. spleen
(j) lymph/o		10. ulcer
(k) -lysis		11. serum
(l) -malacia		12. tonsil
(m) port/o		13. lymph
(n) py/o		14. gland node
(o) -rrhoea (Am. -rrhea)		15. excessive flow
(p) ser/o		16. picture/tracing/ recording
(q) splen/o		17. condition of softening
(r) thym/o		18. disintegration/ breakdown
(s) -tome		19. portal vein
(t) tonsill/o		20. thymus gland

Score

20

Test 6C

Write the meaning of:

(a) lymphorrhoea
(Am. lymphorrhea)

(b) splenic

(c) lymphadenectasis

(d) thymolysis

(e) serologist

Score

5

Test 6D

Build words that mean:

(a) tumour (Am. tumor)
of lymph (tissue)

(b) X-ray examination of the
lymph system

(c) removal of the spleen

(d) condition of bleeding/
bursting forth of the spleen

(e) tumour (Am. tumor) of a
lymph vessel

Score

5

Check answers to Self-Assessment Tests on page 325.

UNIT 7
THE URINARY SYSTEM

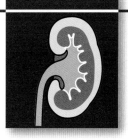

OBJECTIVES

Once you have completed Unit 7 you should be able to:

- understand the meaning of medical words relating to the urinary system

- build medical words relating to the urinary system

- associate medical terms with their anatomical position

- understand medical abbreviations relating to the urinary system.

EXERCISE GUIDE

Use this list of word components and their meanings to complete the word exercises in this unit.

Prefixes

dys-	difficult/painful
hyper-	above normal/excessive
intra-	within/inside
oligo-	deficiency/few/little
poly-	many/much

Roots/Combining forms

albumin/o	albumin/albumen
azot/o	urea
calc/i	calcium
col/o	colon
enter/o	intestine
gastr/o	stomach
haemat/o	blood
hemat/o (Am.)	blood
hydr/o	water
lith/o	stone
metr/o	a measure
proct/o	anus/rectum
py/o	pus
sigmoid/o	sigmoid colon
trigon/o	trigone of the bladder

Suffixes

-al	pertaining to
-algia	condition of pain
-cele	swelling/protrusion/hernia
-clysis	infusion/injection/irrigation
-dynia	condition of pain
-ectasis	dilatation/stretching
-ectomy	removal of
-ferous	pertaining to carrying/bearing

-genesis	capable of causing/pertaining to formation
-gram	X-ray/tracing/recording
-graphy	technique of recording/making an X-ray
-ia	condition of
-iasis	abnormal condition
-ic	pertaining to
-itis	inflammation of
-lapaxy	empty/wash out/evacuate
-lithiasis	abnormal condition of stones
-logist	specialist who studies
-lysis	breakdown/disintegration
-meter	measuring instrument
-metry	process of measuring
-osis	abnormal condition/disease of
-ous	pertaining to/of the nature of
-pathy	disease of
-pexy	surgical fixation/fix in place
-phyma	tumour (Am. tumor)/boil
-plasty	surgical repair/reconstruction
-ptosis	falling/diplacement/prolapse
-rrhagia	condition of bursting forth of blood/bleeding
-rrhaphy	suturing/stitching
-sclerosis	condition of hardening
-scope	instrument to view
-scopy	visual examination
-stenosis	condition of narrowing
-stomy	to form a new opening or outlet
-tome	cutting instrument
-tomy	incision into
-tripsy	act of crushing
-triptor	instrument to crush/fragment (using shock waves)
-trite	instrument to crush/fragment
-uresis	excrete in urine/urinate

ANATOMY EXERCISE

When you have finished Word Exercises 1–11, look at the word components listed below. Complete Figure 32 by writing the appropriate combining form on each line – more than one component may relate to the same position. (You can check their meanings in the Quick Reference box on p. 89.)

Cyst/o	Ren/o	Urin/o
Glomerul/o	Ureter/o	Vesic/o
Nephr/o	Urethr/o	
Pyel/o		

The urinary system

The main components of the urinary system are the kidneys that remove metabolic wastes from the blood by forming them into urine. This yellow liquid is passed from the kidneys through the ureters to the urinary bladder where it is stored. Periodically urine is passed out of the body through the urethra in the process of urination.

Besides removing waste substances that could be toxic to tissue cells, the kidneys maintain the volume of water in the blood and regulate its salt concentration and pH. The kidneys are therefore involved in homeostasis, i.e. maintaining constant conditions within the tissue

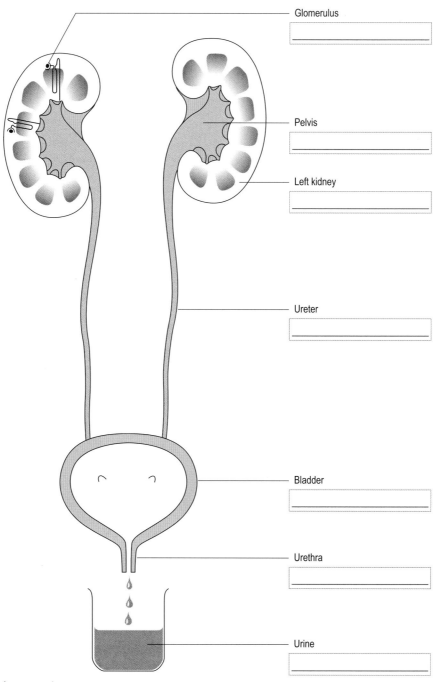

Glomerulus

Pelvis

Left kidney

Ureter

Bladder

Urethra

Urine

Figure 32 The urinary system

fluids of the body. The continuous activity of the kidneys is required to maintain life.

Use the Exercise Guide at the beginning of this unit to complete Word Exercises 1–11 unless you are asked to work without it.

ROOT

Ren
*(A Latin word **ren**, meaning kidney.)*

Combining form   **Ren/o**

WORD EXERCISE 1

Using your Exercise Guide, find the meaning of:

(a) **ren/o**/gastr/ic

(b) **ren/o**/gram

(c) **ren/o**/graphy

Renography may show up a renal calculus (from Latin *calcis* – small stone), i.e. a kidney stone. The presence of a stone in a ureter leads to severe pain and is referred to as **renal colic**. Renal colic can also be caused by disorder and disease within a kidney.

Radioisotope renograms are useful in assessing kidney function. They are made following injection of radioisotopes into the bloodstream. The technique of making this type of recording is discussed in more detail in Unit 18.

ROOT

Nephr
*(From a Greek word **nephros**, meaning kidney.)*

Combining form   **Nephr/o**

WORD EXERCISE 2

Using your Exercise Guide, find the meaning of:

(a) **nephr/o**/ptosis

(b) hydr/o/**nephr**/osis

(c) **nephr/o**/cele

(d) **nephr**/algia

Using your Exercise Guide find the meaning of -ectomy,-lithiasis, -pexy and tomy, then build words that mean:

(e) surgical fixation of a kidney (e.g. floating kidney)

(f) surgical repair of a kidney

(g) incision into a kidney

(h) condition of stones in the kidney

(i) removal of a kidney

Within each kidney there are approximately one million kidney tubules or nephrons that do the work of the kidney. At the beginning of each nephron is a **glomerulus**, a ball of capillaries surrounded by porous membranes that filter metabolic wastes from the blood. When glomeruli undergo pathological change the filtering mechanism of the kidneys is seriously affected, reducing their ability to maintain homeostasis.

Using your Exercise Guide, find the meaning of:

(j) **glomerul**/it is (suppurative)

(k) **glomerul/o**/pathy

(l) **glomerul/o**/sclerosis

Infections and disorders of the kidneys sometimes lead to kidney failure. This results in the waste products of metabolism increasing in concentration within the blood and a failure to regulate water, mineral metabolism and pH; these changes will lead to death. The patient with kidney failure can be kept alive if one of the following procedures is applied.

Haemodialysis (Am. hemodialysis)

This involves diverting the patient's blood through a dialyser, commonly called a kidney machine (Fig. 33). In the dialyser waste products are removed from the blood which is then returned to the body via another blood vessel. The patient must be connected to the dialyser for many hours per week and so cannot lead a normal life. (Dialysis means separating, i.e. separating wastes from the blood.)

CAPD (continuous ambulatory peritoneal dialysis)

The patient is fitted with a peritoneal catheter (tube) (Fig. 34). Every 6 hours approximately 2 litres of dialysing fluid is passed into the peritoneum. Toxic wastes diffuse into the dialysing fluid and are removed from the body when the fluid is changed. This procedure is repeated four times a day, 7 days a week. CAPD has been used on a long-term basis but there is danger from peritonitis caused by infection.

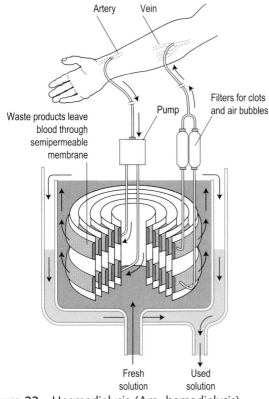

Artery   Vein

Filters for clots
and air bubbles

Pump

Waste products leave
blood through
semipermeable
membrane

Fresh   Used
solution   solution

Figure 33   Haemodialysis (Am. hemodialysis)

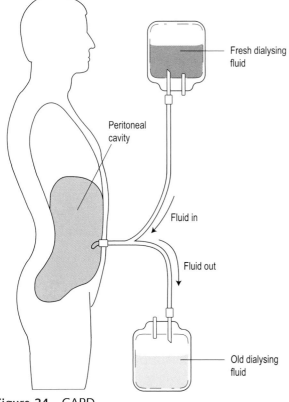

Fresh dialysing
fluid

Peritoneal
cavity

Fluid in

Fluid out

Old dialysing
fluid

Figure 34   CAPD

Kidney transplant

A kidney can be transplanted between two individuals of the same species, i.e. between two humans who are not closely related. This type of transplant or graft is known as a homotransplant or homograft (*homo* meaning the

same, synonymous with allograft). The donor could be living and survive with one remaining kidney, or a victim of a fatal accident. A transplant may keep a patient alive for many years and avoids the inconvenience and dangers associated with CAPD and dialysis. Transplants between genetically identical twins are more successful. These are known as isografts (*iso* means same/equal).

ROOT

Pyel
*(From a Greek word **pyelos**, meaning trough or basin. Here pyel/o means the renal pelvis, the space inside a kidney in which urine collects after its formation.)*

Combining form   **Pyel/o**

(Do not confuse this with py/o, meaning pus.)

WORD EXERCISE 3

Without using your Exercise Guide, write the meaning of:

(a) **pyel/o**/nephr/itis

(This is often due to a bacterial infection ascending from the urinary tract or entering the kidney from the blood.)

(b) **pyel/o**/lith/o/tomy

(c) **pyel/o**/nephr/osis

Without using your Exercise Guide, build words that mean:

(d) surgical repair of the renal pelvis

(e) X-ray picture of the renal pelvis

The technique of making an X-ray of the renal pelvis is known as **pyelo**graphy. It involves filling the pelvis with a radio-opaque dye. There are several ways of doing this:

Intravenous pyelography (Syn. intravenous urography)
Here the dye is injected into the bloodstream and it eventually passes through the kidney pelvis (**intra** – meaning inside, **ven/o** – meaning vein).

Antegrade pyelography
Here the dye is injected into the renal pelvis (**ante** – meaning before/in front; **grad** – meaning take steps/to go (Latin)). It refers to the fact that the dye goes into the pelvis before it leaves the kidney. The dye is injected through a percutaneous catheter, i.e. through the skin.

Retrograde (or ascending) pyelography (Syn. retrograde or ascending urography)
Here the dye is injected into the kidney via the ureter, so it is being forced backwards up the ureter into the urine within the pelvis (**retro** – means backwards).

Note. We have already used cyst/o in Unit 2 with cholecyst/o meaning the gallbladder (bile bladder). Here we are using **cyst/o** alone to mean the urinary bladder, the organ that stores urine until it is expelled from the body.

ROOT

Ureter
*(From a Greek word **oureter**, meaning ureter, the narrow tube that connects each kidney to the bladder. Urine flows through the ureters assisted by the action of smooth muscle.)*

Combining form **Ureter/o**

WORD EXERCISE 4

Without using your Exercise Guide, write the meaning of:

(a) **ureter/o/cele**

(b) **ureter/o/cel/ectomy**

Using your Exercise Guide, find the meaning of:

(c) **ureter/o/rrhagia**

(d) **ureter/o/rrhaphy**

(e) **ureter/ectasis**

(f) **ureter/o/ren/o/scopy**

(Note the difference between -scope and -scopy.)

(g) **ureter/o/stomy**

Using your Exercise Guide look up col/o, enter/o and -stomy, and then build words that mean:

(h) formation of an opening between the intestine and ureter

(i) formation of an opening between the colon and ureter

WORD EXERCISE 5

Without using your Exercise Guide, write the meaning of:

(a) **cyst/itis**

There are many causes of this acute or chronic condition including injury and infection. As the bladder is accessible from outside via the urethra, it is relatively easy for microorganisms to enter. Sometimes infections such as *Neisseria gonorrhoeae* and *Chlamydia* are transmitted into the urinary tract by sexual contact. Cystitis occurs more frequently in women because the female urethra is short and close to the anus (a source of bacteria). Symptoms include pelvic pain, an urge to urinate frequently and haematuria (Am. hematuria).

(b) **cyst/o/lith/ectomy**

(c) **cyst/o/pyel/itis**

(d) **cyst/o/ptosis**

Using your Exercise Guide, find the meaning of:

(e) **cyst/o/scope**

(f) **cyst/o/proct/o/stomy**

Meter and **metr/o** originate from Greek *metron*, meaning a measure, and **metry** from *metrein*, meaning process of measuring. Use these to build words meaning:

(g) instrument used to measure the bladder (capacity or pressure)

(h) technique of measuring the bladder (capacity and changes in pressure)

(i) a trace, or recording of bladder measurements (changes in pressure)

ROOT

Cyst
*(From Greek **kystis**, meaning bladder.)*

Combining form **Cyst/o**

A technique that applies an electric current to tissues, causing them to heat up, is known as **diathermy** (*dia* – meaning through and *thermy* – meaning heat). These can be combined here to make:

Cystodiathermy
The process of applying heat through the bladder. The heat is produced by an electric current and is used to destroy tumours (Am. tumors) in the bladder wall.

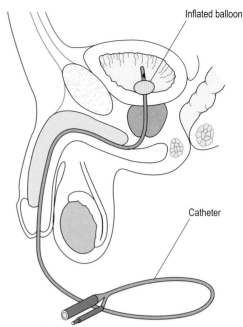

Figure 35   Catheterization

ROOT

Vesic
(From Latin **vesica**, *meaning bladder.)*

Combining form **Vesic/o**

WORD EXERCISE 6

Without using your Exercise Guide, build words that mean:

(a) formation of an opening into the bladder

(b) incision into the bladder

Using your Exercise Guide, find the meaning of:

(c) **vesic/o**/clysis

(d) **vesic**/al

(e) **vesic/o**/sigmoid/o/stomy

Without using your Exercise Guide, write the meaning of:

(f) **vesic/o**/ureter/al

Catheterization of the bladder is required following some surgical operations and when there is difficulty in emptying the bladder owing to a neuromuscular disorder or physical damage to the spinal cord. The procedure involves inserting a catheter through the urethra into the bladder (Fig. 35). A urinary **catheter** consists of a fine tube that allows urine to drain from the bladder into an external container. Some self-retaining catheters are held in position by means of an inflated balloon.

ROOT

Urethr
(From Greek **ourethro**, *meaning urethra, the tube through which urine leaves the body from the bladder.)*

Combining form **Urethr/o**

WORD EXERCISE 7

Without using your Exercise Guide, write the meaning of:

(a) **urethr/o**/metry

(b) **urethr/o**/trigon/itis

(Trigone refers to a triangular area at the base of the bladder, bounded by the openings of the ureters at the back and the urethral opening at the front.)

(c) **urethr/o**/pexy

Without using your Exercise Guide, build words that mean:

(d) condition of pain in the urethra

(e) condition of flow of blood from the urethra

(f) visual examination of the urethra

Using your Exercise Guide, find the meaning of:

(g) **urethr/o**/phyma

(h) **urethr/o**/tome

(i) **urethr/o**/stenosis

(j) **urethr/o**/dynia

ROOT

Urin

*(From a Latin word **urina**, meaning urine, the excretory product of the kidneys.)*

Combining forms   **Urin/a/i/o**

WORD EXERCISE 8

Using your Exercise Guide, find the meaning of:

(a) **urin/i**/ferous

(b) **urin/a**/lysis

(This word refers to the technique of analysing urine. Detailed urinalysis is a valuable aid to the diagnosis of disease, for example detecting the presence of high concentrations of glucose in the urine may indicate diabetes. Other components commonly analysed are pH, specific gravity, ketone bodies, phenylketones, protein, bilirubin and solid casts of varying composition.)

Without using your Exercise Guide, write the meaning of:

(c) **urin/o**/meter
(Used to estimate specific gravity of urine.)

ROOT

Ur

*(From a Greek word **ouron**, meaning urine.)*

Combining form   **Ur/o**

(This combining form is also used to refer to the urinary tract and urination.)

WORD EXERCISE 9

Without using your Exercise Guide, write the meaning of:

(a) **ur/o**/graphy

(The above procedure is also performed by injecting dye directly into the urinary tract rather than into a vein.)

Using your Exercise Guide, find the meaning of:

(b) **ur/o**/logist

(c) **ur/o**/genesis

(d) olig/**ur**/ia

(e) albumin/**ur**/ia

(f) azot/**ur**/ia

(g) poly/**ur**/ia

(h) dys/**ur**/ia

(i) haemat/**ur**/ia
(Am. hemat/ur/ia)

(j) py/**ur**/ia

(k) hyper/calci/**ur**/ia

Note. The act of passing urine is known as micturition (from Latin *micturire*, meaning to pass water).

ROOT

Lith

*(From a Greek word **lithos**, meaning stone.)*

Combining form   **Lith/o**

Here **lith/o** refers to a kidney stone, which is a hard mass composed mainly of mineral matter present in the urinary system. Remember a stone is sometimes called a **renal calculus** (pl. **calculi**). Stones can prevent the passage of urine, causing pain and kidney damage. They need to be passed or removed because they can seriously affect the functioning of the kidneys.

WORD EXERCISE 10

Without using your Exercise Guide, write the meaning of:

(a) **lith/o**/nephr/itis

(b) ur/o/**lith**/iasis

(c) **lith/o**/genesis

Using your Exercise Guide, find the meaning of:

(d) **lith/o**/trite

(e) **lith/o**/lapaxy

(f) **lith/o**/triptor

(This instrument focuses high-energy shock waves generated by a high voltage spark on to a kidney stone. No surgery is required, as the stone disintegrates within the body and is passed in the urine. The procedure for using this instrument is called extra-corporeal shock wave lithotripsy (ECSL), *extra* meaning outside, *corporeal* meaning body.)

(g) **lith/o**/tripsy

(h) **lith**/uresis

Medical equipment and clinical procedures

Before completing Exercise 11, revise the names of all instruments and clinical procedures mentioned in this unit. Make sure you know the meanings of: -meter, -scope, -scopy, -thermy, -tome, -triptor, and -trite.

WORD EXERCISE 11

Match each term in Column A with a description from Column C by placing an appropriate number in Column B.

Column A	Column B	Column C
(a) diathermy		1. an instrument used for crushing stones
(b) cystoscope		2. a device that separates wastes from the blood
(c) lithotriptor		3. an instrument used for cutting the urethra
(d) urinometer		4. visual examination of the ureter
(e) haemodialyser (Am. hemodialyzer)		5. an instrument that measures the pressure and capacity of the bladder
(f) ureteroscopy		6. an instrument used to view the urethra
(g) urethrotome		7. a device that destroys stones using shock waves
(h) cystometer		8. technique of heating a tissue by applying an electric current
(i) urethroscope		9. an instrument used for measuring the specific gravity of urine
(j) lithotrite		10. an instrument used to view the bladder

ANATOMY EXERCISE

Now complete the Anatomy Exercise on page 82.

CASE HISTORY 7

The object of this exercise is to understand words associated with a patient's medical history.

To complete the exercise:

- read through the passage on urolithiasis; unfamiliar words are underlined and you can find their meaning using the Word Help

- write the meaning of the medical terms shown in bold print on the lines that follow the Word Help.

Urolithiasis

Mr G, an engineer recently returned from working in the Middle East, was admitted to Accident and Emergency in pain and clutching his right side. He had been awoken during the night by an excruciating pain in his right flank radiating to the iliac fossa and right testicle. In the past two days, he had developed severe **urethral** pain and **dysuria** associated with **haematuria (Am. hematuria)**. Fluid intake made the pain worse and he had been vomiting. Mr G had recently been treated with antibiotics by his GP for bacteriuria and diagnosed as suffering from obstructive **uropathy**. His condition had become acute whilst waiting for his referral appointment. On admission he required immediate analgesia for severe pain and was administered 10mg morphine i.m. He was kept in overnight for observation and transferred to the Urology Unit the following morning.

The next day a dull pain was still present, and examination revealed loin tenderness and an enlarged palpable hydronephrotic right kidney. A plain abdominal radiograph identified a single calculus in the line of the right ureter. Excretion urography (intravenous **pyelography** IVP) confirmed the calculus to be obstructing the pelviureteric junction. The kidney outline appeared enlarged but smooth with no anatomical abnormalities of the calyces.

Mr G underwent extracorporeal shockwave **lithotripsy** (ESWL) and the calculus was successfully fragmented and excreted. His urinary catheter was left in place for one day, and he was discharged on 50mg diclofenac t.i.d. His recovery was unremarkable and a follow-up KUB was arranged for two weeks through the Lithotripsy reception.

Mr G was advised that he should increase his fluid intake particularly when he returned to the Middle East. It was recommended that a urine output of 2–2.5 litres per day would be appropriate. Urine analysis indicated a slight **hypercalciuria,** and it was recommended that he restricted his intake of calcium and vitamin D. He was referred to the dietician for advice on food intake.

WORD HELP

analgesia condition of pain relief

calculus a stone or abnormal concretion (plural calculi)

calyces cup-shaped divisions of the renal pelvis (sing. calyx)

catheter a tube for introducing or withdrawing fluid from the body

GP general practitioner (family doctor)

hydronephrotic pertaining to hydronephrosis (a kidney swollen with water)

iliac fossa pertaining to the concave, upper and anterior part of the sacropelvic surface of the iliac bone. A fossa is a depression/recess below the general surface of a part

i.m. intramuscular (here meaning an injection into muscle)

KUB kidneys, ureters and bladder (X-ray/examination)

pelviureteric pertaining to a ureter and renal pelvis

radiograph an X-ray picture

t.i.d. three times daily (ter in die)

urography technique of recording/making an X-ray of the urinary tract

urology study of the urinary system (here it refers to a hospital department)

Quick Reference

Combining forms relating to the urinary system:

Albumin/o	albumin/albumen
Azot/o	urea/nitrogen
Cyst/o	bladder
Glomerul/o	glomerulus
Lith/o	stone
Nephr/o	kidney
Pyel/o	pelvis of kidney
Ren/o	kidney
Trigon/o	trigone
Ureter/o	ureter
Urethr/o	urethra
Urin/o	urine
Ur/o	urine/urinary tract
Vesic/o	bladder

Abbreviations

Some common abbreviations related to the urinary system are listed below. Note some are not standard and their meaning may vary from one health care setting to another. There is a more extensive list for reference on page 335.

ARF	acute renal failure
BUN	blood urea nitrogen
CRF	chronic renal failure
CSU	catheter specimen of urine
Cysto	cystoscopy
HD	haemodialysis (Am. hemodialysis)
IVP	intravenous pyelogram
KUB	kidney, ureter, bladder
MSU	midstream urine
PCNL	percutaneous nephrolithotomy
U & E	urea and electrolytes
UTI	urinary tract infection

Now write the meaning of the following words from the case history without using your dictionary lists:

(a) urolithiasis

(b) urethral

(c) dysuria

(d) haematuria
(Am. hematuria)

(e) uropathy

(f) pyelography

(g) lithotripsy

(h) hypercalciuria

(Answers to the case history exercise are given in the Answers to Word Exercises beginning on page 301.)

Medical Notes

Diabetic kidney

Renal failure is the cause of death in approximately ten percent of all diabetics and up to fifty percent of cases of insulin dependent diabetes mellitus (Type 1). In this condition there is damage to large and small blood vessels in many parts of the body. The effects on the kidney include progressive glomerulosclerosis and atrophy of the renal tubules, acute pyelonephritis and nephrotic syndrome.

Glomerulonephritis (GN)

Glomerular disorders, collectively called glomerulonephritis, result from damage to the glomerular-capsular membranes that filter blood in the kidneys. Immune mechanisms, heredity, and other factors can cause this damage. Without successful treatment, glomerular disorders can progress to kidney failure.

Acute glomerulonephritis is the most common form of kidney disease. It may be caused by a delayed immune response to streptococcal infection. If antibiotic treatment is not successful it may progress to a chronic form of glomerulonephritis.

Chronic glomerulonephritis is the general name for various non-infectious glomerular disorders that are characterized by progressive kidney damage leading to renal failure. Immune mechanisms are believed to be the major cause of this condition. Antigen-antibody complexes that form in the blood may lodge in the glomerular capsule membrane triggering a response. Less commonly, antibodies may form that directly attack the glomerular-capsular membranes.

Kidney failure

Kidney failure or renal failure, is simply the failure of the kidney to properly process blood plasma and form urine. Renal failure can be classified as acute or chronic.

Acute renal failure (ARF) is an abrupt reduction in kidney function that is characterized by oliguria and a sharp rise in nitrogenous compounds in the blood. Acute renal failure can be caused by various factors that alter blood pressure or affect glomerular filtration; examples include haemorrhage (Am. hemorrhage), severe burns, or obstruction of the lower urinary tract. If the underlying cause is attended to recovery is usually rapid and complete.

Chronic renal failure (CRF) is a slow progressive condition resulting from the gradual loss of nephrons. There are many diseases that result in a gradual loss of nephron function including infections, diabetes glomerulonephritis, tumours, systemic autoimmune disorders and obstructive disorders.

Nephrotic syndrome

Nephrotic syndrome is not a disease in itself but a collection of signs and symptoms that accompany various glomerular disorders. When glomeruli are damaged, the permeability of the glomerular membrane is increased and plasma proteins pass through into the filtrate. Proteinuria, hypoalbuminaemia (Am. hypoalbuminemia), hyperlipidaemia (Am. hyperlipidemia) and oedema (Am. edema) characterize this syndrome.

Renal calculi

Renal calculi, or kidney stones, are crystallized mineral deposits that develop in the renal pelvis or calyces. Many calculi form when minerals crystallize on the renal papillae and then break off into the urine. The solutes that form calculi include oxalates, phosphates, urates and uric acid, often deposited in layers.

If the stones are small enough, they simply pass through the ureters and urethra and are eventually voided with the urine. Stag-horn calculi are large, branched stones that form in the pelvis and branched calyces. A large stone may obstruct the ureter, causing intense pain (*renal colic*) as rhythmical contractions in the wall of the ureter attempt to dislodge it. Hydronephrosis may occur if the stone does not move from its obstructing position.

Tumours (Am. tumors)

Tumours of the urinary system typically obstruct urine flow causing hydronephrosis in one or both kidneys. Most kidney tumours are malignant neoplasms called renal clear cell carcinomas; they usually occur in one kidney only. Bladder cancer occurs about as frequently as renal cancer. Bladder tumours are often multiple, their cause is unknown but predisposing factors include cigarette smoking and exposure to chemicals used in the manufacture of aniline dyes and rubber.

Urinary incontinence

This is the involuntary voiding of urine due to defective voluntary control of the external urethral sphincter that controls the exit of urine from the body.

Retention and overflow incontinence may be due to disruption of the nerve input into the bladder. Such paralysis results in loss of normal control of micturition (voiding of urine) and is sometimes termed a neurogenic bladder. The condition is characterized by involuntary retention of urine, subsequent distention of the bladder and perhaps a burning sensation or fever. Once the bladder is full, the increased pressure opens the urethral sphincter and urine dribbles from the urethra.

Urge incontinence is characterized by a sudden and intense urge to pass urine, the amounts voided are generally small and are sometimes accompanied by pain. The condition may be due to calculi, tumours and stress.

Wilm's tumour (nephroblastoma)

A highly malignant tumour (Am. tumor) of the kidney arising from embryonic tissue that develops in early childhood.

NOW TRY THE WORD CHECK

WORD CHECK

This self-check exercise lists all the word components used in this unit. First write down the meaning of as many word components as you can. Then check your answers using the Exercise Guide and Quick Reference box or the Glossary of Word Components (pp. 347–371).

Prefixes

ante-

dia-

dys-

hyper-

intra-oligo-

poly-

retro-

Combining forms of word roots

albumin/o

azot/o

calc/i

col/o

cyst/o

enter/o

gastr/o

glomerul/o

haem/o
(Am. hem/o)

hydr/o

lith/o

nephr/o

proct/o

pyel/o

py/o

ren/o

sigmoid/o

sten/o

trigon/o

ureter/o

urethr/o

urin/o

ur/o

ven/o

vesic/o

Suffixes

-al

-algia

-cele

-clysis

-dynia

-ectasis

-ectomy

-ferous

-genesis

-gram

-graphy

-iasis

-ic

-itis

-lapaxy

-lithiasis

-logist

-lysis

-meter

-metry

-osis

-ous

-pexy

-phyma

-plasty

-ptosis

-rrhage

-rrhaphy

-sclerosis

-scope

-scopy

-stomy

-thermy

-tome

-tomy

-tripsy

-triptor

-trite

-uresis

NOW TRY THE SELF-ASSESSMENT

SELF-ASSESSMENT

Test 7A

Below are some combining forms that refer to the anatomy of the urinary system. Indicate which part of the system they refer to by putting a number from the diagram (Fig. 36) next to each word.

(a) ureter/o

(b) nephr/o

(c) glomerul/o

(d) pyel/o

(e) urethr/o

(f) lith/o

(g) cyst/o

(h) urin/o

Score

8

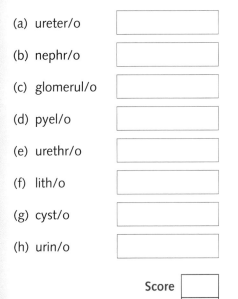

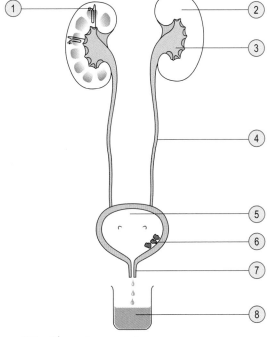

Figure 36 The urinary system

Test 7B

Prefixes and suffixes

Match each prefix or suffix in Column A with a meaning in Column C by inserting the appropriate number in Column B.

Column A	Column B	Column C
(a) ante-		1. technique of breaking stones with shock waves
(b) -cele		2. measuring instrument
(c) -clysis		3. a crushing instrument
(d) dia-		4. abnormal condition of urine
(e) dys-		5. technique of measuring
(f) -ferous		6. backward
(g) -iasis		7. protrusion/swelling/hernia
(h) intra-		8. tumour (Am. tumor)/boil
(i) -lapaxy		9. before
(j) -meter		10. to fall/displace
(k) -metry		11. pertaining to carrying
(l) oligo-		12. abnormal condition of
(m) -phyma		13. too little/few
(n) poly-		14. difficult/painful
(o) -ptosis		15. infusion/injection into
(p) retro-		16. through
(q) -thermy		17. within/inside
(r) -tripsy		18. evacuation/wash out
(s) -trite		19. many
(t) -uresis		20. heat

Score

20

Test 7C

Combining forms of word roots

Match each combining form in Column A with a meaning in Column C by inserting the appropriate number in Column B.

Column A	Column B	Column C
(a) col/o		1. blood
(b) cyst/o		2. kidney (i)
(c) gastr/o		3. kidney (ii)
(d) glomerul/o		4. sigmoid colon
(e) haemat/o (Am. hemat/o)		5. pus
(f) lith/o		6. trigone/base of bladder
(g) nephr/o		7. urethra
(h) proct/o		8. bladder (i)
(i) pyel/o		9. bladder (ii)
(j) py/o		10. vein
(k) ren/o		11. stomach
(l) sigmoid/o		12. pelvis/trough
(m) sten/o		13. urine
(n) trigon/o		14. urine/urinary tract
(o) ureter/o		15. glomeruli (of kidney)
(p) urethr/o		16. ureter
(q) urin/o		17. colon
(r) ur/o		18. anus/rectum
(s) ven/o		19. stone
(t) vesic/o		20. narrowing

Score

20

Test 7D

Write the meaning of:

(a) nephropyelolithotomy

(b) ureterostenosis

(c) cystourethrography

(d) vesicocele

(e) pyelectasis

Score

5

Test 7E

Build words that mean:

(a) dilatation of a ureter

(b) formation of an opening between the ureter and sigmoid colon

(c) technique of making an X-ray of the bladder (use cyst/o)

(d) X-ray picture of the urinary tract

(e) abnormal condition of hardening of the kidney

Score

5

Check answers to Self-Assessment Tests on page 325.

UNIT 8
THE NERVOUS SYSTEM

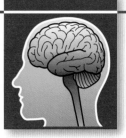

OBJECTIVES

Once you have completed Unit 8 you should be able to:

- understand the meaning of medical words relating to the nervous system

- build medical words relating to the nervous system

- associate medical terms with their anatomical position

- understand medical abbreviations relating to the nervous system.

EXERCISE GUIDE

Use this list of word components and their meanings to complete the word exercises in this unit.

Prefixes

a-	without/not
acro-	extremities/point
agora-	open place
an-	without/not
di-	two/double
dys-	difficult/disordered
epi-	above/upon/on
hemi-	half
hyper-	above
hypo-	below
intra-	within/inside
macro-	large
meso-	middle
micro-	small
para-	beside/near
poly-	many
post-	after/behind
pre-	before/in front of
quadri-	four
sub-	under
tetra-	four

Roots/Combining forms

aqua-	water
cancer/o	cancer
ech/o	echo/reflected sound
electr/o	electrical
fibr/o	fibre
haemat/o	blood
hemat/o (Am.)	blood
hydro-	water

necr/o	death (dead tissue)
polio-	grey matter (of CNS)
py/o	pus
somat/o	body
syring/o	pipe/tube/cavity

Suffixes

-al	pertaining to
-algia	condition of pain
-cele	swelling/protrusion/hernia
-centesis	surgical puncture to remove fluid
-cyte	cell
-ectomy	removal of
-form	having the form of
-genic	pertaining to formation/originating in
-gram	X-ray picture/tracing/recording
-graph	usually an instrument that records
-graphy	technique of recording/making an X-ray
-gyric	pertaining to circular motion
-ia	condition of
-iatr(y)	doctor/medical treatment
-ic	pertaining to/in pharmacology a drug
-itis	inflammation of
-logist	specialist who studies...
-logy	study of
-malacia	condition of softening
-meter	measuring instrument
-metry	process of measuring
-oma	tumour (Am. tumor)/swelling
-osis	abnormal condition/disease of

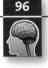

-ous	pertaining to	-stomy	to form a new opening or outlet
-pathy	disease of	-therapy	treatment
-phthisis	wasting away	-tic	pertaining to
-plasia	condition of growth/formation (of cells)	-tomy	incision into
		-trauma	injury/wound
-rrhagia	condition of bursting forth of blood/bleeding	-trophy	nourishment/development
		-tropic	pertaining to affinity for/stimulating/ changing in response to a stimulus
-schisis	cleaving/splitting/parting		
-sclerosis	condition of hardening		
-scopy	visual examination	-us	thing/structure

ANATOMY EXERCISE

When you have finished Word Exercises 1–21, look at the word components listed below. Complete Figures 37 and 38 by writing the appropriate combining form on each line – more than one component may relate to the same position. (You can check their meanings in the Quick Reference box on p. 107.)

Cephal/o	Gangli/o	Psych/o
Cerebr/o	Mening/i/o	Rachi/o
Crani/o	Myel/o	Radicul/o
Encephal/o	Neur/o	Ventricul/o

The nervous system

Humans have a complex nervous system with a brain that is large in proportion to their body size. The brain and spinal cord are estimated to contain at least 10^{10} cells with vast numbers of connections between them. The nervous system performs three basic functions:

- It receives, stores and analyses information from sense organs such as the eyes and ears, making us aware of our environment. This awareness enables us to think and make responses that will aid our survival in changing conditions.
- It controls the physiological activities of the body systems and maintains constant conditions (homeostasis) within the body.
- It controls our muscles, enabling us to move and speak.

Because of its complexity, the nervous system has been difficult to study and progress in understanding its common disorders has been slow. However, recently developed imaging techniques are improving the diagnosis and treatment of nervous disorders.

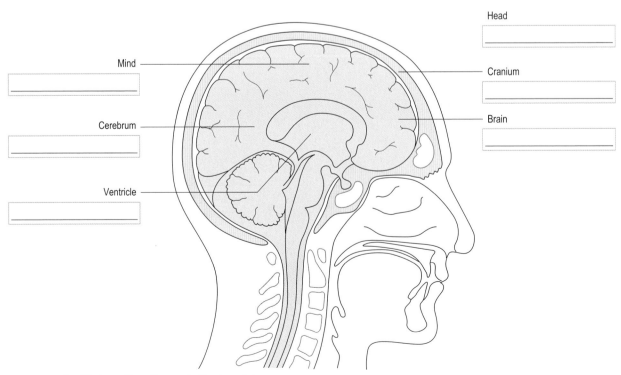

Figure 37 Sagittal section through the head

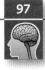

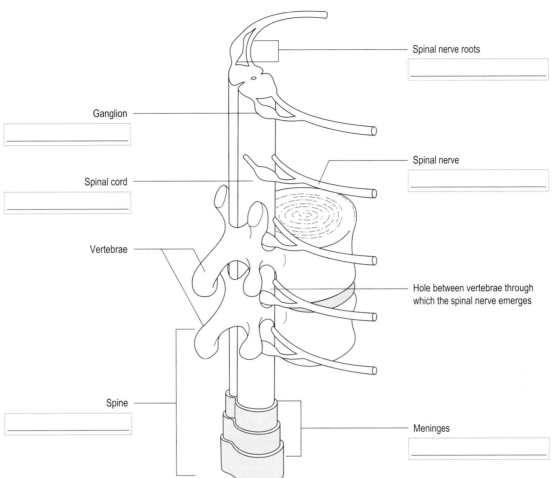

Spinal nerve roots

Ganglion

Spinal cord

Vertebrae

Spinal nerve

Hole between vertebrae through which the spinal nerve emerges

Spine

Meninges

Figure 38 Section through the spine

The structure of the nervous system

For convenience of study medical physiologists have divided the system into the:

Central nervous system (CNS)
The CNS consists of the brain and spinal cord.

Peripheral nervous system (PNS)
The PNS is composed of 12 pairs of cranial nerves and 31 pairs of spinal nerves that connect the CNS with sense organs, muscles and glands.

Autonomic nervous system (ANS)
The ANS describes certain peripheral nerves that send impulses to internal organs and glands.

We begin our study of medical terms by examining the cells that form the system.

ROOT

Neur
(From a Greek word **neuron**, *meaning nerve.)*

Combining form **Neur/o**

Neurons are the basic structural units of the nervous system. They are specialized cells, elongated for the transmission of nerve impulses. Each neuron consists of a cell 'body' plus long extensions known as dendrons or dendrites and axons (Fig. 39). Axons conduct impulses away from the cell 'body' whilst dendrites conduct impulses towards the cell 'body'. A **nerve fibre** is a general term for any process such as a dendrite or axon projecting from a cell 'body'.

A **nerve** is a group of nerve fibres enclosed in a connective tissue sheath; it may contain both sensory and motor fibres.

There are three basic types of neuron:

The sensory neuron
The sensory neuron transmits nerve impulses from sense organs to the central nervous system (CNS) (*sensory* – meaning pertaining to sensation).

The motor neuron
The motor neuron transmits nerve impulses away from the central nervous system to muscle cells or glands (*motor* – meaning pertaining to action).

The interneuron (also called an association neuron or connecting neuron)
The interneuron transmits nerve impulses from sensory neurons to motor neurons in the brain and spinal cord.

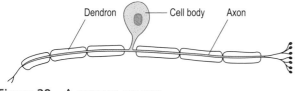

Figure 39 A sensory neuron

Note. As sensory neurons are transferring nerve impulses towards the CNS they are sometimes referred to as **afferent** neurons (from Latin *affere* – to bring). Motor neurons are sometimes referred to as **efferent** neurons because they carry nerve impules away from the CNS (from Latin *effere* – to carry away).

Use the Exercise Guide at the beginning of this unit to complete Word Exercises 1–21 unless you are asked to work without it.

WORD EXERCISE 1

Using your Exercise Guide, find the meaning of:

(a) **neur/o**/logy

(b) **neur/o**/pathy

(c) **neur**/algia

(d) **neur/o**/fibr/oma

(e) poly/**neur**/itis

(f) **neur/o**/genic

Using your Exercise Guide find the meaning of -logist, -malacia and -sclerosis, then build words that mean:

(g) hardening of a nerve

(h) condition of softening of a nerve

(i) a person who specializes in the study of nerves and their disorders

Using your Exercise Guide, find the meaning of:

(j) **neur/o**/phthisis

(k) **neur/o**/tropic

(l) **neur/o**/trauma

The neurons of the central nervous system are supported by another type of cell that sticks to them. These are known as **neuroglia** (glia is from a Greek word *glia*, meaning glue). **Neurogli/o** refers to a neurogliocyte also spelt neurogliacyte. There are four types of glial cell, astrocytes, microglia, oligodendrocytes and ependymocytes.

Without using your Exercise Guide, write the meaning of:

(m) **neurogli/o**/cyte

(n) **neurogli**/oma

ROOT

Plex
*(From a Latin word **plexus**, meaning plait. Here plex/o means a nerve plexus, a network of nerves.)*

Combining form   **Plex/o**

WORD EXERCISE 2

Without using your Exercise Guide, write the meaning of:

(a) **plex/o**/pathy

(b) **plex/o**/genic

ROOT

Cephal
*(From a Greek word **kephale**, meaning head.)*

Combining form   **Cephal/o**

WORD EXERCISE 3

Using your Exercise Guide, find the meaning of:

(a) **cephal/o**/cele

(b) a/**cephal**/ous

(This refers to a condition seen in a dead embryo or fetus.)

(c) **cephal**/haemat/oma
    (Am. **cephal**/hemat/oma)

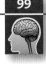

(d) hydro/**cephal**/us

(Fig. 40 shows hydrocephalus, the condition is characterized by an excess of cerebro-spinal fluid in the brain resulting in an enlarged head, compression of the brain and if not corrected, mental retardation.)

Using your Exercise Guide find the meaning of -gram, -ic, micro-, and -metry, then build words that mean:

(e) pertaining to a very small head

(f) X-ray picture of the head

(g) measurement of the head

Using your Exercise Guide, find the meaning of:

(h) macro/**cephal**/us

(i) **cephal**/o/gyric

ROOT

Encephal
*(From a Greek word **encephalos**, meaning brain.)*

Combining form   Encephal/o

Note. **-encephalon** means the brain and is used with prefixes to denote parts of the brain, e.g. the met**encephalon,** the anterior part of the hindbrain

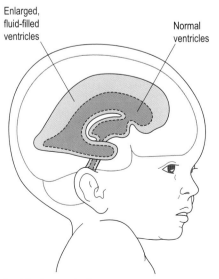

Enlarged, fluid-filled ventricles

Normal ventricles

Figure 40   Hydrocephalus

WORD EXERCISE 4

Without using your Exercise Guide, write the meaning of:

(a) **encephal**/oma

Using your Exercise Guide, find the meaning of:

(b) **encephal**/o/py/osis

(c) an/**encephal**/ic

(d) electr/o/**encephal**/o/graph

(Fig. 41)

This instrument records the electrical activity of the brain through electrodes placed on the surface of the scalp. The electroencephalogram is traced on to a recording paper and appears as a series of waves. Analysis of the waves can be used to diagnose epilepsy, localize intracranial lesions and confirm brain death.

Using your Exercise Guide find the meaning of electr/o and -graphy and then build words that mean:

(e) technique of X-raying/ recording the brain

(f) technique of making a trace/ recording of the electrical activity of the brain

Without using your Exercise Guide, build words that mean:

(g) disease of the brain

(h) protrusion or hernia of brain

Using your Exercise Guide, find the meaning of:

(i) ech/o/**encephal**/o/gram (Ultrasonic soundwaves are used.)

(j) mes/**encephalon**

(k) polio/**encephal**/itis

ROOT

Cerebr
*(From a Latin word **cerebrum**, meaning brain. Here cerebr/o means the cerebrum of the brain or cerebral hemispheres.)*

Combining form   Cerebr/o

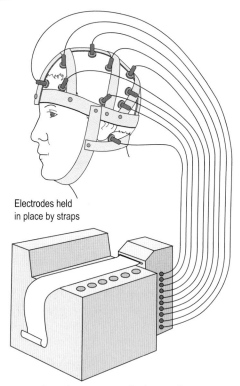

Electrodes held
in place by straps

Figure 41 The electroencephalograph

Note. The outer layer of the cerebrum is known as the cerebral cortex (*cortex* is from Latin, meaning rind/bark). It is extensively folded into fissures, giving it a large surface area. This part of the brain contains motor and sensory areas and is the site of consciousness and intelligence.

WORD EXERCISE 5

Without using your Exercise Guide, build words that mean:

(a) hardening of the cerebrum

(b) condition of softening of the cerebrum

(c) abnormal condition/disease of the cerebrum

Note. Cerebrovascular accident (CVA) or stroke occurs when vascular disease suddenly interrupts the flow of blood to the brain (*vascul/o* meaning vessel and *-ar* meaning pertaining to). An obsolete term apoplexy has also been used to mean stroke or CVA (see the Medical Notes on stroke on page 108).

ROOT

Ventricul
*(From a Latin word **ventriculum**, meaning ventricle or chamber. Here ventricul/o means ventricle, one of the cavities in the brain filled with cerebrospinal fluid.)*

Combining form   Ventricul/o

WORD EXERCISE 6

Using your Exercise Guide find the meaning of -scopy and -tomy, then build words that mean:

(a) visual examination of the ventricles

(b) incision into the ventricles

Without using your Exercise Guide, write the meaning of:

(c) **ventricul/o**/graphy

(Air, gas or radio-opaque dyes are injected into the ventricles during this procedure, it is now rarely performed.)

Use the Latin root **cisterna**, meaning a closed space serving as a reservoir for fluid, and your Exercise Guide, to write the meaning of the word below. The closed space referred to here is the **subarachnoid space** outside the brain.

Using your Exercise Guide, find the meaning of:

(d) **ventricul/o**/cistern/o/stomy
(This is an operation for hydrocephalus.)

ROOT

Crani
*(From Greek **kranion** meaning skull. The bones of the skull protect the soft brain beneath.)*

Combining form   Crani/o

WORD EXERCISE 7

Using your Exercise Guide find the meaning of intra-, metry and -tomy, then build words that mean:

(a) incision into the skull

(b) the measurement of skulls

(c) pertaining to within the cranium (use -al)

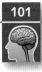

ROOT

Gangli
*(From a Greek word **ganglion**, meaning swelling. Here gangli/o means a ganglion, a knot of nerve cell bodies located outside the central nervous system.)*

Combining form   Gangli/o, note that the root -ganglion- is also used

WORD EXERCISE 8

Without using your Exercise Guide, build a word using **gangli/o** that means:

(a) tumour (Am. tumor) of a ganglion

Using your Exercise Guide, find the meaning of:

(b) pre/**ganglion**/ic

(c) post/**ganglion**/ic

(d) **ganglion**/ectomy

ROOT

Mening
(From a Greek word menigx, meaning membrane. Here mening/o means the meninges, the three membranes that surround the brain and spinal cord.)

Combining forms   Mening/i/o

WORD EXERCISE 9

Without using your Exercise Guide, build words using **mening/o** that mean:

(a) inflammation of the meninges

(b) hernia or protrusion of the meninges

Using your Exercise Guide find the meaning of -rrhagia, then build a word that means:

(c) condition of bursting forth (of blood) from meninges

Without using your Exercise Guide, write the meaning of:

(d) **mening/o**/encephal/o/cele

(e) **mening/o**/encephal/itis

(f) **mening/o**/encephal/o/pathy

(g) **meningi**/oma

The outer of the three membranes of the meninges is known as the **dura mater**. The injection of local anaesthetic into the spine above the dura, i.e. into the epidural space, is known as an epidural block. It is often used for a forceps birth or caesarean (Am. cesarean) section delivery (epi- means above or upon).

Using your Exercise Guide, find the meaning of:

(h) epi/**dur**/al

(i) sub/**dur**/al haemat/oma
   (Am. hemat/oma)
   (See Fig. 42)

This is a common condition seen by neurologists following head injuries. It requires surgery via the cranium to seal leaking blood vessels and remove the blood clot. Surgery also relieves pressure on the brain tissue preventing further damage.

The two inner meninges, the **pia mater** and the **arachnoid membrane**, are thin. When these are inflamed the condition is known as **leptomeningitis** (from a Greek word *leptos*, meaning thin/slender). When the thick outer dura mater is inflamed it is known as **pachymeningitis** (pachy-meaning thick). When meningitis is caused by the bacterial coccus *Neisseria meningitidis*, it is referred to as **meningo**coccal **mening**itis.

ROOT

Radicul
*(From a Latin word **radicula**, meaning root. Here radicul/o means the spinal nerve roots that emerge from the spinal cord.)*

Combining form   Radicul/o

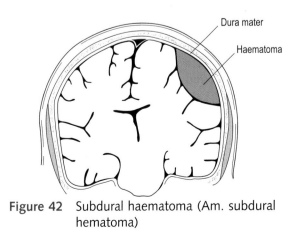

Figure 42   Subdural haematoma (Am. subdural hematoma)

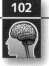

WORD EXERCISE 10

Without using your Exercise Guide, write the meaning of:

(a) **radicul/o**/ganglion/itis

(b) **radicul/o**/neur/itis

Another combining form **radic/o** is also derived from this root, e.g.

(c) **radic/o**/tomy

ROOT

Myel

*(From a Greek word **myelos**, meaning marrow. Here myel/o means the spinal cord i.e. the soft marrow within the spine. Note, myel/o is also used to mean bone marrow and myelocyte.)*

Combining form   Myel/o

WORD EXERCISE 11

Without using your Exercise Guide, write the meaning of:

(a) **myel/o**/mening/itis

(b) mening/o/**myel/o**/cele

(c) **myel/o**/radicul/itis

(d) **myel/o**/encephal/itis

(e) **myel/o**/phthisis

(f) polio/**myel**/itis

Without using your Exercise Guide, build words that mean:

(g) hardening of the spinal marrow

(h) condition of softening of the spinal marrow

(i) technique of making an X-ray of the spinal cord

Using your Exercise Guide, find the meaning of:

(j) **myel/o**/dys/plasia

(k) **myel**/a/trophy

(l) syring/o/**myel**/ia

ROOT

Rachi

*(From a Greek word **rhachis**, meaning spine.)*

Combining form   Rachi/o

WORD EXERCISE 12

Using your Exercise Guide, find the meaning of:

(a) **rachi/o**/meter

(b) **rachi/o**/centesis

Rachiocentesis or rachicentesis (Fig. 43) is performed to obtain a sample of cerebrospinal fluid (CSF) from the subarachnoid space in the lumbar region of the spinal cord. This procedure is commonly known as a **lumbar puncture** or **spinal tap**.

Using your Exercise Guide, find the meaning of:

(c) **rachi**/schisis

(Synonymous with spina bifida, a congenital neural tube defect in which the vertebral arches (laminae) fail to unite in the midline. This leaves the meninges and part of the spinal cord exposed and protruding from the spine; it leads to physical and mental handicap. Spina bifida is associated with folate (vitamin B) deficiency in women of child bearing age. The condition can be detected by testing for alphafetoprotein in the amniotic fluid or by ultrasonography. (Bifida means divided into two equal parts in the midline (from Latin *bi-* meaning two and *findere* meaning to cleave).

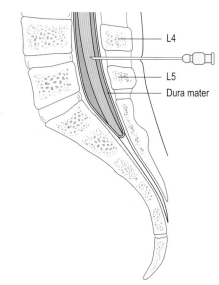

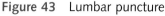

Figure 43   Lumbar puncture

ROOT

Pleg
*(From Greek **plege**, meaning a blow. Here -pleg- means a paralysis. A stroke also called a cerebrovascular accident, is often the cause of this condition when a blockage or haemorrhage (Am. hemorrhage) in the brain leads to destruction of cells that control motor activities.)*

Combining form   -pleg-

WORD EXERCISE 13

Using your Exercise Guide, find the meaning of:

(a) quadri/**pleg**/ia
(paralysis of limbs)

(b) hemi/**pleg**/ia
(paralysis of right or left side of the body)

(c) para/**pleg**/ia
(paralysis of lower limbs)

(d) di/**pleg**/ia
(paralysis of like parts on either side of body)

(e) tetra/**pleg**/ia

Note. The obsolete term **palsy** meaning paralysis is still used in **Bell's palsy** (paralysis of the VIIth cranial nerve commonly called the facial nerve) and in **cerebral palsy.**

ROOT

Aesthesi
*(From Greek **aisthesis**, meaning perception or sensation. Here aesthes/i/o means sensation.)*

Combining forms   Aesthe/s/i/o, Esthe/s/i/o (Am.), aesthet-, esthet- (Am.)

WORD EXERCISE 14

Without using your Exercise Guide, write the meaning of:

(a) an/**aesthes**/ia
(Am. an/**esthes**/ia)

(b) an/**aesthe**/tic
(Am. an/**esthe**/tic)

(c) an/**aesthesi**/o/logy
(Am. an/**esthesi**/o/logy)

(d) an/**aesthesi**/o/logist
(Am. an/**esthesi**/o/logist)

(e) hemi/an/**aesthes**/ia
(Am. hemi/an/**esthes**/ia; refers to one side of the body)

Using your Exercise Guide, find the meaning of:

(f) hypo/**aesthes**/ia
(Am. hypo/**esthes**/ia)

(g) hyper/**aesthes**/ia
(Am. hyper/**esthes**/ia)

The term par**aesthes**ia (Am. par**esthes**ia) is used to mean any abnormal sensations, such as 'pins and needles' (from Greek word *para*, meaning near).

Without using your Exercise Guide, build words that mean:

(h) pertaining to following/ after anaesthesia
(Am. anesthesia)

(i) pertaining to before anaesthesia
(Am. anesthesia)

ROOT

Narc
*(From a Greek word **narke**, meaning stupor. Here narc/o means narcosis, an abnormally deep sleep induced by a drug (a narcotic). This is a different level of consciousness from anaesthesia (Am. anesthesia); patients are not oblivious to pain and can be woken up.)*

Combining form   Narc/o

WORD EXERCISE 15

Without using your Exercise Guide, write the meaning of:

(a) **narc**/osis

Using your Exercise Guide, find the meaning of:

(b) **narc**/o/therapy

ROOT

Alges
*(From a Greek word **algesis**, meaning a sense of pain.)*

Combining forms   Alges/i/o

WORD EXERCISE 16

Without using your Exercise Guide, write the meaning of:

(a) **alges**/ia

(b) an/**alges**/ia

(c) hyper/**alges**/ia

(d) an/**alges**/ic (a drug)

Note. Psychoses originate in the mind itself, in contrast to neuroses which are mental conditions believed to arise because of stresses and anxieties in the patient's environment. Neurotic comes from *neur/o* meaning nerves and *tic*, meaning pertaining to; in psychiatry it means pertaining to a neurosis.

(e) **psych/o**/tropic (drug)

Using your Exercise Guide, find the meaning of:

(f) **psych/o**/somat/ic

(g) **psych**/iatry

Psychiatry

Disorders that interfere with the normal functioning of the brain may affect behaviour and personality, i.e. the mind. The study of the mind and treatment of its disorders is a specialist branch of medicine known as psychiatry. A psychiatrist is a person with medical qualifications who has specialized in the study and treatment of mental disease. Psychiatrists use the following terms:

ROOT

Phob
*(From a Greek word **phobos**, meaning fear. Here -phob- means an irrational fear or aversion to something.)*

Combining form   -phob-

WORD EXERCISE 18

Using your Exercise Guide, find the meaning of:

(a) acro/**phob**/ia

(b) agora/**phob**/ia

(c) aqua/**phob**/ia

(d) cancer/o/**phob**/ia

(e) necr/o/**phob**/ia

ROOT

Psych
*(From Greek **psyche**, meaning soul or mind. Here psych/o means the mind.)*

Combining form   Psych/o

WORD EXERCISE 17

Without using your Exercise Guide, write the meaning of:

(a) **psych/o**/logy

Note. A psychologist is not usually medically qualified and cannot treat disorders by means of drugs or surgery. Psychologists study human behaviour: for example, an educational psychologist may study intelligence and behaviour of school children.

(b) **psych**/ic

(c) **psych/o**/pathy

Note. A psychopath is a person with a specific type of personality disorder in which he/she lacks empathy and may display aggressive and antisocial behaviour. The term has a complex meaning in psychiatry.

(d) **psych**/osis

ROOT

Epilept
*(From Greek **epileptikos**, meaning a seizure. Here epilept/o means epilepsy, a state of disordered electrical activity in the brain that produces a 'fit' and unconsciousness.)*

Combining forms   Epilept/i/o

WORD EXERCISE 19

Without using your Exercise Guide, write the meaning of:

(a) **epilept/o**/genic

(b) post/**epilept**/ic

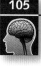

Using your Exercise Guide, find the meaning of:

(c) **epilept/i/form**

Modern treatments of mental disease involve drug treatments and occasionally surgery. One of the most useful physical methods of treatment that brings about improvement in depressive states, mania and stupor is **electroconvulsive therapy** (ECT). This involves the application of a high voltage to the head via electrodes placed on its surface.

Medical equipment and clinical procedures

A patient showing signs and symptoms of disease of the nervous system will be referred to a neurologist. Much information about the state of health of the nervous system can be gained from relatively simple tests that assess the response of the body to various stimuli. One such test you are probably familiar with is the knee jerk reflex where the sensory nerve endings in the patella (knee cap) are tapped with a hammer (Fig. 44). In a healthy patient the response will be that muscles in the thigh will contract, causing the leg to jerk upwards. A normal reflex action will indicate that the nerve pathway from the knee through the spinal cord is working normally.

More detailed examinations of the nervous system require specialized equipment, described below.

Computerized tomography

This is a technique of making a recording using a **tomograph**, an X-ray machine that produces images of cross-sections through the body.

Positron emission tomography (PET)

This is a technique of imaging the distribution of positron emitting radioisotopes administered to the body. Active brain cells take up some isotopes used in PET; this makes the technique particularly useful for studying brain metabolism. More information about PET is included in Unit 18.

Electroencephalography

This is the technique of making a recording using an **electroencephalograph**, a machine that produces a tracing of the electrical activity of the brain. This

Figure 44 A tendon hammer

procedure is used to aid diagnosis of epilepsy, brain tumours (Am. tumors) and other disorders of the brain (see Fig. 41).

Magnetic resonance imaging (MRI)

This recently developed technique using nuclear magnetic resonance is particularly useful for imaging the soft tissue of the brain and spinal cord. The patient is placed in an intense magnetic field where hydrogen atoms in the nerve tissue are excited with radio waves and signals from them are detected and computed into a picture. The procedure does not have the risks associated with X-rays.

The stereotaxic instrument

This is a device used in neurosurgery to locate precise positions within the brain by three-dimensional measurement. The stereotaxic instrument is fixed to the skull and is used to guide probes that destroy or stimulate brain tissue in patients with serious neurological or psychological problems.

Revise the names of all instruments and clinical procedures mentioned in this unit, and then try Exercises 20 and 21.

WORD EXERCISE 20

Match each term in Column A with a description from Column C by placing an appropriate number in Column B.

Column A	Column B	Column C
(a) encephalography		1. an instrument used for testing reflexes
(b) positron emission tomography		2. an instrument that images serial sections of body using X-rays
(c) ventriculoscopy		3. measurement of the cranium
(d) tendon hammer		4. technique of imaging a section through the body using radioisotopes that emit positrons
(e) tomograph		5. technique of making X-ray/recording of the brain
(f) craniometry		6. technique of viewing ventricles

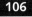
WORD EXERCISE 21

Match each term in Column A with a description from Column C by placing an appropriate number in Column B.

Column A	Column B	Column C
(a) magnetic resonance imaging		1. technique of resonance imaging serial sections of body using X-rays
(b) lumbar puncture		2. technique of making a recording of the electrical activity of the brain
(c) myelography		3. technique of imaging soft tissues of the brain and spinal cord without using X-rays
(d) computed axial tomography		4. technique of making an X-ray/recording of brain ventricles
(e) electroen-cephalography		5. technique of making an X-ray/recording of the spinal cord
(f) ventriculog-raphy		6. technique of removing cerebrospinal fluid from spinal cord

ANATOMY EXERCISE

Now complete the Anatomy Exercise on page 96.

CASE HISTORY 8

The object of this exercise is to understand words associated with a patient's medical history.

To complete the exercise:

- read through the passage on cerebrovascular accident; unfamiliar words are underlined and you can find their meaning using the Word Help

- write the meaning of the medical terms shown in bold print on the lines that follow the Word Help.

Cerebrovascular accident (stroke)

Mr H, a single 56-year-old white male, became ill early in the day of admission whilst eating his breakfast. He had felt dizzy, developed a headache and complained of impaired vision in one eye. Signs of a right-sided **hemiplegia, hemiparaesthesia** and aphasia followed these symptoms. Three weeks prior to his illness he had suffered a TIA in which he developed mild, right **hemisensory loss** in his arm and a sudden, transient hemianopia. His GP suspected a **cerebral** infarction or **intracranial** haemorrhage (Am. hemorrhage) and he was referred to the **neurology** unit for assessment.

On admission in the evening, Mr H's right arm and leg were flaccid and **hyper-reflexic**. A CT scan demonstrated a low density area (an infarct) without a mass effect. There was a loud localized bruit in his neck and digital subtraction angiography (DSA) detected a tight stenosis of the left internal carotid artery. Following diagnosis of a stroke caused by internal carotid artery occlusion; he was given anticoagulant therapy. Two weeks later he underwent a successful internal carotid endarterectomy.

The long term prognosis of Mr H's neurological deficit is uncertain. Three weeks following surgery he showed signs of recovery and had sufficient language to be intelligible. He maintained a rigorous programme of physiotherapy (Am. physical therapy) and speech therapy following initial recovery. The occupational therapist visited his home and advised on the installation of aids that will assist his rehabilitation. Unfortunately, Mr H is severely depressed following his resignation as a structural engineer with a building company.

WORD HELP

aphasia condition of being without speech

bruit abnormal sound upon auscultation (listening to body sounds)

CT computerized tomography, a technique of imaging a 'slice' through the body using X-rays

DSA digital subtraction angiography. A technique of making two X-rays, one taken before an injection of dye into a blood vessel. A computerized image of the first X-ray is subtracted from the second producing a clear image.

endarterectomy removal of the inside of a blood vessel to remove a blockage and open its lumen

flaccid relaxed, flabby and soft

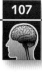

GP general practitioner (family doctor)

haemorrhage (Am. hemorrhage) bursting forth of blood from a vessel

hemianopia loss of half the vision in each eye (loosely used to mean half the vision in one eye)

infarction process of forming an infarct, a piece of dead tissue formed by the failure of its blood supply

neurological pertaining to neurology

occlusion state of being closed up

occupational therapist specialist in providing treatment/assistance aimed at helping people with physical and/or mental disability to become independent

physiotherapy (Am. physical therapy) employment of physical measures (massage/exercise etc.) to restore function following injury or disease

rehabilitation re-education that allows a sick or injured person to take his or her place in the world or gain some independence

stenosis abnormal condition of narrowing

TIA transient ischaemic (Am. ischemic) attack (i.e. insufficient blood supply to the brain)

Now write the meaning of the following words from the case history without using your dictionary lists:

(a) cerebrovascular

(b) hemiplegia

(c) hemiparaesthesia
   (Am. hemiparesthesia)

(d) hemisensory loss

(e) cerebral

(f) intracranial

(g) neurology

(h) hyper-reflexic

(Answers to the case history exercise are given in the Answers to Word Exercises beginning on page 301.)

Quick Reference

Combining forms relating to the nervous system:

Aesthesi/o	sensation (Am. esthesi/o)
Alges/i	sense of pain
Cephal/o	head
Cerebr/o	cerebrum/brain
Cistern/o	cistern/subarachnoid space
Crani/o	cranium
Dur/o	dura mater
Encephal/o	brain
Epilept/o	epilepsy
Esthesi/o (Am.)	sensation
Gangli/o	ganglion
Gli/a/o	gluelike/neuroglial cells
Mening/o	meninges
Motor	action/moving/set in motion
Myel/o	marrow/spinal cord
Narc/o	stupor/numbness
Neur/o	nerve
Plex/o	network, e.g. of nerves
Polio-	grey matter (of CNS)
Psych/o	mind
Rachi/o	spine
Radicul/o	nerve root
Somat/o	body
Syring/o	tube/cavity
Ventricul/o	ventricle (of the brain)

Abbreviations

Some common abbreviations related to the nervous system and psychiatry are listed below. Note some are not standard and their meaning may vary from one health care setting to another. There is a more extensive list for reference on page 335.

CT	computerized tomography
CN	cranial nerve
CSF	cerebrospinal fluid
CVA	cerebrovascular accident
ECT	electroconvulsive therapy
EEG	electroencephalogram
ICP	intracranial pressure
KJ	knee jerk
MRI	magnetic resonance imaging
NCVs	nerve conduction velocities
PR	plantar reflex
SDH	subdural haematoma (Am. hematoma)

Medical Notes

Alzheimer's disease

This is the commonest form of dementia and was previously known as presenile dementia. It is characterized by progressive atrophy of the cerebral cortex accompanied by deteriorating mental functioning. The degeneration can progress to adversely affect memory, attention span, intellectual capacity, personality and motor control. Death usually occurs between two and five years after onset; Alzheimer's disease is responsible for over seventy-five percent of all cases of dementia in people over sixty-five years of age.

Creutzfeldt–Jakob Disease (CJD)

CJD is a poorly understood condition caused by an infectious heat-resistant particle known as a prion protein. Infection produces a rapidly progressive form of dementia that is always fatal. New variant CJD has been transmitted to humans from cattle meat infected with bovine spongiform encephalitis (BSE).

Epilepsy

There are a number of seizure disorders known as epilepsies that result from disordered electrical activity of the brain. They are characterized by seizures or fits caused by a sudden abnormal electrical discharge by neurons.

Generalized seizures may be *tonic-clonic* (grand mal) or *absences* (petit mal). Tonic-clonic seizures are the commonest type with loss of consciousness and convulsions. Absence seizures occur mainly in children and are characterized by a brief loss of consciousness without abnormal movements.

Partial seizures occur when the electrical disturbance is limited to a particular focus of the brain; they are manifested in a variety of ways. Consciousness is maintained but there is an abnormal twitching movement, tingling sensations and hallucinations of vision, smell or taste. In *Jacksonian epilepsy* the twitching movements may spread from one part of the body to another.

Huntington's chorea

Huntington's chorea is an inherited disease characterized by involuntary, purposeless movements (chorea) that progresses to dementia and death. The initial symptoms of this disease first appear between the ages of thirty and forty with death generally occurring by the age of fifty-five

Manic depressive psychosis (manic depression)

A type of mental illness in which the patient's mood alternates between phases of intense excitement and phases of depression. In between these phases there can be periods of normality. The condition is also known as bipolar depression or bipolar affective disorder because of the alternation of the two states.

Motor neuron disease

A group of disorders in which there is chronic progressive degeneration of the motor neurons. The most common type is amyotrophic lateral sclerosis (ALS) also called Lou Gehrig's disease after a famous American baseball player who became a victim of the disease. The lesions develop in the cerebral cortex, brain stem and anterior horns of the spinal cord. It usually presents after the age of fifty and the cause is unknown; early signs are weakness and twitching of the small muscles of the hand, arm and shoulder girdle. The legs are affected later. As the disease progresses, the patient has difficulty eating and speaking and becomes immobile. Death is usually due to involvement of neurons in the respiratory centre of the medulla oblongata or from respiratory infection.

Multiple sclerosis

Multiple sclerosis is characterised by destruction of the myelin in the sheaths that surround neurons of the central nervous system and death of oligodendrocytes. Hard plaque-like lesions replace the destroyed myelin, and inflammatory cells invade affected areas. As demyelination occurs nerve conduction is impaired and this leads to weakness, loss of coordination, visual impairment and speech disturbance. In most cases the disease is prolonged with remissions and relapses occurring over many years.

Parkinson's disease

Parkinson's disease is progressive disease of the central nervous system with an unknown cause. Typically it affects victims around the age of sixty who show degeneration of dopamine producing neurons in the substantia nigra region of the midbrain. Severe loss of dopamine results in symptoms of muscle tremor of the extremities, expressionless facial features, rigidity of voluntary muscles, a slow shuffling gait and stooping posture.

Schizophrenia

Schizophrenia is a general term for a group of psychotic disorders and is one of the major diagnostic categories of mental illness. Disintegration of personality, progressive loss of emotional stability, poor judgement and loss of contact with reality characterize the illness. A list of positive and negative symptoms called Schneider's first rank symptoms is used in the diagnosis and classification of schizophrenia. Positive symptoms for the disease include hallucinations and delusions or hearing voices and having strange thoughts. Negative symptoms include apathy, paucity of speech and social withdrawal. Types of schizophrenia include:

Catatonic schizophrenia characterized by prolonged rigid postures interspersed with outbursts of motor activity such as repeated movements.

Paranoid schizophrenia characterized by hallucinations and paranoid delusions, patients may suffer delusions of grandeur, persecution or jealousy.

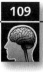

Hebephrenic schizophrenia a form that occurs suddenly in young adults characterized by a general disintegration of the personality. There is thought disorder, meaningless behaviour, incoherence, giggling, peculiar mannerisms and delusions.

Sciatica

A type of neuritis characterized by severe pain along the path of the sciatic nerve and its pathways. A common cause is a prolapsed intervertebral disc.

Stroke (cerebrovascular accident)

A stroke or cerebrovascular accident (CVA) occurs when vascular (vessel) disease suddenly interrupts the flow of blood to the brain. There are two main causes *cerebral infarction* and *spontaneous intracranial haemorrhage (Am. hemorrhage)*. Cerebral infarction is a result of atheroma complicated by thrombosis or blockage of an artery by an embolus. Spontaneous intracranial haemorrhage is commonly associated with a ruptured aneurysm or with high blood pressure (hypertension). Lack of oxygen to the brain tissue (hypoxia) often results in paralysis on one side of the body and disturbances of speech and vision. As cells in the cerebrum control voluntary movements of many parts of the body, paralysis of limbs and loss of speech are common symptoms of strokes. The severity of symptoms depends on the area of brain tissue damaged. Sometimes there is partial recovery and the patient may be left with slight paralysis (paresis).

NOW TRY THE WORD CHECK

WORD CHECK

This self-check exercise lists all the word components used in this unit. First write down the meaning of as many word components as you can. Then check your answers using the Exercise Guide and Quick Reference box or the Glossary of Word Components (pp. 347–371).

Prefixes

a-

acro-

agora-

an-

di-

dys-

epi-

hemi-

hyper-

hypo-

lepto-

macro-

meso-

micro-

pachy-

para-

poly-

post-

pre-

quadri-

sub-

tetra-

Combining forms of word roots

aesthesi/o
(Am. esthesi/o)

alges/i

cancer/o

cephal/o

cerebr/o

cistern/o

crani/o

cyt/o

dur/o

ech/o

electr/o

encephal/o

epilept/o

fibr/o

gangli/o

gli/a/o

haemat/o
(Am. hemat/o)

hist/o

hydro-

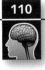
iatr/o

mening/o

motor

myel/o

narc/o

necr/o

neur/o

plex/o

pneum/o

polio-

psych/o

py/o

rachi/o

radicul/o

somat/o

syring/o

ventricul/o

Suffixes

-al

-algia

-cele

-centesis

-cyte

-ectomy

-form

-genic

-gram

-graph

-graphy

-gyric

-ia

-ic

-ical

-itis

-logist

-logy

-malacia

-meter

-metry

-oma

-osis

-ous

-pathy

-phobia

-phthisis

-plasia

-plegia

-rrhagia

-schisis

-sclerosis

-scopy

-stomy

-therapy

-tomy

-tic

-trauma

-trophy

-tropic

-us

NOW TRY THE SELF-ASSESSMENT

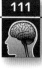

SELF-ASSESSMENT

Test 8A

Below are some combining forms that refer to the anatomy of the nervous system. Indicate which part of the system they refer to by putting a number from the diagrams (Figs 45 and 46) next to each word.

(a) crani/o

(b) encephal/o

(c) meningi/o

(d) neur/o

(e) rachi/o

(f) gangli/o

(g) ventricul/o

(h) radicul/o

(i) cephal/o

(j) myel/o

Score 10

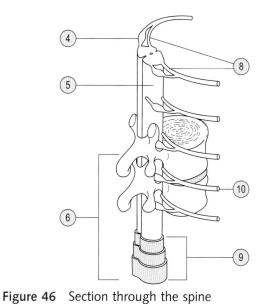

Figure 45 Sagittal section through the head

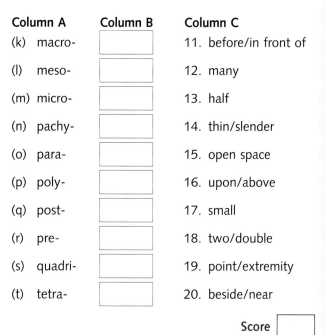

Figure 46 Section through the spine

Test 8B

Prefixes

Match each prefix in Column A with a meaning in Column C by inserting the appropriate number in Column B.

Column A	Column B	Column C
(a) a-		1. after/behind
(b) acro-		2. middle
(c) agora-		3. water (i)
(d) an-		4. water (ii)
(e) aqua-		5. thick
(f) di-		6. large
(g) epi-		7. without/not (i)
(h) hemi-		8. without/not (ii)
(i) hydro-		9. four (i)
(j) lepto-		10 four (ii)

Column A	Column B	Column C
(k) macro-		11. before/in front of
(l) meso-		12. many
(m) micro-		13. half
(n) pachy-		14. thin/slender
(o) para-		15. open space
(p) poly-		16. upon/above
(q) post-		17. small
(r) pre-		18. two/double
(s) quadri-		19. point/extremity
(t) tetra-		20. beside/near

Score 20

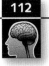
Test 8C

Combining forms of word roots

Match each combining form in Column A with a meaning in Column C by inserting the appropriate number in Column B.

Column A	Column B	Column C
(a) aesthesi/o (Am. esthesi/o)		1. spine
(b) cephal/o		2. mind
(c) cistern/o		3. grey matter (of CNS)
(d) crani/o		4. stupor/deep sleep
(e) dur/o		5. body
(f) encephal/o		6. membranes of CNS
(g) epilept/o		7. ganglion
(h) gangli/o		8. cranium/skull
(i) gli/a/o		9. ventricles of brain
(j) mening/o		10. head
(k) motor		11. dura mater
(l) myel/o		12. fit/seizure/epilepsy
(m) narc/o		13. cistern/ reservoir/ subarachnoid space
(n) neur/o		14. root (of spinal nerve)
(o) polio-		15. nerve
(p) psych/o		16. marrow (of spine)
(q) rachi/o		17. pertaining to action
(r) radicul/o		18. glue (cell)
(s) somat/o		19. brain
(t) ventricul/o		20. sensation

Score ☐

20

Test 8D

Suffixes

Match each suffix in Column A with a meaning in Column C by inserting the appropriate number in Column B.

Column A	Column B	Column C
(a) -centesis		1. condition of paralysis
(b) -form		2. abnormal condition/disease of
(c) -genic		3. technique of recording/making an X-ray
(d) -gram		4. pertaining to the body
(e) -graphy		5. pertaining to affinity for/stimulating
(f) -gyric		6. formation of an opening into
(g) -malacia		7. having form of
(h) -osis		8. condition of increase in cell formation/ number of cells
(i) -phobia		9. nourishment
(j) -phthisis		10. hardening
(k) -plasia		11. wasting away/decay
(l) -plegia		12. condition of softening
(m) -schisis		13. recording/tracing/ X-ray
(n) -sclerosis		14. puncture
(o) -somatic		15. treatment
(p) -stomy		16. splitting
(q) -therapy		17. condition of fear
(r) -trauma		18. pertaining to movement around a centre
(s) -trophy		19. formation/originating in
(t) -tropic		20. injury/shock

Score ☐

20

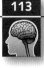

Test 8E

Write the meaning of:

(a) neuromyelitis

(b) rachiotomy

(c) meningomalacia

(d) encephalomyelopathy

(e) ventriculoscope

Score

5

Test 8F

Build words that mean:

(a) disease of the meninges

(b) instrument for measuring the head

(c) inflammation of the spinal cord and spinal nerve roots

(d) condition of bursting forth (of blood) from the brain

(e) study of cells of the nervous system

Score

5

Check answers to Self-Assessment Tests on page 325.

UNIT 9
THE EYE

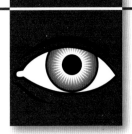

OBJECTIVES

Once you have completed Unit 9 you should be able to:

- understand the meaning of medical words relating to the eye
- build medical words relating to the eye
- associate medical terms with their anatomical position
- understand medical abbreviations relating to the eye.

EXERCISE GUIDE

Use this list of word components and their meanings to complete the word exercises in this unit.

Prefixes

a-	without
ambly-	dull/dim
an-	without
an-iso-	not equal/unequal
bin-	two each/double
dia-	through
diplo-	double
dys-	difficult/painful
en-	in/within
ex-	out/out of/away from
hemi-	half
iso-	same/equal
mono-	one
pan-	all
presby-	old man/old age
uni-	one
xero-	dry

Roots/Combining forms

aden/o	gland
aesthesi/o	sensation
blast/o	immature germ cell/cell that forms . . .
blenn/o	mucus
chromat/o	colour
cyst/o	bladder
electr/o	electrical
esthesi/o (Am.)	sensation
helc/o	ulcer
lith/o	stone
motor	action

my/o	muscle
myc/o	fungus
nas/o	nose
neur/o	nerve
py/o	pus
rhin/o	nose
ton/o	tone/tension

Suffixes

-agogic	pertaining to inducing/stimulating
-al	pertaining to
-algia	condition of pain
-ar	pertaining to
-cele	swelling/protrusion/hernia
-centesis	puncture
-chalasis	slackening/loosening
-conus	cone-like protrusion
-dialysis	separating
-ectasis	dilatation/stretching
-ectomy	removal of
-edema (Am.)	swelling due to fluid
-erysis	drag/draw/suck out
-gram	X-ray/tracing/recording
-graph	usually an instrument that records
-graphy	technique of recording/making an X-ray
-gyric	pertaining to circular motion
-ia	condition of
-itis	inflammation of
-kinesis	movement
-logist	specialist who studies . . .

-malacia	condition of softening	-ptosis	falling/displacement/prolapse
-meter	measuring instrument	-rrhaphy	suturing/stitching
-metrist	specialist who measures	-rrhea (Am.)	excessive flow
-metry	process of measuring	-rrhoea	excessive flow (Am. rrhea)
-mileusis	to carve	-schisis	cleavage/splitting/parting
-nyxis	perforation/pricking/puncture	-sclerosis	condition of hardening
-oedema	swelling due to fluid (Am. edema)	-scope	viewing instrument
		-scopy	visual examination
-oma	tumour (Am. tumor)/swelling	-spasm	involuntary muscle contraction
-osis	abnormal condition/disease/ abnormal increase	-stenosis	condition of narrowing
		-stomy	formation of an opening into . . .
-pathy	disease of	-synechia	condition of adhering together
-pexy	fixation (by surgery)	-thermy	heat
-plasty	surgical repair/reconstruction	-tome	cutting instrument
-plegia	condition of paralysis	-tomy	incision into

ANATOMY EXERCISE

When you have finished Word Exercises 1–21, look at the word components listed below. Complete Figures 47 and 48 by writing the appropriate combining form on each line – more than one component may relate to the same position. (You can check their meanings in the Quick Reference box on p. 125.)

Blephar/o	Ir/o	Papill/o
Choroid/o	Lacrim/o	Pupill/o
Corne/o	Irid/o	Phac/o
Cor/e/o	Kerat/o	Phak/o
Cycl/o	Ocul/o	Retin/o
Dacry/o	Ophthalm/o	Scler/o

The eye

The eyes are our main sense organs. Light enters the eye through the pupil and transparent cornea, it passes through the lens and is focused on to the light-sensitive retina. In the retina light stimulates receptors (rods and cones) to generate nerve impulses in sensory neurons; these impulses travel via neurons in the optic nerve to areas of the brain concerned with vision. In the visual cortex of the brain the impulses are interpreted as an image.

Use the Exercise Guide at the beginning of this unit to complete Word Exercises 1–21 unless you are asked to work without it.

ROOT

Ophthalm
*(From a Greek word **ophthalmos**, meaning eye.)*

Combining form **Ophthalm/o**

(Be careful with spelling ophth.)

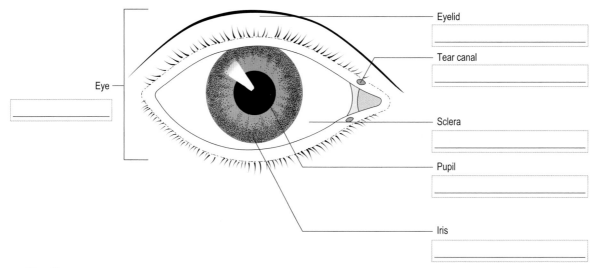

Figure 47 The eye

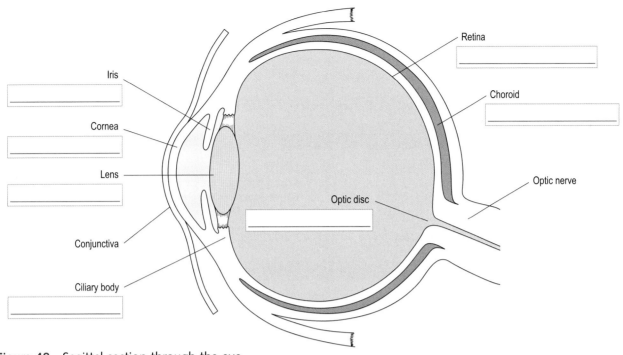

Figure 48   Sagittal section through the eye

WORD EXERCISE 1

Using your Exercise Guide, find the meaning of -itis, -logist, myc/o, -osis, -plegia and -scope, then build words that mean:

(a) an instrument to view the eye

(b) a medically qualified person who specializes in the study of the eye and its disorders

(c) condition of paralysis of the eye

(d) inflammation of the eye (synonymous with ophthalmia)

(e) abnormal condition of fungal infection of the eye

Using your Exercise Guide, find the meaning of:

(f) **ophthalm**/algia

(g) **ophthalm**/o/gyric

(h) **ophthalm**/o/neur/itis

(i) pan/**ophthalm**/itis

(j) **ophthalm**/o/ton/o/meter

(This instrument is used to detect raised pressure within the eye and is used in the diagnosis of glaucoma. Sometimes **tonometer** is used alone and **tonography** is used to mean the technique of using a tonometer.)

(k) blenn/**ophthalm**/ia

(l) xer/**ophthalm**/ia

(m) en/**ophthalmos**

(n) ex/**ophthalmos**

ROOT

Ocul

(From Latin **oculus**, meaning of the eye.)

Combining form   Ocul/o

WORD EXERCISE 2

Using your Exercise Guide, find the meaning of:

(a) mon/**ocul**/ar

(b) uni/**ocul**/ar

(c) bin/**ocul**/ar

ROOT

(d) ocul/o/motor nerve

(e) ocul/o/nas/al

(f) electr/o-ocul/o/gram

(This is produced from an electrodiagnostic test; it also records eye position and movement.) Without using your Exercise Guide, write the meaning of:

(g) ocul/o/gyric

ROOT

Opt
(From optikos, a Greek word meaning sight. The words optical and optician are derived from this root. Optical means pertaining to sight; optician refers to a person who makes and sells spectacles in accordance to an ophthalmic prescription.)

Combining form   Opt/o

WORD EXERCISE 3

Without using your Exercise Guide, write the meaning of:

(a) opt/o/meter

Using your Exercise Guide, find the meaning of:

(b) opt/o/metry

(c) opt/o/metrist

(d) opt/o/my/o/meter

(e) opt/o/aesthes/ia
(Am. opt/o/esthes/ia)

Orthoptics is the science of studying and treating muscle imbalances of the eye (squints). *Ortho* means straight or correct, therefore orthoptic means pertaining to straight or correct sight.

The combining form **optic/o** is also derived from the same root as **opt/o**. It also means pertaining to sight but it is sometimes used to mean optic nerve, e.g. optico-pupillary – pertaining to the pupil and optic nerve.

ROOT

Op
(From Greek ops, also meaning eye. Here -op- is usually used in the suffix -opia to mean a condition of defective vision. Many focusing defects can be corrected by prescribing appropriate spectacles.)

Combining form   -op-, used in the suffixes -opia and -opsia

WORD EXERCISE 4

Using your Exercise Guide, find the meaning of:

(a) dipl/op/ia

(b) presby/op/ia

(refers to a condition in which the lens loses its elasticity; near point approximately 1 m)

(c) ambly/op/ia

(d) hemi/a/chromat/ops/ia

(e) dys/op/ia

(f) hemi/an/op/ia

Focusing a clear image on to the retina is essential for good vision. In the normal eye, light rays enter the eye and are focused into a clear upside down image on the retina. Our brain can easily invert the image in our conscious perception but it cannot correct an image that is out of focus. There are several common words relating to errors of refraction using the suffix -opia that are difficult to understand from their word components, for example:

Hypermetropia
A condition of long-sightedness in which light rays are focused beyond the retina (*hyper* – beyond/above). The light rays when measured focus beyond the retina (*metr* – measure). This results in distant objects appearing in focus but near objects out of focus.

Myopia
A condition of short-sightedness. *My* comes from *myein*, meaning to close. Presumably the eye tends to close when trying to view a distant object. Myopia is a condition in which the eyeball is elongated causing images of distant objects to focus in front of the retina rather than on it. Distant objects appear fuzzy but near objects are seen in focus as the eye accommodates normally.

Emmetropia
A condition of normal/ideal vision Here, light falls directly on to the retina in its correct position, with no errors. (*em* meaning in, *metr* meaning measure).

ROOT

Blephar
*(From a Greek word **blepharon**, meaning eyelid.)*

Combining form   **Blephar/o**

WORD EXERCISE 5

Without using your Exercise Guide, build a word that means:

(a) condition of paralysis of the eyelid

Using your Exercise Guide look up the meaning of -ptosis, -rrhaphy and -spasm and then build words that mean:

(b) involuntary muscle contraction of the eyelid

(c) falling/displacement of the eyelid

(d) stitching/suturing of an eyelid

Using your Exercise Guide, find the meaning of:

(e) **blephar/o/py/o/rrhoea**
   (Am. **blephar/o/py/o/rrhea**)

(f) **blephar/o/aden/itis**

(refers to meibomian glands lying in grooves on inner surface of eyelids)

(g) **blephar/o/synechia**

(h) **blephar/o/chalasis**

ROOT

Scler
*(From Greek **skleros**, meaning hard. Here scler/o means the sclera, the tough, outer white part of the eye. The sclera is continuous with the transparent cornea at the front of the eye.)*

Combining forms   **Scler/o**

WORD EXERCISE 6

Using your Exercise Guide, find the meaning of:

(a) **scler/o/tomy**

(b) **scler/ectasis**

(c) **scler/o/tome**

ROOT

Kerat
*(From a Greek word **keras**, meaning horn. Here kerat/o means the cornea, the transparent, avascular membrane covering the front of the eye; it provides strength, refractive power and transmits light into the eye.)*

Combining form   **Kerat/o**

WORD EXERCISE 7

Without using your Exercise Guide, write the meaning of:

(a) **scler/o/kerat/itis**

(b) **kerat/o/metry**

(c) **kerat/o/tome**

Using your Exercise Guide, find the meaning of:

(d) **kerat/o/plasty**

(e) **kerat/o/centesis**

(f) **kerat/o/helc/osis**

(g) **kerat/o/nyxis**

(h) **kerat/o/mileusis**

(actually an operation for correction of myopia or short-sightedness)

(i) **kerat/o/conus**

(See Fig. 49)

The word cornea comes from the Latin word *corneus*, also meaning horny. Corneoplasty is synonymous with keratoplasty, an operation performed to replace a diseased or damaged cornea with a corneal graft.

Abnormal curvatures of the cornea cause light rays to focus on the retina unevenly. This is known as **astigmatism**.

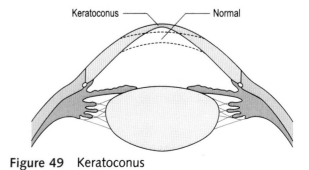

Figure 49   Keratoconus

The sclera and cornea are covered at the front of the eye with a delicate, transparent membrane that also lines the inner surface of the eyelids. This membrane is the **conjunctiva**; it is prone to irritation and infection, giving rise to **conjunctivitis**.

ROOT

Ir

*(From a Greek word **iris**, meaning rainbow. Here irid/o means the iris, a circular, coloured membrane surrounding the pupil of the eye. Contraction of its muscle fibres regulates the size of the aperture (pupil) within the iris, thereby regulating the amount of light entering the eye.)*

Combining forms   **Ir/o, irid/o**

WORD EXERCISE 8

Without using your Exercise Guide, build words using irid/o that mean:

(a) falling/displacement of the iris

(b) inflammation of the cornea and iris (use kerat/o)

Using your Exercise Guide, find the meaning of:

(c) **irid/o**/kinesis

(d) **irid/o**/dialysis

(e) **irid/o**/cele

Without using your Exercise Guide, write the meaning of:

(f) scler/o/**irid/o**/dialysis

(g) scler/o/**irid/o**/tomy

(h) kerat/o/**ir**/itis

ROOT

Cycl
*(From a Greek word **kyklos**, meaning circle. Here cycl/o means the ciliary body of the eye.)*

Combining form   **Cycl/o**

The ciliary body is a structure composed of smooth muscle fibres and secretory epithelial cells that lies behind the iris (see Fig. 48). It connects the circumference of the iris to the choroid (the middle layer of the eyeball), changes the shape of the lens and secretes

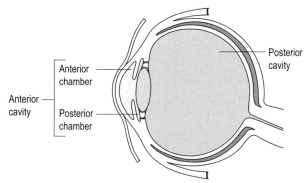

Figure 50   Sagittal section through the eye

a watery fluid, aqueous humor, into the anterior chamber. Study Figure 50 showing the anterior cavity in front of the lens and the posterior cavity behind the lens. The anterior cavity is sub-divided into the anterior chamber in front of the lens and iris, and the posterior chamber between the iris and lens. The ciliary body continuously secretes aqueous humor into the anterior chamber. The fluid is drained into veins in the sclera at the same rate that it is produced. A raised intraocular pressure due to the accumulation of excess aqueous humor may result in **glaucoma,** a common disorder that causes pain and damage to the eye. The posterior cavity is filled with vitreous humor, a soft jelly-like material that maintains the spherical shape of the eyeball.

WORD EXERCISE 9

Without using your Exercise Guide, write the meaning of:

(a) irid/o/**cycl**/itis

(b) **cycl**/o/plegia

Using your Exercise Guide, find the meaning of:

(c) **cycl**/o/dia/thermy

ROOT

Goni
*(From a Greek word **gonia**, meaning angle. Here goni/o means the peripheral angle of the anterior chamber. This angle is observed when evaluating types of glaucoma.)*

Combining form   **Goni/o**

WORD EXERCISE 10

Without using your Exercise Guide, build words that mean:

(a) an instrument used to measure the angle of the anterior chamber

(b) an instrument used to view the angle of the anterior chamber

(c) an operation to make an incision into the angle of the anterior chamber (for glaucoma)

ROOT

Pupill

(From a Latin word pupilla, meaning little girl. Here pupill/o means the pupil, the small aperture that allows light to enter the eye.)

Combining form   Pupill/o

WORD EXERCISE 11

Without using your Exercise Guide, write the meaning of:

(a) **pupill**/o/plegia

(b) **pupill**/o/metry

ROOT

Cor
(From a Greek word kore, meaning the pupil of the eye.)

Combining forms   Cor/e/o

WORD EXERCISE 12

Using your Exercise Guide, find the meaning of:

(a) iso/**cor**/ia

(b) an/iso/**cor**/ia

(c) **core**/o/pexy

Without using your Exercise Guide, write the meaning of:

(d) **core**/o/plasty

ROOT

Choroid
(From a Greek word choroeides, meaning like a skin. Here choroid/o means the choroid, the middle pigmented vascular coat of the posterior five-sixths of the eyeball. The choroid absorbs light and stops reflections within the eye.)

Combining form   Choroid/o

WORD EXERCISE 13

Without using your Exercise Guide, write the meaning of:

(a) **choroid**/o/cycl/itis

(b) scler/o/**choroid**/itis

The word **uvea** from Latin *uva*, meaning grape, is used when referring to the pigmented parts of the eye. These parts include the iris, ciliary body and choroid. **Uveitis** refers to inflammation of all pigmented parts of the eye.

ROOT

Retin
(From a Medieval/Latin word retina, probably derived from rete, meaning net. Here retin/o means the retina, the light-sensitive area of the eye. Light is focused on to the retina by the lens.)

Combining form   Retin/o

WORD EXERCISE 14

Using your Exercise Guide, find the meaning of:

(a) **retin**/o/blast/oma

(b) **retin**/o/malacia

(c) **retin**/o/schisis

(d) **retin**/o/pathy

(e) **retin**/o/scopy

Without using your Exercise Guide, build words that mean:

(f) picture/recording of the electrical activity of the retina

(g) inflammation of the choroid and retina

(h) inflammation of the retina and choroid

Note. The words in (g) and (h) above are synonymous. Remember, when building words, we add the components as we read the meaning, e.g. in (g) we begin with **-itis**, then add **choroid/o**, followed by **retin/o**; in (h) we begin with **-itis**, but then add **retin/o**, followed by **choroid/o**, thus making two different words that have the same meaning.

ROOT

Papill
(From a Latin word **papilla**, meaning nipple-shaped. Here papill/o means the optic disc or optic papilla.)

Combining form   **Papill/o**

Sensory neurons leaving the retina travel through the optic nerve at the back of the eye. Where the sensory neurons collect and form the optic nerve there is a disc-shaped area in the retina (visible through the pupil). This area is known as the optic disc or optic papilla. **Papill/o** refers to the optic disc.

WORD EXERCISE 15

Using your Exercise Guide, find the meaning of:

(a) **papill**/oedema
    (Am. **papill**/edema)

Without using your Exercise Guide, build a word that means:

(b) inflammation of the optic
    disc and retina

A common disorder of the lens is the development of a cataract, an opacity of the lens or lens capsule. There are many types of cataract. Two common ones are hard cataracts, that tend to form in the elderly, and soft cataracts, that occur at any age. The lens can be removed by **phako**-emulsification. In this process ultrasonic vibrations liquefy the lens and it is then sucked out. The lens is replaced with an intraocular implant, i.e. a plastic lens.

ROOT

Phak
(From a Greek word **phakos**, meaning lentil. Here phac/o means the lens of the eye. The lens is a lentil-shaped crystalline structure surrounded by the lens capsule. The shape of the lens and its focus are changed by ligaments connected to muscles in the ciliary body. The ability to change focus of the lens is known as accommodation.)

Combining forms   **Phac/o or phak/o**

WORD EXERCISE 16

Without using your Exercise Guide, build words using phac/o that mean:

(a) condition of softening of a
    lens (i.e. a soft cataract)

(b) instrument to view
    the lens (actually to view
    changes in its shape)

Using your Exercise Guide find the meaning of a-, -sclerosis and -ia, then build words that mean:

(c) hardening of a lens
    (i.e. a hard cataract)

(d) condition of without
    a lens (use phak/o)

Using your Exercise Guide, find the meaning of:

(e) **phac/o**/cyst/ectomy

(f) **phac/o**/erysis

ROOT

Scot
(From a Greek word **skotos**, meaning darkness. Here scot/o means a scotoma, a normal or abnormal blind spot in the visual field where vision is poor.)

Combining forms   **Scot/o**, also used as **scotoma-**

WORD EXERCISE 17

Without using your Exercise Guide, write the meaning of:

(a) **scot/o**/meter

(b) **scot/o**/metry

Using your Exercise Guide, find the meaning of:

(c) **scotoma**/graph

ROOT

Lacrim

(From a Latin word **lacrima**, *meaning tear. Here lacrim/o means tear or lacrimal apparatus.)*

Combining form **Lacrim/o**

The eye is cleansed and lubricated by the lacrimal apparatus (Fig. 51) consisting of a gland, sac and ducts. The gland produces lacrimal fluid that washes over the eyeball and drains into the lacrimal sac through lacrimal ducts. The lacrimal sac in turn drains the fluid into the nose through the nasolacrimal duct.

WORD EXERCISE 18

Without using your Exercise Guide, build words that mean:

(a) incision into the lacrimal apparatus

(b) pertaining to the lacrimal apparatus and nose (use nas/o)

ROOT

Dacry

(From a Greek word **dakryon**, *meaning tear. Here dacry/o means tear or lacrimal apparatus.)*

Combining form **Dacry/o**

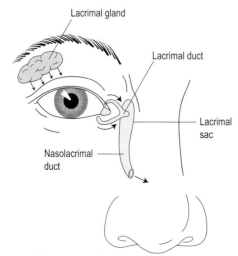

Figure 51 The lacrimal apparatus

Lacrimal gland

Lacrimal duct

Lacrimal sac

Nasolacrimal duct

WORD EXERCISE 19

Using your Exercise Guide, find the meaning of:

(a) **dacry/o**/cyst (the lacrimal sac)

(b) **dacry/o**/cyst/o/graphy

(c) **dacry/o**/cyst/o/rhino/stomy

(d) **dacry/o**/lith

(e) **dacry/o**/stenosis

(f) **dacry**/agogic

Without using your Exercise Guide, write the meaning of:

(g) **dacry/o**/cyst/o/blenn/o/rrhoea
    (Am. **dacry/o**/cyst/o/blenno/
    rrhea)

(h) **dacry/o**/cyst/o/py/osis

Medical equipment and clinical procedures

Revise the names of all instruments and clinical procedures mentioned in this unit and the try Exercises 20 and 21.

WORD EXERCISE 20

Match each term in column A with a description from column C by placing an appropriate number in Column B.

Column A	Column B	Column C
(a) ophthalmoscope		1. an X-ray picture of the lacrimal apparatus
(b) dacryocystogram		2. measurement of scotomas
(c) keratome		3. an instrument that measures tension within the eye
(d) pupillometry		4. an instrument used for visual examination of the eye
(e) optometry		5. an instrument used to cut the cornea

(f) scotometry ☐ 6. an instrument used for measuring the power of ocular muscles

(g) ophthalmotono- ☐ 7. technique of meter measuring sight

(h) optomyometer ☐ 8. technique of measuring pupils (width)

WORD EXERCISE 21

Match each term in column A with a description from Column C by placing an appropriate number in Column B.

Column A	Column B	Column C
(a) sclerotome	☐	1. visual examination of the retina
(b) optometer	☐	2. technique of recording raised pressure/tension in the eye
(c) keratometry	☐	3. technique of making an X-ray of the lacrimal (tear) sac
(d) pupillometer	☐	4. an instrument used to measure sight
(e) phacoscope	☐	5. an instrument used to cut the sclera
(f) retinoscopy	☐	6. measurement of the cornea (its curvature)
(g) tonography	☐	7. an instrument used to view the lens
(h) dacryocys-tography	☐	8. an instrument that measures pupils (width)

ANATOMY EXERCISE

Now complete the Anatomy Exercise on page 116.

CASE HISTORY 9

The object of this exercise is to understand words associated with a patient's medical history.

To complete the exercise:

• read through the passage on optic neuritis; unfamiliar words are underlined and you can find their meaning using the Word Help

• write the meaning of the medical terms shown in bold print on the lines that follow the Word Help.

Optic neuritis

Mr I, a 22-year-old physics researcher, consulted his **optometrist** complaining of **diplopia** whilst driving and reading. He had also experienced dizziness and **ophthalmalgia** when moving his eyes. He thought his inappropriate, old spectacles caused his symptoms. The optometrist observed **optic neuritis** involving the head of the optic disc (**papillitis**) and perimetry detected a central **scotoma**. She contacted Mr I's GP and he was sent to the neurologist.

Examination revealed the pupils were equal, round and reactive to light but there was a mild paradoxic dilation of the left pupil to the swinging flashlight test. Vertical gaze was normal. There was an abnormal **ocular** movement on lateral gaze, when he attempted to look left, his right eye failed to adduct and although the left eye abducted, it showed a coarse horizontal nystagmus. When he looked to the right, there was no abnormality in the movement of the left eye but the right eye failed to abduct. His abdominal reflexes were absent and his gait was unsteady and wide.

Clinical examination indicated Mr I had lesions in the right medial longitudinal fasciculus (MLF) of the midbrain producing an internuclear **ophthalmoplegia** and sixth nerve palsy. This was confirmed with an MRI scan that revealed small periventricular foci within the pons in the region of the MLF.

Mr I was informed that he had multiple sclerosis (MS) and received appropriate counselling for his condition.

WORD HELP

abducted to move away from the median line (an imaginary line running down the centre of the body)

adduct to move towards the median line or midline of the body

foci centre of disease process (visible on the MRI scan)

gait manner of walking

GP general practitioner (family doctor)

internuclear between nuclei (here nucleus refers to a collection of nerve cells that control eye movement)

lateral gaze looking to the side

MLF medial longitudinal fasciculus, a region of the midbrain that controls eye movement

MRI magnetic resonance imaging

multiple sclerosis nervous system disease characterized by loss of the myelin sheaths of nerve fibres and their replacement with scar tissue; the sclerotic (hard) patches being found at numerous sites in the brain, spinal cord and optic nerves (synonymous with disseminated sclerosis)

nystagmus involuntary rapid jerky eye movement

palsy paralysis

paradoxic dilation contradictory occurrence (here the left pupil dilates in response to light)

perimetry measuring acuity (clearness of vision) throughout the visual field

periventricular pertaining to around a ventricle (a fluid-filled cavity in the brain)

pons part of the hind brain above the medulla

swinging flashlight test a test in which a flashlight is used to detect a pupillary defect

vertical gaze looking up and down

Quick Reference

Combining forms relating to the eye:

Blephar/o	eyelid
Choroid/o	choroid
Chromat/o	colour
Conjunctiv/o	conjunctiva
Cor/e/o	pupil
Corne/o	cornea
Cycl/o	ciliary body
Dacry/o	tear/lacrimal apparatus/lacrimal ducts
Goni/o	angle (of anterior chamber)
Ir/o	iris
Irid/o	iris
Kerat/o	cornea
Lacrim/o	tear/lacrimal apparatus/lacrimal ducts
Ocul/o	eye
Ophthalm/o	eye
Optic/o	optic nerve
Opt/o	sight
Papill/o	optic disc
Phac/o	lens
Phak/o	lens
Pupill/o	pupil
Retin/o	retina
Scler/o	sclera
Scot/o	dark
Ton/o	tone/tension
Uve/o	uvea (pigmented part of eye)

Now write the meaning of the following words from the case history without using your dictionary lists:

(a) optometrist

(b) diplopia

(c) ophthalmalgia

(d) optic neuritis

(e) papillitis

(f) scotoma

(g) ocular

(h) ophthalmoplegia

(Answers to the case history exercise are given in the Answers to Word Exercises beginning on page 301.)

Abbreviations

Some common abbreviations related to the eye are listed below. Note some are not standard and their meaning may vary from one health care setting to another. There is a more extensive list for reference on page 335.

Accom	accommodation of eye
Astigm	astigmatism of eye
Em	emmetropia/good vision
IOFB	intraocular foreign body
My	myopia/short sight
OD	oculus dexter/right eye
OS	oculus sinister/left eye
OU	oculus unitas/both eyes together
POAG	primary open angle glaucoma
PERLAC	pupils equal, react to light, accommodation consensual
VA	visual acuity
VF	visual field

Medical Notes

Cataract

A cataract is a loss of transparency of the lens of the eye and is considered to be part of the aging process. Cataracts form because of changes to the protein fibres within the lens making it appear white and opaque. With increasing loss of transparency the detail and clarity of the image produced by the retina is lost and focusing becomes difficult. Age related cataracts develop because of long exposure to a variety of predisposing factors such as cigarette smoke, UV light, diabetes mellitus and systemic drug treatments with for example, corticosteroids.

Chalazion

A cyst on the edge of the eye-lid formed by retained secretion of the Meibomian glands (tarsal glands).

Glaucoma

Glaucoma is an excessive intraocular pressure caused by an abnormal accumulation of aqueous humor within the eye. The condition is due to impaired drainage of fluid through the scleral venous sinus (canal of Schlemm) in the angle between the iris and cornea in the anterior chamber. As pressure against the retina and optic nerve increases, there is mechanical pressure against neurons in the optic nerve and compression of their blood vessels. Damage to the optic nerve impairs vision and can lead to permanent blindness.

Chronic open-angle glaucoma occurs mostly in people over forty years of age and is usually bilateral. There is a gradual rise in intraocular pressure with progressive loss of vision; peripheral vision is lost first and may not be noticed until only central tunnel vision remains. As the optic disc atrophies due to damage to its neurons vision is reduced. The condition eventually results in permanent blindness.

Acute closed angle glaucoma occurs mostly in people over forty years of age and usually affects one eye. A sudden obstruction in the outflow of aqueous humor from the eye and a consequent rise in pressure characterize the condition. Symptoms of an acute attack include sudden pain, photophobia, lacrimation and loss of vision. As the pupil constricts in bright light the pressure on the scleral venous sinus may be relieved leading to recovery, however repeated attacks may be incomplete and vision is progressively impaired.

Congenital glaucoma may be due to abnormal development of the anterior chamber because of genetic abnormality or maternal infection, for example with rubella virus (German measles).

Macular degeneration

Age related macular degeneration (ARMD) is a leading cause of blindness in the elderly that causes loss of central and colour vision. The macula lutea is the central part of the retina that produces the clearest central vision. Age related degeneration involves loss of retinal pigment cells and damage to the macula

Retinal detachment

Damage to the retina impairs vision because even a well-focused image cannot be perceived if some or all of the light receptors do not function properly. Retinal detachment is a painless condition that forms when a tear or hole in the retina allows fluid to accumulate between the layers of retinal cells or the retina and its supporting layers. Once a hole forms, more fluid collects and the detachment spreads. Patients experience floating spots and flashes of light when the eye moves due to random stimulation of light receptors. Causes include trauma to the head or eye, tumours (Am. tumors), haemorrhage (Am. hemorrhage) and cataract surgery. If left untreated the retina may detach completely and cause total blindness in the affected eye. Retinal detachment is more common in patients with myopia.

Strabismus (squint)

A manifest (visible) condition in which the visual axes of the eyes are misaligned and one eye deviates from the point of fixation when uncovered. This gives one the appearance of being cross-eyed because the eyes fail to move together. (The visual axis of the eye is an imaginary line passing from the object being looked at to the fovea centralis of the retina.)

Stye (hordeolum)

A stye is an acute bacterial infection of sebaceous or tarsal glands at the eyelid margin. The most common infectious organism is *Staphylococcus aureus*. Infection of the tarsal glands (Meibomian glands) may block their ducts leading to the formation of a cyst called a chalazion that may damage the cornea.

Trachoma

A chronic inflammation of the eye caused by the coccoid bacterium *Chlamydia trachomatis*. In this condition, fibrous tissue forms in the conjunctiva and cornea leading to eyelid deformity and blindness. It is common in tropical regions where it is spread by flies and communal use of washing water, towels and clothing.

Retinopathy

Diabetic retinopathy occurs in Type I and Type II diabetes mellitus and is characterized by small haemorrhages (Am. hemorrhages) and microaneurysms in retinal blood vessels that disrupt the supply of oxygen to the photoreceptors. The eye responds by building new abnormal blood vessels that can block vision and cause retinal detachment. Over a long period diabetes mellitus may result in degeneration of the retina and permanent blindness.

Vascular retinopathy occurs when the central retinal artery or vein becomes blocked causing sudden pain and unilateral loss of vision. Arterial occlusion is often due to an embolism. Venous occlusion is usually associated with arteriosclerosis or with venous thrombosis at another site. The retinal veins become distended and retinal haemorrhage occurs.

NOW TRY THE WORD CHECK

WORD CHECK

This self-check exercise lists all the word components used in this unit. First write down the meaning of as many word components as you can. Then check your answers using the Exercise Guide and Quick Reference box or the Glossary of Word Components (pp. 347–371).

Prefixes

a-

ambly-

an-

bin-

dia-

diplo-

dys-

em-

en-

ex-

hemi-

hyper-

iso-

mono-

ortho-

pan-

presby-

uni-

xero-

Combining forms of word roots

aesthesi/o

(Am. esthesi/o)

aden/o

blast/o

blenn/o

blephar/o

choroid/o

chromat/o

conjunctiv/o

cor/e/o

cycl/o

cyst/o

dacry/o

electr/o

goni/o

helc/o

ir/o

irid/o

kerat/o

lacrim/o

lith/o

-motor-

myc/o

my/o

my- (from myein)

nas/o

neur/o

ocul/o

ophthalm/o

optic/o

opt/o

papill/o

phak/o, phac/o

pupill/o

py/o

retin/o

rhin/o

scler/o

scot/o

sten/o

ton/o

uve/o

Suffixes

-agogic

-al

-algia

-cele

-centesis

-chalasis

-conus

-desis

-dialysis

-ectasis

-ectomy

-erysis

-gram

-graph

-graphy

-gyric

-ia

-itis

-kinesis

-logist

-malacia

-meter

-metrist

-metry

-mileusis

-nyxis

-oedema
(Am. -edema)

-oma

-opia

-osis

-pathy

-pexy

-phobia

-plasty

-plegia

-ptosis

-rrhaphy

-rrhoea
(Am. -rrhea)

-schisis

-sclerosis

-scope

-scopy

-spasm

-synechia

-thermy

-tome

-tomy

NOW TRY THE SELF-ASSESSMENT

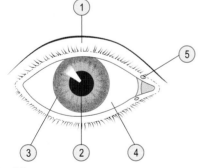

SELF-ASSESSMENT

Test 9A

Below are some combining forms that refer to the anatomy of the eye. Indicate which parts of the eye they refer to by putting a number from the diagrams (Figs 52 and 53) next to each word:

(a) irid/o

(b) scler/o

(c) pupill/o

(d) lacrim/o

(e) blephar/o

(f) phac/o

(g) papill/o

(h) retin/o

(i) kerat/o

(j) ophthalmoneur/o

Score

10

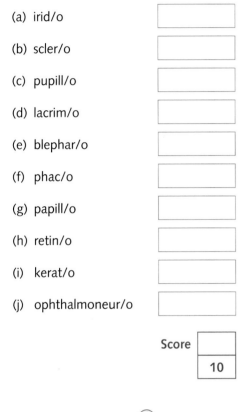

Figure 52   The eye

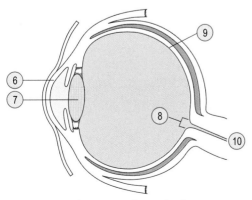

Figure 53   Sagittal section through the eye

Test 9B

Prefixes and suffixes

Match each prefix or suffix in Column A with a meaning in Column C by inserting the appropriate number in Column B.

Column A	Column B	Column C
(a) -agogic		1. dragging/drawing/ sucking out
(b) ambly-		2. splitting
(c) -dialysis		3. swelling (due to fluid)
(d) diplo-		4. one (i)
(e) -erysis		5. one (ii)
(f) -graph		6. person who measures
(g) -gyric		7. old man, old age
(h) hemi-		8. all
(i) -kinesis		9. condition of sticking together
(j) -metrist		10. dulled/made dim
(k) -mileusis		11. condition of vision (defective)
(l) mono-		12. pertaining to inducing/ stimulating
(m) -oedema (Am. -edema)		13. pertaining to a turning or circular movement
(n) -opia		14. instrument that records
(o) pan-		15. movement
(p) presby-		16. to carve
(q) -rrhaphy		17. suturing/stitching
(r) -schisis		18. separating
(s) -synechia		19. double
(t) uni-		20. half

Score

20

Test 9C

Combining forms of word roots

Match each combining form in Column A with a meaning in Column C by inserting the appropriate number in Column B.

Column A	Column B	Column C
(a) blephar/o		1. cone (shaped)
(b) choroid/o		2. cornea
(c) chromat/o		3. optic disc
(d) conjunctiv/o		4. iris (rainbow)
(e) -conus		5. pupil
(f) cycl/o		6. sight/vision
(g) dacry/o		7. pigmented area of eye (uvea)
(h) helc/o		8. retina
(i) irid/o		9. colour
(j) kerat/o		10. ulcer
(k) lacrim/o		11. lens
(l) ocul/o		12. ciliary body
(m) ophthalm/o		13. darkness/blind spot
(n) optic/o		14. choroid
(o) papill/o		15. eye (i)
(p) phak/o		16. eye (ii)
(q) pupill/o		17. eyelid
(r) retin/o		18. conjunctiva
(s) scotom/o		19. tear (i)
(t) uve/o		20. tear (ii)

Score [ ] / 20

Test 9D

Write the meaning of:

(a) ophthalmoplasty

(b) retinopexy

(c) dacryopyorrhoea (Am. dacryopyorrhea)

(d) sclero-iritis

(e) oculomotor nerve

Score [ ] / 5

Test 9E

Build words that mean:

(a) visual examination of the eye

(b) inflammation of the eyelid

(c) any disease of the cornea

(d) an instrument used to view the retina

(e) condition of paralysis of the iris

Score [ ] / 5

Check answers to Self-Assessment Tests on page 325.

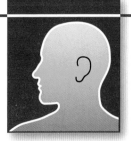

OBJECTIVES

Once you have completed Unit 10 you should be able to:

- understand the meaning of medical words relating to the ear
- build medical words relating to the ear
- associate medical terms with their anatomical position
- understand medical abbreviations relating to the ear.

EXERCISE GUIDE

Use this list of word components and their meanings to complete the word exercises in this unit.

Prefixes

bin-	two of each/double
endo-	within/inside
macro-	large
micro-	small

Roots/Combining forms

electr/o	electrical
laryng/o	larynx
myc/o	fungus
pharyng/o	pharynx
py/o	pus
rhin/o	nose
ten/o	tendon

Suffixes

-al	pertaining to
-algia	condition of pain
-ar	pertaining to
-centesis	puncture to remove fluid
-eal	pertaining to
-ectomy	removal of
-emphraxis	blocking/stopping up
-genic	pertaining to formation/originating in
-gram	X-ray tracing/picture/recording
-graphy	technique of recording/making an X-ray
-ia	condition of
-itis	inflammation of
-logy	study of
-meter	measuring instrument
-metry	process of measuring
-osis	abnormal condition/disease/ abnormal increase
-plasty	surgical repair/reconstruction
-rrhea (Am.)	excessive discharge/flow
-rrhoea	excessive discharge/flow (Am. -rrhea)
-sclerosis	condition of hardening
-scope	instrument to view
-scopy	technique of viewing/examining
-stomy	formation of an opening/an opening
-tome	cutting instrument
-tomy	incision into

ANATOMY EXERCISE

When you have finished Word Exercises 1–14, look at the word components listed below. Complete Figure 54 by writing the appropriate combining form on each line – more than one component may to the same position. (You can check their meanings in the Quick Reference box on p. 138.)

Auricul/o	Mastoid/o	Salping/o
Cochle/o	Myring/o	Tympan/o
Labyrinth/o	Ot/o	Vestibul/o

The ear

The ear is a major sense organ concerned with two important functions:

1. hearing
2. balance.

The ear provides an auditory input into the brain. Sound waves in the air cause vibrations in the ear drum and these are transmitted to the fluid-filled cochlea in the inner ear. The cochlea is the organ of hearing and contains special receptor cells that generate nerve impulses in response to sound. Nerve impulses from the cochlea are relayed via sensory neurons to auditory areas in the brain where they are interpreted as sounds. The possession of two ears enables us to sense the direction of sound.

The vestibular apparatus of the inner ear contains receptors that detect changes in velocity and position of the body. Sensory impulses from the vestibular apparatus are relayed via sensory neurons to centres in the cerebellum and other regions of the brain where they are used in the neural processes that allow us to maintain our balance and upright posture.

Use the Exercise Guide at the beginning of this unit to complete Word Exercises 1–14 unless you are asked to work without it.

ROOT

Ot
(From Greek word **ous**, meaning ear.)

Combining forms   Ot/o

WORD EXERCISE 1

Using your Exercise Guide find the meaning of -logy, -osis, py/o, -sclerosis and -scope, then build words that mean:

(a) the study of the ear

(b) instrument to view the ear

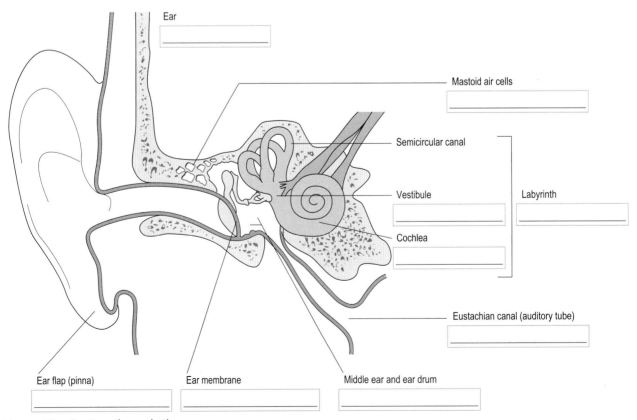

Figure 54   Section through the ear

(c) condition of hardening of the ear

(An inherited bone disorder that leads to progressive hearing loss. Conductive deafness results from hard bone formation around the footplate of the stapes reducing its ability to transmit vibrations across the middle ear to the oval window.)

(d) condition of pus in the ear

Using your Exercise Guide, find the meaning of:

(e) **ot/o**/scopy

(f) **ot/o**/rhin/o/laryng/o/logy

(g) **ot/o**/myc/osis

(h) **ot/o**/py/o/rrhoea
(Am. **ot/o**/py/o/rrhea)

(i) micr/**ot**/ia

(j) macr/**ot**/ia

The ear can be divided into three areas, the external, middle and inner ear. Infection and inflammation (**otitis**) can occur in any of these areas. The following terms are used to describe the position of the inflammation:

Otitis externa
inflammation of the external ear.

Otitis media
inflammation of the middle ear.

Otitis interna
inflammation of the inner ear.

Infection commonly begins in the middle ear because it is connected to the **nasopharynx** by a short tube known as the **Eustachian tube** (**auditory tube** or **pharyngotympanic tube**). This tube functions to equalize the pressure on either side of the ear drum by allowing air into the middle ear but in doing so it also provides an entrance for microorganisms from the nose. See otitis in the Medical Notes on page 139.

ROOT

Aur
(From a Latin word **auris**, *meaning ear.)*

Combining forms **Aur/i**

WORD EXERCISE 2

Without using your Exercise Guide, build a word that means:

(a) instrument used to view the ear (see Fig. 55)

Viewing of the ear canal and tympanic membrane is improved by using an **aural speculum** (Fig. 56), a device that is inserted into the external ear before examining with an **auriscope**.

The auriscope is used to examine the external ear canal and the ear membrane. Occasionally, the ear canal can become blocked by excessive amounts of wax produced by the ceruminous (wax) glands in its lining. Earwax (cerumen) can be removed by washing the ear with warm water using an aural syringe (Fig. 57) or using wax solvents to bring about ceruminolysis.

Using your Exercise Guide, find the meaning of:

(b) bin/**aur**/al

(c) end/**aur**/al

The Latin word *auricula* refers to the ear flaps (pinnae) of the external ear.

(d) bin/**auricul**/ar

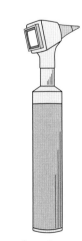

Figure 55 Otoscope / auriscope

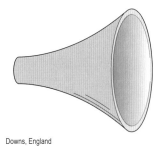

Downs, England

Figure 56   Aural speculum

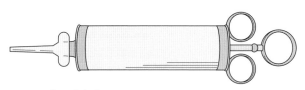

Downs, England

Figure 57   Aural syringe

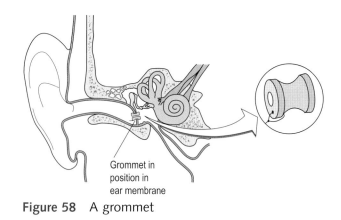

Grommet in
position in
ear membrane

Figure 58   A grommet

ROOT

Tympan
*(From a Greek word **tympanon**, meaning drum. Here
tympan/o means the tympanum, the name for the
cavity of the middle ear and tympanic membrane
combined.)*

Combining forms   Tympan/o

ROOT

Myring
*(A New Latin word **myringa**, meaning membrane.
Here myring/o means the tympanic membrane or ear
drum.)*

Combining forms   Myring/o

WORD EXERCISE 3

Using your Exercise Guide find the meaning of
-tome and -tomy, then build words that mean:

(a) incision into the ear membrane
     (allows air to enter to aid drainage)

(b) instrument used to cut the ear membrane

Without using your Exercise Guide, build a word
that means:

(c) abnormal condition of fungal infection of the
     ear membrane

WORD EXERCISE 4

Using your Exercise Guide, build words that mean:

(a) reconstructive surgery of the tympanum

(b) puncture of the tympanum

(c) opening into the tympanum

Without using your Exercise Guide, write the
meaning of:

(d) **tympan**/itis

(e) **tympan**/o/tomy

Sometimes the ear membrane is surgically punctured to
assist the drainage of fluid from the middle ear (as in
glue ear). Once an opening is made in the membrane,
fluid drains through the Eustachian tube (auditory
tube) into the nasopharynx. A small plastic grommet
(Fig. 58) can be fixed into the membrane to equalize
the air pressure on either side of the membrane and
allow drainage through the Eustachian tube for an
extended period. The grommet eventually falls out and
the membrane heals.

ROOT

Salping
*(From Greek **salpigx**, meaning trumpet tube. Here
salping/o means Eustachian tube, the trumpet-shaped
tube that connects the middle ear to the
nasopharynx. The Eustachian tube is also called the
auditory tube or pharyngotympanic tube.)*

Combining forms   Salping/o

WORD EXERCISE 5

Using your Exercise Guide, find the meaning of:

(a) **salping**/emphraxis

(b) **salping**/**o**/**pharyng**/eal

Within the middle ear we find the smallest bones in the body, the ear ossicles (Fig. 59). These have been named **malleus**, **incus** and **stapes**. Their function is to transmit vibrations from the tympanic membrane to the oval window of the inner ear. Behind the oval window is a fluid-filled structure known as the **cochlea**, the organ of hearing. Within the cochlea are sensory hair cells (receptors) that respond to vibrations in the fluid by producing nerve impulses. The auditory area of the brain interprets nerve impulses from the cochlea as sound, enabling us to hear.

ROOT

Stapedi
(From a Latin word **stapes***, meaning stirrup. Here stapedi/o means the stapes, the stirrup-shaped ear ossicle.)*

Combining forms **Staped/i/o**

WORD EXERCISE 6

Using your Exercise Guide find the meaning of -ectomy and then build a word that means:

(a) removal of the stapes

Using your Exercise Guide, find the meaning of:

(b) **stapedi**/**o**/ten/**o**/tomy

ROOT

Malle
(From a Latin word **malleus***, meaning hammer. Here malle/o means the malleus, the hammer-shaped ear ossicle.)*

Combining form **Malle/o**

WORD EXERCISE 7

Without using your Exercise Guide, write the meaning of:

(a) **malle**/**o**/tomy

ROOT

Incud
(From a Latin word **incus***, meaning anvil. Here incud/o means the incus, the anvil-shaped ear ossicle.)*

Combining forms **Incud/o**

WORD EXERCISE 8

Without using your Exercise Guide, write the meaning of:

(a) **incud**/**o**/mall/eal

(b) **incud**/**o**/stapedi/al

(c) malle/**o**/**incud**/al

ANATOMY EXERCISE

Write the appropriate combining form for each ossicle on the lines of Figure 59. Sometimes the small ear bones are referred to in a more general way, using **ossicul/o**, to mean ossicles, e.g. **ossicul**ectomy for removal of one or more ossicles, **ossiculo**tomy for incision into the ear ossicles. The ossicles can be replaced by a plastic prosthesis that will transmit vibrations to the inner ear and restore hearing.

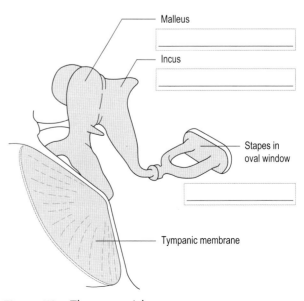

Malleus

Incus

Stapes in oval window

Tympanic membrane

Figure 59 The ear ossicles

ROOT

Cochle
*(From a Latin word **cochlea**, meaning snail. Here cochle/o means the cochlea, the snail-shaped anterior bony labyrinth of the inner ear.)*

Combining form   Cochle/o

WORD EXERCISE 9

Using your Exercise Guide find the meaning of electr/o, -graphy and -stomy, then build words that mean:

(a) an opening into the cochlea

(b) technique of recording the cochlea's electrical activity

ROOT

Labyrinth
*(From a Greek word **labyrinthos**, meaning maze or anything twisted or spiral-shaped. Here labyrinth/o means the labyrinth of the inner ear.)*

Combining form   Labyrinth/o

The inner ear consists of bony and membranous labyrinths. The bony labyrinth is a series of canals in the temporal bone filled with fluid. It consists of the cochlea (organ of hearing), vestibule and semicircular canals (organs of equilibrium).

The membranous labyrinth lies within the bony labyrinth and is also filled with fluid. Distension of the membranous labyrinth with excess fluid gives rise to **Ménière's** disease, symptoms of which include vertigo (dizziness) and deafness (see the Medical Notes on page 139).

The portions of the inner ear concerned with balance are collectively known as the **vestibular apparatus**.

WORD EXERCISE 10

Without using your Exercise Guide, build words that mean:

(a) inflammation of a labyrinth

(b) removal of a labyrinth

ROOT

Vestibul
*(From the Latin word **vestibulum**, meaning entrance. Here vestibul/o means the vestibule, the oval cavity in the middle of the bony labyrinth.)*

Combining form   Vestibul/o

WORD EXERCISE 11

Without using your Exercise Guide, write the meaning of:

(a) **vestibul/o**/tomy

Using your Exercise Guide, find the meaning of:

(b) **vestibul/o**/genic

ROOT

Mast
*(From a Greek word **mastos**, meaning breast. Here mastoid/o means the mastoid process or mastoid bone containing nipple-shaped air cells or air spaces. The mastoid process is a bone located behind the external ear.)*

Combining form   Mastoid/o

WORD EXERCISE 12

Using your Exercise Guide, look up the meaning of -algia and build a word that means:

(a) condition of pain in the mastoid region

Without using your Exercise Guide, build words that mean:

(b) incision into the mastoid bone

(c) removal of tissue from the mastoid process

(d) inflammation of the mastoid process and tympanum

ROOT

Audi
*(From a Latin word **audire**, meaning to hear.)*

Combining forms   Audi/o

WORD EXERCISE 13

Without using your Exercise Guide, build a word that means:

(a) the science dealing with the study of hearing

_____

Using your Exercise Guide, find the meaning of:

(b) **audio**/meter _____

(c) **audio**/gram _____

(d) **audio**/metry _____

Note. An **audiometrist** is a technician specialized in the study of hearing. He or she tests and measures a patient's hearing ability (-*ist* meaning a specialist who . . .).

Medical equipment and clinical procedures

Revise the names of all instruments and clinical procedures mentioned in this unit before completing Exercise 14.

WORD EXERCISE 14

Match each term in Column A with a description in Column C by placing an appropriate number in Column B.

Column A	Column B	Column C
(a) audiometer		1. technique of measuring hearing
(b) audiometry		2. an instrument for viewing the ear
(c) aural speculum		3. technique of viewing the ear
(d) auriscope		4. a device for removing wax from the ear
(e) otoscopy		5. a device to aid drainage of fluid from the ear
(f) aural syringe		6. an instrument that measures hearing
(g) grommet		7. a device that holds the ear canal open

ANATOMY EXERCISE

Now complete the Anatomy Exercise on page 132.

CASE HISTORY 10

The object of this exercise is to understand words associated with a patient's medical history.

To complete the exercise:

• read through the passage on otitis media with effusion; unfamiliar words are underlined and you can find their meaning using the Word Help

• write the meaning of the medical terms shown in bold print on the lines that follow the Word Help.

Otitis media with effusion (OME, 'glue ear')

Miss J, a 5-year old infant, presented to her GP with persistent **otalgia**. She had a previous history of acute otitis media with perforation in the left ear and had been treated with broad-spectrum antibiotics. Her parents were concerned that her hearing and speech were impaired. Miss J's nursery teacher reported that she was inattentive in class and seemed 'in a world of her own'. Her mother had also noticed her snoring and had been worried about her breathing during a recent cold. Her tonsils were very large, she had a poor nasal airway and was breathing through her mouth, signs consistent with hypertrophy of the adenoid tissue.

Pneumatic **otoscopy** by her GP revealed bilateral otitis media with effusion (non-suppurative OM) and she was referred to the **audiometrist** for a hearing assessment. She cooperated well and a pure-tone **audiogram** was obtained indicating a mild loss of 20–30 decibels in hearing threshold. Over the next 6 months she received several courses of antibiotic therapy. Initially, there were signs of improvement but her condition did not resolve and she was referred to the paediatric **otology** clinic.

The consultant otologist confirmed the diagnosis. Her tympanic membranes were dull, retracted and lacked mobility. Fluid containing air bubbles was visible in the right ear, and she had a negative Rinne test.

Tympanometry revealed a flat tympanogram characteristic of glue ear with reduced compliance and a negative middle ear pressure. Her audiogram indicated conductive deafness across the entire frequency range of 35–40 decibels.

Miss J underwent adenoidectomy and anterior, bilateral **myringotomy** under general anaesthesia. A thick mucoid secretion was aspirated from both ears and grommets (**tympanostomy** tubes) inserted into her tympanic membranes. Six months later the grommets were still in position and her hearing and speech were much improved.

WORD HELP

acute symptoms/signs of short duration

adenoid resembling a gland (here it refers to the adenoids seen in the nasopharynx of children)

adenoidectomy removal of the adenoids (an enlarged pharyngeal tonsil)

anterior pertaining to towards the front

aspirated withdrawal by suction of fluid

bilateral pertaining to two sides

broad-spectrum affecting a wide range (of infective organisms)

compliance quality of yielding to pressure (here referring to the movement of the ear drum in relation to pressure)

conductive deafness deafness caused by impairment of conduction of sound waves through the normal route

decibel unit used for measurement of intensity of sound

effusion a fluid discharge into a part/escape of fluid into an enclosed space

GP general practitioner (family doctor)

grommet plastic tube inserted into the ear drum to ventilate the middle ear

hypertrophy increase in size of cells in a tissue (above normal growth/nourishment)

mucoid resembling mucus

otitis media condition of inflammation of the middle ear

otologist a specialist who studies the ear and its disorders

paediatric pertaining to medical care and treatment of children

perforation a hole made through a membrane or similar tissue

pneumatic pertaining to air (pneumatic otoscopy refers to viewing the ear membrane whilst stimulating it with a puff of air to observe its movement)

Rinne test a test using a tuning fork for diagnosis of conductive deafness

suppurative having a tendency to produce pus

tympanogram a recording of the compliance and impedance of the tympanic membrane

(a) otalgia

(b) otoscopy

(c) audiometrist

(d) audiogram

(e) otology

(f) tympanometry

(g) myringotomy

(h) tympanostomy

(Answers to the case history exercise are given in the Answers to Word Exercises beginning on page 301.)

Quick Reference

Combining forms relating to the ear:

Audi/o	hearing
Aur/i	ear
Auricul/o	pinna ear flap
Cochle/o	cochlea
Incud/o	incus (an ear ossicle)
Labyrinth/o	labyrinth (of inner ear)
Malle/o	malleus (an ear ossicle)
Mastoid/o	mastoid process/mastoid air cells
Myring/o	ear membrane (drum)
Ossicul/o	ossicle
Ot/o	ear
Salping/o	Eustachian/auditory tube
Stapedi/o	stapes (an ear ossicle)
Tympan/o	ear drum/middle ear
Vestibul/o	vestibular apparatus (of inner ear)

Abbreviations

Some common abbreviations related to the ear are listed below. Note some are not standard and their meaning may vary from one health care setting to another. There is a more extensive list for reference on page 335.

AC	air conduction
AD	auris dextra (right ear)
AS	auris sinistra (left ear)
ASOM	acute suppurative otitis media
aud	audiology
BC	bone conduction
CSOM	chronic suppurative otitis media
ENT	ear, nose and throat
ETF	Eustachian tube function
OE	otitis externa
OM	otitis media
oto	otology

Now write the meaning of the following words from the case history without using your dictionary lists:

Medical Notes

Cholesteatoma

Cholesteatoma is an uncommon but serious condition in which skin cells and purulent debris (including cholesterol) accumulate in the middle ear. The condition may be a result of chronic otitis media (middle ear infection) with perforation of the eardrum. During the healing process, skin from the ear canal grows into the middle ear and may damage the ossicles and surrounding bone. If left untreated, it can erode the roof of the middle ear and lead to inner ear infection and possibly meningitis. The cholesteatoma is removed by mastoidectomy or through the eardrum but the procedure may result in conduction deafness.

Deafness

Hearing impairment can be classified into two main categories:

Conductive deafness due to impaired transmission of sound waves through the external and middle ear to the sensory receptors of the inner ear (the conduction pathway).

Sensorineural deafness also known as **nerve deafness or perceptive deafness** is the result of disease in the cochlea, vestibular nerve or in the area of the brain concerned with hearing. Those affected usually perceive sound but cannot discriminate between different frequencies or understand what is being said. Sometimes patients have both conductive and sensorineural deafness in one ear, it is then known as **mixed deafness**.

Glue ear

Glue ear is an accumulation of thick, mucoid fluid behind the tympanic membrane in the middle that impairs hearing. Persistent glue ear is most common in children and is often accompanied by enlargement of the adenoids; it usually develops following an upper respiratory tract infection. Glue ear is also known as otitis media with effusion or as serous otitis media (see otitis below).

Ménière's disease

Ménière's disease is a chronic inner ear disease characterized by recurrent tinnitus, deafness and vertigo, in eighty-five percent of cases only one ear is affected. Nausea, vomiting and nystagmus (jerky eye movements) often accompany vertigo. The symptoms are caused by an increase in the amount of fluid in the membranous labyrinth of the inner ear. The accumulating fluid damages the part of the ear that controls balance (the labyrinth) and sometimes organ of hearing (the cochlea) as well. The cause of the increased fluid accretion is unknown but it tends to occur after fifty years of age.

Otitis

Otitis is an inflammation of the ear often caused by infection in one of its main regions:

Otitis externa or *external otitis* is usually due to an infection in the ear canal (external auditory meatus) often caused by the bacterium *Staphylococcus aureus*. More generalized inflammation may be due to fungi or allergic reactions to shampoos, hair dyes and dandruff.

Otitis media is an inflammation of the middle ear cavity between the eardrum and inner ear. *Acute otitis media* is usually caused by spread of micro-organisms from an upper respiratory infection through the auditory tube or through a ruptured tympanic membrane. Infection leads to the accumulation of pus in the middle ear causing the eardrum to bulge and rupture; when the eardrum bursts, the purulent material is discharged. The condition is common in children and is accompanied by severe earache.

Serous otitis media also known as *glue ear* or *secretory otitis media*, is a condition in which fluid collects in the cavity of the middle ear. It can be caused by blockage in the auditory tube by enlargement of the adenoids, swelling in the pharynx, tumours (Am.tumors), barotrauma and untreated otitis media. When the auditory tube becomes blocked, air in the middle ear is absorbed and a negative pressure develops causing the eardrum to bulge inwards. The reduced pressure causes a clear serous fluid to form in the cavity of the middle ear. In adults the condition causes discomfort and conductive hearing loss but in young children speech development is also delayed and as a result behavioural problems may develop.

Otitis interna or *labyrinthitis* is the inflammation of the vestibular structures in the internal ear. The condition causes vertigo and is almost always caused by bacterial or viral infection. Other causes include or head injury, development of cholesteatoma, and inadequately treated otitis media.

Presbycusis

Presbycusis is a form of hearing impairment associated with the ageing process. Degeneration of the sensory cells that detect sounds result in sensorineural deafness, this means the patient has difficulty perceiving certain frequencies. Perception of high frequencies is impaired first and later low frequencies. Patients have difficulty in following conversations as some frequencies are not perceived.

Tinnitus

Tinnitus is a ringing, buzzing or whistling noise heard in the ear in the absence of noise in the environment. In this condition the acoustic nerve transmits nerve impulses to the brain in the absence of vibrations from external sources. The condition is a symptom of many ear disorders including presbycusis, otosclerosis and exposure to continuous loud noise.

Vertigo

Vertigo is a sensation that one's self or one's surroundings are rotating or spinning in any plane. It results from a disturbance of the semicircular canals and/or their nerves in the inner ear. Labyrinthitis and Ménière's disease can cause sudden vertigo that is often accompanied by vomiting and unsteadiness.

NOW TRY THE WORD CHECK

WORD CHECK

This self-check exercise lists all the word components used in this unit. First write down the meaning of as many word components as you can. Then check your answers using the Exercise Guide and Quick Reference box or the Glossary of Word Components (pp. 347–371).

Prefixes

bin-

endo-

macro-

micro-

Combining forms of word roots

audi/o

aur/i

auricul/o

cochle/o

electr/o

incud/o

labyrinth/o

laryng/o

malle/o

mastoid/o

myc/o

myring/o

ossicul/o

ot/o

pharyng/o

py/o

rhin/o

salping/o

stapedi/o

ten/o

tympan/o

vestibul/o

Suffixes

-al

-algia

-ar

-aural

-centesis

-eal

-ectomy

-emphraxis

-externa

-genic

-gram

-ia

-interna

-ist

-itis

-media

-logy

-meter

-metry

-osis

-plasty

-rrhoea (Am. -rrhea)

-sclerosis

-scope

-stomy

-tome

-tomy

NOW TRY THE SELF-ASSESSMENT

SELF-ASSESSMENT

Test 10A

Below are some combining forms that refer to the anatomy of the ear. Indicate which part of the system they refer to by putting a number from the diagram (Fig. 60) next to each word.

(a) ot/o

(b) myring/o

(c) tympan/o

(d) nasopharyng/o

(e) ossicul/o

(f) labyrinth/o

(g) cochle/o

(h) mastoid/o

(i) salping/o

(j) vestibul/o

Score

10

Test 10B

Prefixes and suffixes

Match each prefix or suffix in Column A with a meaning in Column C by inserting the appropriate number in Column B.

Column A	Column B	Column C
(a) -al		1. incision into
(b) -ar		2. flow/discharge
(c) -aural		3. external
(d) bin-		4. instrument that cuts
(e) -eal		5. condition of hardening
(f) -emphraxis		6. inner/internal
(g) endo-		7. middle
(h) -externa		8. pertaining to (i)
(i) -gram		9. pertaining to (ii)
(j) -ia		10. pertaining to (iii)
(k) -interna		11. small
(l) macro-		12. in/within
(m) -media		13. abnormal condition/ disease of
(n) -metry		14. pertaining to the ear
(o) micro-		15. picture/X-ray/ tracing
(p) -osis		16. two of each/double
(q) -rrhoea (Am. -rrhea)		17. condition of
(r) -sclerosis		18. large
(s) -tome		19. to block/stop up
(t) -tomy		20. measurement

Score

20

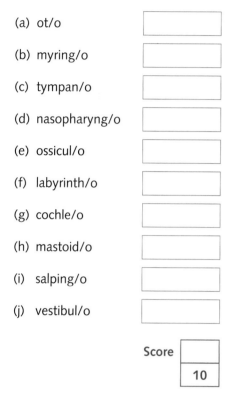

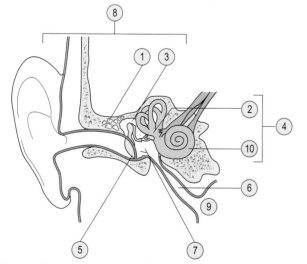

Figure 60 Section through the ear

Test 10C

Combining forms of word roots

Match each combining form in Column A with a meaning in Column C by inserting the appropriate number in Column B.

Column A	Column B	Column C
(a) audi/o		1. stapes
(b) aur/i		2. larynx
(c) auricul/o		3. nose
(d) incud/o		4. Eustachian tube
(e) labyrinth/o		5. ear (i)
(f) laryng/o		6. ear (ii)
(g) malle/o		7. ear flap (pinna)
(h) mastoid/o		8. ear drum/middle ear
(i) myc/o		9. vestibular apparatus
(j) myring/o		10. malleus
(k) ossicul/o		11. fungus
(l) ot/o		12. hearing
(m) pharyng/o		13. ear membrane
(n) py/o		14. tendon
(o) rhin/o		15. incus
(p) salping/o		16. pharynx
(q) stapedi/o		17. mastoid
(r) ten/o		18. ear bones/ossicles
(s) tympan/o		19. pus
(t) vestibul/o		20. labyrinth of inner ear

Score

20

Test 10D

Write the meaning of:

(a) otolaryngology

(b) tympanosclerosis

(c) stapediovestibular

(d) tympanomalleal

(e) vestibulocochlear

Score

5

Test 10E

Build words that mean:

(a) puncture of the mastoid process

(b) removal of the ear membrane

(c) surgical repair of the ear

(d) condition of pain in the ear

(e) originating in the middle ear

Score

5

Check answers to Self-Assessment Tests on page 325.

> **Test** your recall of the meanings of word components in Units 6–10 by completing the appropriate self-assessment tests in Unit 22 on page 293.

UNIT 11
THE SKIN

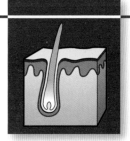

OBJECTIVES

Once you have completed Unit 11 you should be able to:

- understand the meaning of medical words relating to the skin

- build medical words relating to the skin

- associate medical terms with their anatomical position

- understand medical abbreviations relating to the skin.

EXERCISE GUIDE

Use this list of word components and their meanings to complete the word exercises in this unit.

Prefixes

a-	without
an-	without/not
auto-	self
crypto-	hidden
dys-	difficult/painful
epi-	above/upon/on
hyper-	above/excessive
hypo-	below/deficient
intra-	within/inside
pachy-	thick
para-	beside/near
sub-	under/below
xantho-	yellow
xero-	dry

Roots/Combining forms

aden/o	gland
aesthe/s/i/o	sensation/sensitivity (Am. esthesi/o)
esthe/s/i/o (Am.)	sensation/sensitivity
lith/o	stone
motor	action
myc/o	fungus
phyt(e)	plant (fungus)
schiz/o	split/cleft

Suffixes

-al	pertaining to
-auxis	increase
-cyte	cell
-ia	condition of
-ic	pertaining to
-itis	inflammation of
-logist	specialist who studies
-lysis	breakdown/disintegration
-oma	tumour (Am. tumor)/swelling
-osis	abnormal condition/disease/ abnormal increase
-phagia	condition of eating
-plasty	surgical repair/reconstruction
-poiesis	formation
-rrhexis	break/rupture
-rrhea (Am.)	excessive discharge/flow
-rrhoea	excessive discharge/flow (Am. -rrhea)
-schisis	splitting/parting/cleaving
-tic	pertaining to
-tome	cutting instrument
-trophy	nourishment/development
-tropic	pertaining to stimulating/affinity for

ANATOMY EXERCISE

When you have finished Word Exercises 1–9, look at the word components listed below. Complete Figure 61 by writing the appropriate combining form on each line – more than one component may relate to the same position. (You can check their meanings in the Quick Reference box on p. 150.)

Derm/o	Melan/o	Seb/o
Hidraden/o	Pil/o	Trich/o
Kerat/o		

The skin

The skin can be regarded as the largest organ in the body; it consists of two layers, the outer **epidermis** and the inner **dermis**. The skin protects us from the environment and plays a major role in thermoregulation. In its protective role, it prevents the body dehydrating, resists the invasion of microorganisms and provides protection from the harmful effects of ultraviolet light. Cells in the epidermis enable the surface of the skin to continuously regenerate, and the presence of elastic fibres and collagen fibres in the dermis make the skin tough and elastic.

Use the Exercise Guide at the beginning of this unit to complete Word Exercises 1–9 unless you are asked to work without it.

ROOT

Derm
(From a Greek word **derma***, meaning skin.)*

Combining forms **Derm/o, derm/a/t/o,** *also used as the suffix* -derma

The medical speciality concerned with the diagnosis and treatment of skin disease is known as **dermatology** (-logy meaning study of).

WORD EXERCISE 1

Using your Exercise Guide, find the meaning of:

(a) **dermat**/osis

_____

Actinic dermatoses are conditions in which the skin is abnormally sensitive to light (from a Greek word *aktis*, meaning ray).

(b) epi/**dermis**

_____

The **epidermis** forms the outer layer of the body and it functions to protect the underlying layer called the **dermis**. Note the dermis and epidermis form the skin; the underlying (subcutaneous) fatty tissue often studied with them is not regarded as part of the true skin.

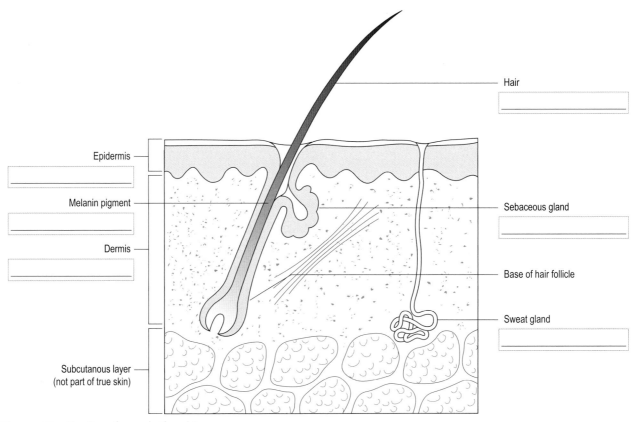

Figure 61   Section through the skin

The epidermis can be subdivided into five distinct layers, the outermost forming a layer of tough dead cells (scales), known as the stratum corneum. At the surface, the cells of the epidermis fit together like the scales of a fish; for this reason it is known as a stratified **squamous** epithelium (squamous from Latin *squama*, meaning scale of a fish or reptile). The word epithelium (combining form epitheli/o) refers to a type of tissue formed from one or more layers of cells that cover and line internal and external surfaces of the body. As the epidermis consists of many layers of cells it is described as a stratified epithelium.

(c) **dermat/o**/phyte

(d) pachy/**derma**

(e) xanth/o/**derma**

(f) **dermat/o**/auto/plasty

(g) xer/o/**derm**/ia

(h) **dermat/o**/logist

Using your Exercise Guide look up -al, hypo-,-ic, intra-, myc/o, -osis and -tome, then build words that mean:

(i) abnormal condition of fungi in the skin (use dermat/o)

(j) an instrument to cut skin for grafts (use derm/a)

(k) pertaining to below the skin (use derm/a)

(l) pertaining to within the skin (use derm/a)

Note. There are a few words in use derived from *cutis*, the Latin for skin, for example cutaneous – pertaining to the skin (from cutane/o meaning skin and -ous meaning pertaining to); The word cuticle means a small skin (from cuti- meaning skin and -cle meaning small) but it is used to mean the epidermis.

ROOT

Kerat
*(From a Greek word **keras**, meaning horn. Here kerat/o means the epidermis, the outer, horny layer of the skin. Note that kerat/o is also used to mean the cornea of the eye.)*

Combining form   Kerat/o

WORD EXERCISE 2

Without using your Exercise Guide, write the meaning of:

(a) actinic **kerat**/osis (actinic means pertaining to the sun's rays)

Using your Exercise Guide, find the meaning of:

(b) hyper/**kerat/o**/tic

(c) **kerat**/oma

(d) **kerat/o**/lysis

Note. There is no way of telling whether a medical term containing the root *kerat* refers to the cornea or epidermis except by noting the context in which it is written.

The cells of the outer layer of the epidermis are said to be **keratinized** because they contain the waterproof protein **keratin** that gives the epidermis its ability to protect the underlying dermis. (The combining form **keratin/o** refers to the protein keratin.)

Other disorders of the epidermis include:

Ichthyosis
A condition in which there is abnormal keratinization, giving rise to a dry, scaly skin that has the appearance of fish skin (from Greek **ichthy/o** meaning fish or fish-like).

Acanthosis
A condition of thickening of the prickle cell layer of the epidermis (**acanth/o** from Greek, meaning spike).

The skin appendages

The multiplication of cells in the basal layer of the epidermis gives rise to the appendages of the skin: hairs, sebaceous glands, sweat glands and nails. Here we use terms associated with each appendage:

ROOT

Pil
*(From a Latin word **pilus**, meaning hair. Hairs grow from depressions in the epidermis and dermis known as hair follicles.)*

Combining form **Pil/o**

WORD EXERCISE 3

Using your Exercise Guide, find the meaning of:

(a) **pil/o**/motor nerve

(This nerve stimulates the arrector pili muscles to contract, causing erection of the hair in cold conditions.)

A technique known as electrolysis is used to destroy hairs permanently by heating the base of a hair to destroy its dividing cells. The heating is achieved by passing an electric current through the hair follicle. This technique is also used by beauty therapists for the removal of excess hair and is known as e**pil**ation (e-meaning out from, i.e. the hair out of its follicle).

Hairs can also be removed by using a de**pil**atory paste that dissolves hair (de- meaning away). The hairs regrow following depilation as the base of the hair is not destroyed.

Alopecia or baldness may be hereditary as in the case of male-pattern baldness or due to disease or damage caused by drug treatment such as chemotherapy. (From a Greek word *alopex* meaning fox, the disease resembling the mange of foxes).

ROOT

Trich
*(From a Greek word **trichos**, meaning hair.)*

Combining form **Trich/o**

WORD EXERCISE 4

Without using your Exercise Guide, write the meaning of:

(a) **trich/o**/phyt/osis

(b) **trich**/osis

Using your Exercise Guide, find the meaning of:

(c) **trich/o**/aesthes/ia
    (Am. tricho/esthes/ia)

(d) schiz/o/**trich**/ia

(e) **trich/o**/rrhexis

ROOT

Seb
*(From a Latin word **sebum**, meaning fat or grease. Here seb/o means sebum, the oily secretion of the sebaceous glands, or sebaceous gland.)*

Combining form **Seb/o**

The sebaceous glands open directly on to the skin or more usually into the side of a hair follicle (a pilose-baceous follicle). They produce an oily secretion, known as sebum, that lubricates and waterproofs the hair and skin. Sebum is mildly bacteriostatic and fungistatic enabling the skin to resist infection.

Excessive production of sebum at puberty gives rise to **acne vulgaris**, a condition in which the skin becomes inflamed and develops pus-filled pimples.

WORD EXERCISE 5

Using your Exercise Guide, find the meaning of:

(a) **seb/o**/rrhoea
    (Am. **seb/o**/rrhea)

(b) **seb/o**/lith

(c) **seb/o**/tropic

ROOT

Hidr
*(From a Greek word **hidros**, meaning sweat.)*

Combining form **Hidr/o**

WORD EXERCISE 6

Without using your Exercise Guide, write the meaning of:

(a) **hidr**/osis

(b) hyper/**hidr**/osis

Using your Exercise Guide, find the meaning of:

(c) **hidr/o**/poiesis

(d) an/**hidr**/osis

(e) **hidr**/aden/itis

Sweat glands are also known by their Latin name of sudoriferous glands (*sudor* meaning sweat, *ferous* meaning pertaining to carrying).

ROOT

Onych
*(From a Greek word **onychos**, meaning nail.)*

Combining form   Onych/o

WORD EXERCISE 7

Using your Exercise Guide, find the meaning of:

(a) **onych**/o/crypt/osis

(b) **onych**/auxis

(c) **onych**/o/dys/trophy

(d) **onych**/a/trophy

(e) par/**onych**/ia

(f) **onych**/o/schisis

(g) **onych**/o/phagia

Without using your Exercise Guide, build words that mean:

(h) breaking down/disintegration of nails

   (In this condition, the nail comes away from the nail bed.)

(i) fungal condition of nails

(j) inflammation of nails
   (synonymous with **onych**ia)

Without using your Exercise Guide, write the meaning of:

(k) **onych**/o/rrhexis

(l) an/**onych**/ia

(m) pachy/**onych**/ia

ROOT

Melan
*(From a Greek word **melas**, meaning black. Here melan/o means melanin, a black pigment found in skin, hair and the choroid of the eye.)*

Combining form   Melan/o

WORD EXERCISE 8

Without using your Exercise Guide, build words that mean:

(a) a pigment cell

(b) abnormal condition of excessive black/pigment

Without using your Exercise Guide, write the meaning of:

(c) **melan**/oma

Malignant melanoma is on the increase, and this is believed to be mainly the effect of solar damage caused by excessive sunbathing. Sometimes a melanoma develops from a pigmented naevus (mole). Melanomas are highly malignant, and once the tumour (Am. tumor) cells have spread, they become difficult to eradicate. Malignant melanoma can be fatal unless treated early in its development. Five-year survival rate is related to the depth of the tumour in the skin at first presentation.

> **Note.** Naevus (pl. naevi; Am. nevus, pl. nevi) is the medical name for a mole or birthmark on the body. Naevi arise from melanocytes or developmental abnormalities of blood vessels.

Medical equipment and clinical procedures

Suspicious lesions of skin need to be examined microscopically for signs of malignancy. Small samples of skin are removed during an excision **biopsy** (*bio* meaning life, *opsis* meaning vision, therefore biopsy means observation of living tissue). These are then sectioned and stained in the histology laboratory. The biopsy tissue is examined by a histologist or pathologist to determine whether the cells are **benign** or **malignant** (benign means innocent or harmless; malignant means virulent and dangerous to life).

Benign lesions can be removed if they are causing a problem or are unsightly. Malignant lesions threaten life and are treated by surgical excision, radiotherapy and chemotherapy.

Other terms used for lesions that appear in skin disease are listed in the following table:

Bulla	a large watery blister (plural-bullae)
Comedone/comedo	an accumulation of sebum in the outlet of a hair folliclei; comedones may be closed forming whiteheads or open forming blackheads
Cyst	a sac with a membranous wall enclosing fluid or semi-solid matter
Fissure	a split, crack or crack-like sore in the skin
Keloid	an overgrowth of scar tissue that occurs after injury or surgery
Macula	a non-palpable flat area of skin showing a change in colour (often red)
Papule	a small circular, solid elevation of the skin (Syn. pimple)
Polyp	a stalked (pedunculated) tumour (Am. tumor) arising from a mucous membrane
Pustule	a small swelling of the skin containing pus
Ulcer	an open sore in the skin often suppurating (forming pus)
Vesicle	a small blister containing clear fluid (serum)
Weal/wheal	a smooth superficial swelling (red or white) characteristic of urticaria or nettle stings
Wen	a sebaceous cyst filled with sebum due to a blocked opening of a sebaceous gland

Treatment of skin disorders using lasers

Developments in physics have led to the development of medical **lasers** which are playing a prominent role in the treatment of skin disorders. Here we examine a selection of their applications to dermatology. First we need to understand the meaning of the acronym laser.

LASER is built from the first letter of each of the following words: Light Amplification by Stimulated Emission of Radiation.

A laser is a device that produces an intense, coherent beam of monochromatic light in the visible region. All the light waves in the beam are in phase and do not diverge so it can be targeted precisely (see Fig. 62). The beam is capable of focusing intense heat and power when focused at close range.

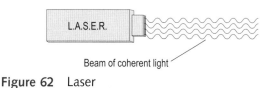

Figure 62 Laser

The medical laser transfers energy in the form of light to the tissues. When the laser beam strikes living tissue it is heated and destroyed (**thermolysis**) in a fraction of a second. Some lasers can heat tissues to over 100°C, resulting in their complete vaporization.

The extent of destruction of a tissue depends on the presence of chemicals in cells that absorb the light. These are known as **chromatophores**. There are three main chromatophores found in tissues: water, melanin and haemoglobin. A skin lesion containing a large amount of melanin, such as a mole, can be specifically targeted and destroyed by a laser with little destruction of the surrounding tissue.

There are many types of medical laser, each one emitting a beam of specific wavelength. The wave-length of the radiation emitted depends on the medium used by the laser, which may be a gas, liquid or solid. In the laser, the atoms of the medium are excited electrically and are stimulated to emit energy in the form of light. Besides laser light, other forms of radiation are used to treat chronic skin disorders. Here are three examples of lasers used by dermatologists:

Type of laser	Medium	Wavelength	Chromatophore	Use
CO_2	Carbon dioxide gas	Infrared 10–600 nm	Water	Vaporizes/cuts tissue. Coagulates blood vessels. Bloodless surgery as it seals up cut vessels. Used to incise tissue and excise a variety of lesions
Argon	Ionized argon gas	Blue–green 488–514 nm	Melanin Haemoglobin	Penetrates epidermis. and coagulates underlying pigments. Used to remove vascular and pigmented navei (Am. nevi)
Dye removing	Various synthetic dyes	Can be tuned to any required wavelength	Melanin Haemoglobin	Removing tattoos, pigmented tattoo inks, vascular lesions, moles, port wine stains, etc.

Treatment of psoriasis

Psoriasis is a common chronic skin condition in which there is an increased rate of production of skin cells. The excess skin cells form plaques of silvery scales that continuously flake off, exposing erythematous (reddened) skin that shows pinpoint bleeding. A large proportion of a dermatologist's time may be concerned with this disorder as it affects approximately 2% of the population. There is no cure and therapies are aimed at reducing the scaling and inflammation. A recent innovation is the technique known as:

PUVA (**P**soralen **U**ltra **V**iolet **A** light)

This is a form of **photochemotherapy** that uses a **psoralen** to sensitize the skin to light before it is irradiated with ultraviolet light (long wave A). After administration of the psoralen (taken orally) the patient is placed in a chamber illuminated with ultraviolet light. The treatment is convenient for patients; their skin shows dramatic improvement and the effect lasts for several months. Unfortunately, there is a risk of developing skin cancer because of excessive exposure to UVA; this risk is being evaluated.

Revise the names of all instruments and clinical procedures mentioned in this unit and then try Exercise 9.

WORD EXERCISE 9

Match each term in Column A with a description in Column C by placing an appropriate number in Column B.

Column A	Column B	Column C
(a) excision biopsy		1. removal of hair
(b) dermatome		2. an instrument that destroys tissue using a beam of coherent light
(c) medical laser		3. destruction of tissue by heating with an electric current
(d) PUVA		4. removal of living tissue from the body
(e) epilation		5. an instrument used for cutting a thin layer of skin (for grafts)
(f) electrolysis		6. technique of exposing photo-sensitized skin to light

ANATOMY EXERCISE

Now complete the Anatomy Exercise on page 144.

CASE HISTORY 11

The object of this exercise is to understand words associated with a patient's medical history.

To complete the exercise:

- read through the passage on psoriasis; unfamiliar words are underlined and you can find their meaning using the Word Help

- write the meaning of the medical terms shown in bold print on the lines that follow the Word Help.

Psoriasis

Mrs K, a 48-year-old woman, presented at the **dermatology** clinic with chronic plaque psoriasis and accompanying arthropathy. She had developed guttate psoriasis at the age of 12 following severe tonsillitis. This was self-limiting but shortly after psoriatic patches appeared on her legs and arms and then on the trunk. Since then the condition has persisted with exacerbations on her scalp, knees and arms, and over the last 5 years she has developed arthritis in her distal interphalangeal finger joints.

Mrs K's condition was reviewed by the **dermatologist**. She had developed large **hyperkeratotic** plaques on her trunk and extremities. Her scalp was also affected with some degree of erythema extending beyond the hair margin. Mrs K indicated that the severity of her arthritis seemed to parallel the worsening of her **cutaneous** lesions.

Her nails were pitted with opaque yellow areas within the nail plates. Several nails were showing signs of **onycholysis** with **keratinous** debris under their free edges. Following assessment, Mrs K underwent a course of PUVA using 8-methoxypsoralen twice weekly for 6 weeks. She experienced drying of the skin and pruritus but showed considerable improvement. At the present she is receiving a single maintenance treatment every 3 weeks and her fair skin is being examined for presence of malignant **epitheliomas** (non-**melanoma** skin cancer being the major, slight, long-term risk factor).

WORD HELP

arthritis inflammation of the joints

arthropathy diseased joints

chronic pertaining to long term, continued

distal further away from point of attachment

erythema relating to erythema (reddening of the skin)

exacerbations increased severity of symptoms

guttate marked or covered with drop-like spots

interphalangeal pertaining to between the bones of the fingers or toes

lesion a pathological change in a tissue

malignant dangerous, life threatening

8-methoxypsoralen a psoralen (drug) that sensitizes the skin to light

plaque a flat area, a patch

pruritus itching

psoriasis a chronic inflammatory disease of the skin exhibiting red patches in the epidermis covered with silvery scales

psoriatic pertaining to psoriasis

PUVA administration of a **p**soralen (a drug that sensitizes the skin to light) followed by exposure to **u**ltra**v**iolet light **A**

Quick Reference

Combining forms relating to the skin:

Acanth/o	spiny
Cutane/o	skin
Derm/at/o	skin/dermis
Epitheli/o	epithelium
Hidr/o	sweat
Hidraden/o	sweat gland
Ichthy/o	fish/fish-like
Kerat/o	epidermis
Keratin/o	keratin
Melan/o	melanin
Onych/o	nail
Pil/o	hair
Seb/o	sebum/sebaceous gland
Squam/o	scaly
Trich/o	hair

Abbreviations

Some common abbreviations related to the skin are listed below. Note some are not standard and their meaning may vary from one health care setting to another. There is a more extensive list for reference on page 335.

bx	biopsy
Derm	dermatology
Ez	eczema
KS	Karposi's sarcoma
SCC	squamous cell carcinoma
SED	skin erythema dose
SPF	sun protection factor
ST	skin test
STD	skin test dose
STU	skin test unit
Subcu	subcutaneous
ung	ointment (unguentum)

Now write the meaning of the following words from the case history without using your dictionary lists:

(a) dermatology

(b) dermatologist

(c) hyperkeratotic

(d) cutaneous

(e) onycholysis

(f) keratinous

(g) epithelioma

(h) melanoma

(Answers to the case history exercise are given in the Answers to Word Exercises beginning on page 301).

Medical Notes

Acne vulgaris

A common condition in adolescents caused by increased levels of sex hormones after puberty. It develops when sebaceous glands in hair follicles become blocked and infected leading to inflammation and the formation of pustules. In severe cases permanent scarring may result. The most common sites are the face, chest and upper back.

Decubitus ulcer

Decubitus ulcers are also known as *pressure sores* or *bedsores* and are caused by lying in one position for long periods. They occur in areas where the skin is compressed between a bony prominence and a hard surface such as a bed or chair. When this occurs blood flow to a local area is reduced causing necrosis, ulcer formation and sloughing of the skin. If infection occurs this can result in septicaemia. Frequent changes in body position and soft support cushions help prevent decubitus ulcers.

Dermatitis

Dermatitis is used synonymously with the term *eczema* and describes inflammation of the skin that can be acute or chronic. In acute dermatitis there is redness, swelling and exudation of serous fluid usually accompanied by itching, crusting and scaling. If the condition becomes chronic, the skin thickens and may become leathery due to excessive scratching and infection may complicate the condition.

Atopic dermatitis a predisposition that brings about hypersensitivity to allergens, often affecting children who also suffer from hay fever or asthma.

Contact dermatitis is caused by direct contact of the skin with irritants such as cosmetics, detergents, synthetic rubber, nickel and other chemicals.

Eczema

Eczema is used synonymously with the term dermatitis and describes an inflammation of the skin that can be acute or chronic. See dermatitis above.

Furuncle

Furuncles are also known as boils, they are localized staphylococcal infections of hair follicles characterized by large, inflamed, pus-filled lesions. A group of untreated boils may fuse into an even larger lesion called a *carbuncle*.

Impetigo

This is a highly contagious bacterial condition that results from staphylococcal or streptococcal infection and occurs most often in young children. Impetigo starts as a reddish discolouration called erythema, but soon develops into vesicles (blisters) with yellowish crusts. Impetigo is most commonly caused by *Staphylococcus aureus*. Superficial pustules develop, usually around the nose and mouth; occasionally the infection becomes systemic and life threatening.

Karposi's sarcoma

A viral-induced malignant disease characterized by the growth of new blood vessels. The lesions appear as red, blue or brown nodules that are common on the ankle, trunk and nose. Originally common in tropical Africa it is now seen in individuals who are immunologically compromised, such as those with AIDS.

Tumours (Am. tumors)

Excessive exposure to the sun can result in skin cancer; there are three basic forms:

Basal cell carcinoma (BCC) also called *rodent ulcer* accounts for over seventy-five percent of all skin cancers. It occurs on exposed parts especially those of the face, nose eyelids and cheek. It begins as a small, firm, flat nodule and grows slowly, eventually forming a shallow ulcer with raised edges. The ulcer is locally destructive destroying deeper tissue as it grows. Fortunately basal cell carcinomas do not spread (metastasize) to other parts of the body.

Squamous cell carcinoma (SCC) also begins in the epidermis and is derived from keratinocytes. High proportions of squamous carcinomata arise on skin damaged by sunlight or chemicals. Initially, the skin thickens and the lesion becomes hyperkeratotic and ulcerated. If the tumour is not promptly removed, there will be metastatic spread into local lymph nodes and beyond.

Malignant melanoma is a malignant tumour of epidermal melanocytes; it is the leading cause of death from skin disease because it can spread rapidly. Melanoma is most common in white females over the age of thirty and its development may be related to severe sun exposure, genetic factors and unknown chemical carcinogens.

Urticaria (hives)

Urticaria is also known as *nettlerash* because the itching and weals that develop on the skin resemble the effects of the stinging nettle (*Urtica dioica*). It is often due to allergic reaction to certain foods, food additives or drugs such as antibiotics.

Verruca

A wart for example *verruca plana*, the common wart that infects the hands, knees and face and *verruca plantaris* a flat wart infecting the sole of the foot (see wart below).

Vitiligo

A skin disease characterized by loss of pigment (depigmentation). There is an absence of melanocytes in affected areas producing white patches. It is associated with autoimmune disease of the endocrine system and in some cases there is an inherited component.

Wart

Warts or verrucas are nipple-like neoplasms of the epidermis caused by infection with the human papilloma virus. Common sites of infection are the hands, face and soles of the feet. Transmission of warts generally occurs through direct contact with warts on the skin of an infected person. Freezing, drying, laser therapy or application of chemicals (keratolytics) can remove them. (see verruca)

NOW TRY THE WORD CHECK

WORD CHECK

This self-check exercise lists all the word components used in this unit. First write down the meaning of as many word components as you can. Then check your answers using the Exercise Guide and Quick Reference box or the Glossary of Word Components (pp. 347–371).

Prefixes

a-

an-

auto-

crypto-

dys-

epi-

hyper-

hypo-

intra-

pachy-

para-

sub-

xantho-

xero-

Combining forms of word roots

acanth/o

aden/o

aesthesi/o
(Am. esthesi/o)

cutane/o

cyt/o

dermat/o

epitheli/o

hidr/o

ichthy/o

kerat/o

keratin/o

lith/o

melan/o

-motor-

myc/o

onych/o

phyt(e)

pil/o

schiz/o-

seb/o

squam/o

trich/o

Suffixes

-auxis

-ia

-ic

-itis

-logist

-logy

-lysis

-oma

-osis

-ous

-phagia

-plasty

-poiesis

-rrhexis

-rrhoea
(Am. -rrhea)

-schisis

-tic

-tome

-trophy

-tropic

NOW TRY THE SELF-ASSESSMENT

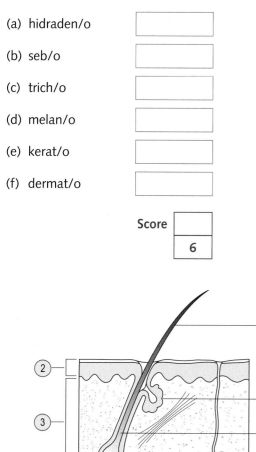

SELF-ASSESSMENT

Test 11A

Below are some combining forms that refer to the anatomy of the skin. Indicate which part of the system they refer to by putting a number from the diagram (Fig. 63) next to each word:

(a) hidraden/o ⬜

(b) seb/o ⬜

(c) trich/o ⬜

(d) melan/o ⬜

(e) kerat/o ⬜

(f) dermat/o ⬜

Score ⬜
6

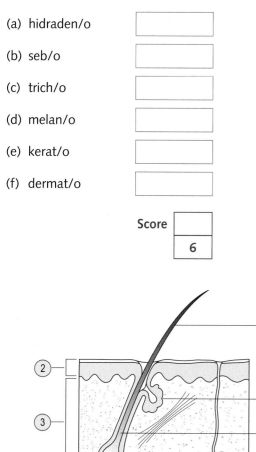

Figure 63 Section through the skin

Column A	Column B	Column C
(e) dys-	⬜	5. condition of eating/swallowing
(f) hyper-	⬜	6. thick
(g) hypo-	⬜	7. nourishment
(h) intra-	⬜	8. hidden/concealed
(i) -lysis	⬜	9. dry
(j) -oma	⬜	10. formation/making
(k) pachy-	⬜	11. break/rupture
(l) -phagia	⬜	12. pertaining to affinity for/stimulating
(m) -poiesis	⬜	13. difficult/painful
(n) -rrhexis	⬜	14. tumour (Am. tumor)/swelling
(o) -schisis	⬜	15. yellow
(p) -tome	⬜	16. below
(q) -trophy	⬜	17. increase
(r) -tropic	⬜	18. without/not
(s) xantho-	⬜	19. self
(t) xero-	⬜	20. splitting

Score ⬜
20

Test 11B

Prefixes and suffixes

Match each prefix or suffix in Column A with a meaning in Column C by inserting the appropriate number in Column B.

Column A	Column B	Column C
(a) a-	⬜	1. cutting instrument
(b) auto-	⬜	2. above
(c) -auxis	⬜	3. breakdown/disintegration
(d) crypto-	⬜	4. within

Test 11C

Combining forms of word roots

Match each combining form in Column A with a meaning in Column C by inserting the appropriate number in Column B.

Column A	Column B	Column C
(a) aden/o	⬜	1. horny/epidermis
(b) dermat/o	⬜	2. pertaining to action
(c) hidr/o	⬜	3. fungus
(d) kerat/o	⬜	4. hair (i)

Column A	Column B	Column C
(e) lith/o		5. hair (ii)
(f) -motor-		6. nail
(g) myc/o		7. skin
(h) onych/o		8. plant
(i) phyt/o		9. sweat
(j) pil/o		10. sebum
(k) seb/o		11. gland
(l) trich/o		12. stone

Score

12

Test 11D

Write the meaning of:

(a) dermatophytosis

(b) keratinocyte

(c) trichoanaesthesia
(Am. trichoanesthesia)

(d) hidradenoma

(e) epidermomycosis

Score

5

Test 11E

Build words that mean:

(a) inflammation of the skin

(b) abnormal condition of nails

(c) condition of nails
blackened with melanin

(d) study of skin

(e) condition of thick nails

Score

5

Check answers to Self-Assessment Tests on page 325.
Check answers to Self-Assessment Tests on page 325.

UNIT 12
THE NOSE AND MOUTH

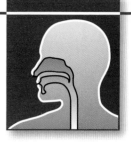

EXERCISE GUIDE

Use this list of word components and their meanings to complete the word exercises in this unit.

Prefixes

a-	without
dys-	difficult/painful
endo-	within/inside
intra-	inside
macro-	large
ortho-	straight/correct/normal
peri-	around
poly-	many
post-	after
prosth-	adding (replacement part)

Roots/Combining forms

aden/o	gland
aer/o	air/gas
angi/o	vessel
bronch/o	bronchi/bronchial tree
bucc/o	cheek
dynam/o	force
laryng/o	larynx
man/o	pressure
myc/o	fungus
nas/o	nose
ot/o	ear
pharyng/o	pharynx
trich/o	hair
tympan/o	middle ear/ear drum

Suffixes

-agogue	agent that induces/promotes
-al	pertaining to
-algia	condition of pain
-cele	swelling/protrusion/hernia
-dynia	condition of pain
-eal	pertaining to
-ectomy	removal of
-genic	pertaining to formation/originating in
-gram	X-ray tracing/picture/recording
-graphy	technique of recording/making an X-ray
-ia	condition of
-ic	pertaining to
-ics	pertaining to a speciality
-ist	specialist
-itis	inflammation of
-lith	stone
-logy	study of
-meter	measuring instrument
-metry	process of measuring
-osis	abnormal condition/disease of
-pathy	disease of
-phagia	condition of eating
-phonia	condition of having voice
-phyma	tumour (Am. tumor)/boil
-plasty	surgical repair/reconstruction
-plegia	condition of paralysis
-rrhagia	condition of bursting forth (of blood)
-rrhaphy	stitching/suturing
-rrhea (Am.)	excessive flow
-rrhoea	excessive flow (Am. -rrhea)
-schisis	cleaving/splitting/parting
-scope	viewing instrument
-scopy	technique of viewing/examining
-stomy	formation of an opening into . . .
-tomy	incision into
-us	thing/structure/anatomical part

ANATOMY EXERCISE

When you have finished Word Exercises 1–18, look at the word components listed below. Complete Figures 64 and 65 by writing the appropriate combining form on each line – more than one component may relate to the same position. (You can check their meanings in the Quick Reference box on p. 163.)

Antr/o	Labi/o	Sial/o
Cheil/o	Nas/o	Sin/o
Faci/o	Odont/o	Stomat/o
Gingiv/o	Palat/o	Uvul/o
Gloss/o	Ptyal/o	
Gnath/o	Rhin/o	

The nose and mouth

Receptors for the sense of smell are located in the olfactory epithelium which is in the roof of the nasal cavity. In order for us to smell a substance it must be volatile so it can be carried into the nose and then it must dissolve in the mucus covering the receptors. Humans can distinguish between 2000 and 4000 different odours.

Receptors for taste are located on the taste buds of the tongue. When a substance is eaten, four types of receptor can be stimulated, producing sensations for sweet, bitter, salty and sour. The sense of taste is known as gustation.

In this unit we will look at terms associated with the mouth and nose.

Use the Exercise Guide at the beginning of this unit to complete Word Exercises 1–18 unless you are asked to work without it.

ROOT

Stomat
(From a Greek word **stomatos**, *meaning mouth.)*

Combining form **Stomat/o**

WORD EXERCISE 1

Using your Exercise Guide, find the meaning of:

(a) **stomat/o**/logy

(b) **stomat/o**/rrhagia

(c) **stomat/o**/pathy

Using your Exercise Guide find the meaning of -dynia, myc/o and -osis, then build words that mean:

(d) condition of pain in the mouth

(e) abnormal condition of fungi in the mouth

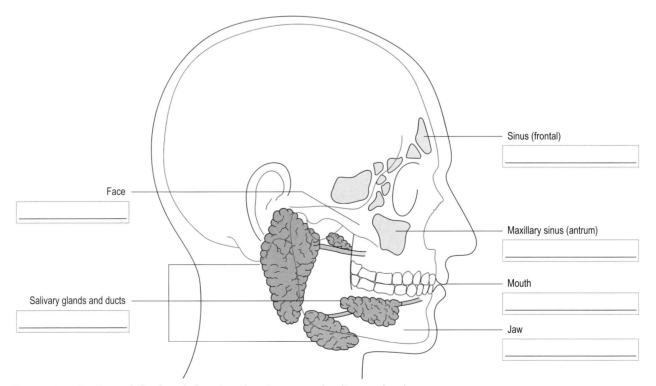

Figure 64 Section of the head showing the sinuses and salivary glands

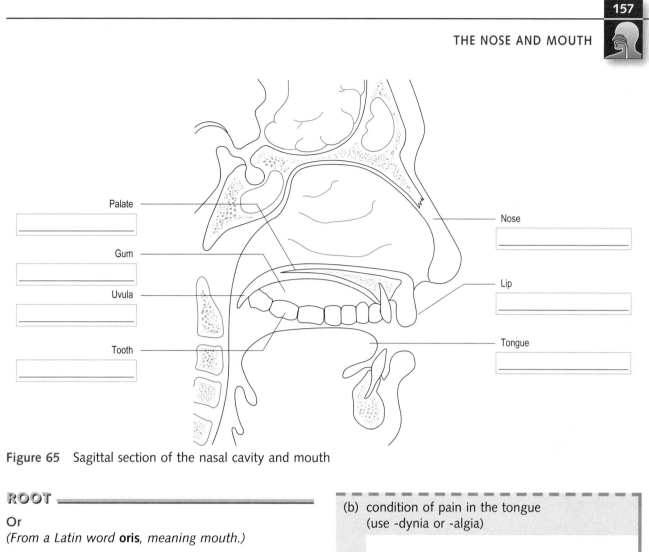

Figure 65 Sagittal section of the nasal cavity and mouth

Palate

Gum

Uvula

Tooth

Nose

Lip

Tongue

ROOT

Or
*(From a Latin word **oris**, meaning mouth.)*

Combining form   Or/o

WORD EXERCISE 2

Using your Exercise Guide, find the meaning of:

(a) **or**/al

(b) intra/-**or**/al

(c) **or/o**/pharyng/eal

(d) **or/o**/nas/al

ROOT

Gloss
*(From a Greek word **glossa**, meaning tongue.)*

Combining form   Gloss/o

WORD EXERCISE 3

Without using your Exercise Guide, build words that mean:

(a) the study of the tongue

(b) condition of pain in the tongue
(use -dynia or -algia)

(c) pertaining to the pharynx and tongue (use -eal)

Using your Exercise Guide, find the meaning of:

(d) **gloss/o**/plegia

(e) **gloss/o**/trich/ia

(f) **gloss/o**/cele

(g) macro/**gloss**/ia

(h) **gloss/o**/plasty

A Latin combining form lingu/o is also used to mean tongue, language or relationship to the tongue, e.g. lingual – pertaining to the tongue, sublingual – under the tongue.

Disorders of the mouth, tongue, pharynx and palate give rise to problems with eating, swallowing and talking, e.g.

Dysphagia
A condition of difficulty in eating (from Greek *phagein* to eat).

Dyslalia
A condition of difficulty in talking (from Greek *lalein* to talk).

ROOT

Sial
*(From a Greek word **sialon**, meaning saliva. Here sial/o means saliva, salivary gland or salivary duct. Three pairs of salivary glands secrete saliva into the mouth. Saliva lubricates the food and contains amylase, an enzyme that begins the digestion of starch.)*

Combining form   **Sial/o**

WORD EXERCISE 4

Using your Exercise Guide, find the meaning of:

(a) **sial**/aden/ectomy

(b) **sial**/angi/o/graphy

(c) poly/**sial**/ia

(d) **sial**/o/gram

Using your Exercise Guide look up -lith, then build a word that means:

(e) a stone in the saliva (salivary duct or salivary gland)

Using your Exercise Guide, find the meaning of:

(f) **sial**/agogue
(a drug)

(g) **sial**/aer/o/phagia

ROOT

Ptyal
*(From a Greek word **ptyalon**, meaning saliva.)*

Combining form   **Ptyal/o**

WORD EXERCISE 5

Using your Exercise Guide, find the meaning of:

(a) **ptyal**/o/genic

(b) **ptyal**/o/rrhoea
(Am. **ptyal**/o/rrhea)

Without using your Exercise Guide, write the meaning of:

(c) **ptyal**/o/lith

ROOT

Gnath
*(From a Greek word **gnathos**, meaning jaw.)*

Combining form   **Gnath/o**

WORD EXERCISE 6

Without using your Exercise Guide, build words that mean:

(a) condition of pain in the jaw

(b) plastic surgery of the jaw

(c) study of the jaw (and chewing apparatus)

(d) pertaining to the jaw and mouth (use -ic)

Using your Exercise Guide, find the meaning of:

(e) **gnath**/o/dynam/o/meter

(f) **gnath**/o/schisis
(refers to the upper jaw and palate – a cleft palate)

(g) **gnath**/itis

ROOT

Cheil
*(From a Greek word **cheilos**, meaning lip.)*

Combining form   **Cheil/o**

WORD EXERCISE 7

Without using your Exercise Guide, write the meaning of:

(a) **cheil/o**/stomat/o/plasty

(b) **cheil/o**/schisis

Using your Exercise Guide, find the meaning of:

(c) **cheil/o**/rrhaphy

Without using your Exercise Guide, build a word that means:

(d) inflammation of the lip

ROOT

Labi
(From a Latin word **labium**, meaning lip.)

Combining form   Labi/o

WORD EXERCISE 8

Using your Exercise Guide, find the meaning of:

(a) **labi/o**/gloss/o/laryng/eal

Without using your Exercise Guide, build a word that means:

(b) pertaining to pharynx, tongue and lips (use -eal)

ROOT

Gingiv
(From a Latin word **gingiva**, meaning gum.)

Combining form   Gingiv/o

WORD EXERCISE 9

Without using your Exercise Guide, build words that mean:

(a) inflammation of the gums

(b) removal of gum
(usually performed for
pyorrhoea (Am. pyorrhea), the flow of pus a result of periodontal disease)

Without using your Exercise Guide, write the meaning of:

(c) labi/o/**gingiv**/al

ROOT

Palat
(From Latin **palatum**, meaning the palate.)

Combining form   Palat/o

WORD EXERCISE 10

Without using your Exercise Guide, build words that mean:

(a) condition of paralysis of the soft palate

(b) pertaining to the jaw and palate (use -ic)

(c) a split palate (cleft palate)

Using your Exercise Guide, find the meaning of:

(d) post/**palat**/al

ROOT

Uvul
(From a Latin word **uvula**, meaning grape. Here uvul/o means the uvula, the central tag-like structure extending downwards from the soft palate.)

Combining form   Uvul/o

WORD EXERCISE 11

Without using your Exercise Guide, build words that mean:

(a) removal of the uvula

(b) incision into the uvula

ROOT

Phas
(From a Greek word **phasis**, meaning speech.)

Combining form   Phas/i/o

WORD EXERCISE 12

Using your Exercise Guide, find the meaning of:

(a) a/**phas**/ia

(b) dys/**phas**/ia

There are many varieties and causes of aphasia. Common types are:

Motor aphasia
A condition due to an inability to move muscles involved in speech. (The word **aphonia** is also used to refer to a loss of voice.)

Sensory aphasia
A condition in which there is an inability to recognize spoken (or written) words.

ROOT

Odont
(From a Greek word **odontos**, meaning tooth.)

Combining form   Odont/o

WORD EXERCISE 13

Without using your Exercise Guide, build words that mean:

(a) the scientific study of teeth (dentistry)

(b) any disease of teeth

(c) condition of pain in a tooth (toothache)

Using your Exercise Guide, find the meaning of:

(d) peri/**odont**/ics (includes all tissues supporting teeth)

(e) end/**odont**/o/logy (includes the tooth pulp and roots)

(f) orth/**odont**/ics

(g) orth/**odont**/ist

(h) prosth/**odont**/ics

A prosthesis is an artificial replacement for a body part (Plural -prostheses). Prosthodontics is the branch of dentistry that specializes in the replacement of lost teeth and associated structures.

ROOT

Rhin
(From a Greek word **rhinos**, meaning nose.)

Combining form   Rhin/o

We have already used rhin/o when studying the breathing system. Here we use the same combining form with new suffixes.

WORD EXERCISE 14

Using your Exercise Guide, find the meaning of:

(a) **rhin**/o/phonia

(b) **rhin**/o/man/o/metry

(c) **rhin**/o/phyma

(d) **rhin**/o/scopy

(e) ot/o/**rhin**/o/laryng/o/logy

Without using your Exercise Guide, write the meaning of:

(f) **rhin**/o/rrhagia
(also known as epistaxis)

Note. There is also a Latin word **nasus** meaning nose; its combining form nas/o is used in several exercises in this unit.

ROOT

Sinus
(A Latin word meaning a hollow or a cavity. Here sin/o means a sinus, a cavity in a bone of the skull.)

Combining forms   Sin/o, sinus-

WORD EXERCISE 15

Using your Exercise Guide, find the meaning of:

(a) **sin**/us

(b) **sin**/o/bronch/itis

Without using your Exercise Guide, write the meaning of:

(c) **sinus**/itis

This condition affects the membrane lining the paranasal sinuses (the air-filled cavities surrounding the nose). Micro-organisms spread from the nose or pharynx to infect the mucous membranes lining the sinuses of the maxillary, sphenoidal, ethmoidal and frontal bones of the skull. The primary viral infection is often followed by secondary bacterial infection *with Staphylococcus aureus, Streptococcus pyogenes* or *Streptococcus pneumoniae*. The congested linings may block the drainage channels from the sinuses preventing the expulsion of the accumulating pus. When this occurs there is a feeling of tension and pain in the affected area. Other symptoms include fever, stuffy nose and loss of the sense of smell. If there are repeated attacks or if recovery is not complete, the infection may become chronic.

(d) **sin/o**/gram

ROOT

Antr
*(From a Greek word **antron**, meaning cave. Here antr/o means antrum, in particular the antrum of Highmore also known as the superior maxillary sinus.)*

Combining form **Antr/o**

WORD EXERCISE 16

Using your Exercise Guide, build words that mean:

(a) an instrument used to view the antrum

(b) inflammation of the tympanum and antrum

Without using your Exercise Guide, write the meaning of:

(c) **antr/o**/tomy
(usually performed
to drain out infected fluid)

(d) **antr/o**/nas/al

(e) **antr/o**/cele

Using your Exercise Guide, find the meaning of:

(f) **antr/o**/bucc/al

(g) **antr/o**/stomy

ROOT

Faci
*(From a Latin word **facies**, meaning face.)*

Combining form **Faci/o**

WORD EXERCISE 17

Without using your Exercise Guide, write the meaning of:

(a) **faci**/al

(b) **faci/o**/plegia

(c) **faci/o**/plasty

Medical equipment and clinical procedures

Revise the names of all instruments and clinical procedures mentioned in this unit before completing Exercise 18.

WORD EXERCISE 18

Match each term in Column A with a description from Column C by placing an appropriate number in Column B.

Column A	Column B	Column C
(a) antroscope		1. an instrument that measures the force of the jaws
(b) sialan-giography		2. technique of recording the tongue (movement in speech)
(c) gnatho dynamometer		3. an instrument for viewing the maxillary sinus (antrum)
(d) rhino-manometer		4. an artificial part of the body, e.g. a false tooth
(e) prosthesis		5. technique of making an X-ray/ recording of salivary ducts
(f) glossography		6. an instrument that measures air pressure in the nose

ANATOMY EXERCISE

Now complete the Anatomy Exercise on page 156.

CASE HISTORY 12

The object of this exercise is to understand words associated with a patient's medical history.

To complete the exercise:

- read through the passage on acute sinusitis; unfamiliar words are underlined and you can find their meaning using the Word Help

- write the meaning of the medical terms shown in bold print on the lines following the Word Help.

Acute sinusitis

Mrs. L, a 28-year-old mother, was brought into Accident and Emergency late at night; her husband was concerned that she was seriously ill. She was recovering from a viral rhinitis when, on the morning of admission she was stricken with an excruciating frontal headache with pain in her cheek and upper teeth. She felt dizzy, and her right cheek was hot and tender to touch. There was no immediate history of any dental problems.

She was examined by the casualty registrar and found to have an elevated temperature and pulse. Rhinoscopy demonstrated reddened, oedematous mucous (Am. edematous) membranes and signs of a mucopurulent discharge from the middle meatus. Questioning of the patient revealed she had hyposmia and in the previous three days had become embarrassed by a cacosmia emanating from her nose.

A CT scan demonstrated fluid in her right maxillary sinus and excluded any orbital or intracranial involvement. A diagnosis of acute maxillary sinusitis was made by the registrar and she was prescribed decongestants and started on a course of antibiotic therapy. A sample of the discharge from her nose was sent to the microbiology laboratory for culture and sensitivity testing. Before leaving A and E she was given appropriate analgesia for her headache and referred to the department of Otorhinolaryngology.

Mrs L's follow up medical treatment with antibiotics and decongestants had limited success and her condition became chronic with a purulent nasal and post-nasal discharge. Pus from the maxillary sinus was removed by antral washout (antral lavage) following proof puncture through the nasal wall of the maxillary antrum. This was repeated on four occasions before the consultant advised surgery and the formation of an intranasal antrostomy. Functional endoscopic sinus surgery (FESS) was used to improve drainage of the maxillary sinus through its natural ostium.

Following her operation Mrs L showed great improvement; mucosal activity and the self-cleaning mechanism of her sinuses was restored.

WORD HELP

acute symptoms/signs of short duration

analgesia condition of without pain/prescribing of drugs that reduce pain

cacosmia condition of stench or unpleasant odour

chronic lasting/lingering for a long time

CT computed tomography

culture and sensitivity testing growing microorganisms in the laboratory and testing them for sensitivity to antibiotics

decongestant a drug used for the relief of congestion

endoscopic pertaining to (using) an endoscope i.e. an instrument used to visually examine the body cavities

intracranial pertaining to within the cranium

hyposmia condition of reduced sense of smell (below normal)

maxillary sinus the sinus/antrum (air space) in the facial bone known as the maxilla

meatus a passage or opening

mucopurulent containing pus and mucus

mucosal pertaining to the mucosa (here the mucous membrane lining the maxillary sinus)

mucous pertaining to or containing mucus (a viscous secretion)

oedematous pertaining to accumulation of fluid in a tissue (Am. edematous)

orbital pertaining to the orbit of the eye (bony eye-socket)

ostium a natural mouth or opening

proof evidence (here proving the antrum is infected)

purulent containing pus

Now write the meaning of the following words from the case history without using your dictionary lists:

(a) rhinitis

(b) rhinoscopy

(c) sinusitis

(d) otorhinolaryngology

(e) post-nasal

(f) antral

(g) intranasal

[   ]

(h) antrostomy

[   ]

(Answers to the case history exercise are given in the Answers to Word Exercises beginning on page 301.)

Quick Reference

Combining forms relating to the nose and mouth:

Aden/o	gland
Antr/o	antrum/maxillary sinus
Bucc/o	cheek
Cheil/o	lip
Faci/o	face
Gingiv/o	gum
Gloss/o	tongue
Gnath/o	jaw
Labi/o	lip
Laryng/o	larynx
Lingu/o	tongue
Nas/o	nose
Odont/o	tooth
Or/o	mouth
Palat/o	palate
Phag/o	eating/consuming
Pharyng/o	pharynx
Ptyal/o	saliva/salivary gland/salivary duct
Rhin/o	nose
Sial/o	saliva/salivary gland/salivary duct
Sin/o	sinus
Sinus-	sinus
Stomat/o	mouth
Uvul/o	uvula

Abbreviations

Some common abbreviations related to the nose and mouth are listed below. Note some are not standard and their meaning may vary from one health care setting to another. There is a more extensive list for reference on page 335.

dmft	decayed missing filled teeth (deciduous)
DMFT	decayed missing filled teeth (permanent)
ging	gingiva (gums)
La	labial (lips)
LaG	labia and gingiva (lips and gums)
NAS	nasal
NP	nasopharynx
NPO	non per os/nothing by mouth
odont	odontology
Os	mouth
po/PO	per os/by mouth
Subling	sublingual/under the tongue

Medical Notes

Allergic rhinitis (hay fever)

Allergic rhinitis is an allergy triggered by air borne substances that cause inflammation of the mucous membrane lining the nasal cavity. In this condition atopic (immediate) hypersensitivity develops to foreign proteins (antigens) that have been inhaled. Allergens commonly associated with allergic rhinitis include scales, hair and feathers from animals, pollen grains and mites in house dust. The exaggerated immune response triggers the release of histamine and other chemicals that cause inflammation, rhinorrhoea (Am. rhinorrhea), reddening of the eyes and excessive secretion of tears.

Aphthae

Aphthae are small ulcers that occur singly or in groups on the inside of the cheek or lip or underneath the tongue. The cause is uncertain but they have been associated with streptococcal infection, minor injury, vitamin B deficiency and iron deficiency. Recurrent mouth ulceration with accompanying inflammation is known as aphthous stomatitis.

Angular chelitis

Angular chelitis is an inflammation in the fold of tissue at the corner of the mouth that develops into a painful crack. The condition usually develops in the elderly or debilitated people if they do not wear their dentures and the folds remain moist. The moisture allows the growth of micro-organism such as *Candida albicans* and *Staphylococcus aureus* that cause inflammation.

Cleft lip

Cleft lip is a vertical split, usually off centre in the upper lip; it may be a minor notch in the lip or a substantial split extending up to the nose. In some cases the upper gum may also be cleft and the nose crooked. The term harelip is used in the rare cases that the cleft is in the midline of the upper lip. Cleft lip is often associated with failure of the two halves of the palate to join, see cleft palate below.

Cleft palate

During embryonic development the roof of the mouth (hard palate) develops as two separate halves. Before birth the right and left halves fuse along the midline of the body. If fusion is incomplete, a cleft palate occurs, the opening can be minor or substantial. A cleft palate creates a gap between the mouth and nasal cavity.

Dental caries (tooth decay)

Formation of dental caries is a result of gradual softening (demineralization) of the dentine and enamel of a tooth. If untreated, bacteria and other organisms will infect the tooth causing inflammation and death of its pulp. This may lead to the formation of an abscess in the bone surrounding the roots and the pain of toothache. Demineralization of teeth is caused by the action of acid formed by bacteria breaking down sugars in the mouth or by ingested fruit acid.

Epistaxis
Bleeding from the nose, usually due to rupture of small blood vessels in the anterior part of the nasal septum.

Leukoplakia
Thick white patches occurring on the tongue, lips and other areas covered with mucous membranes. The hyperplasia (increase in growth of cells) in the patch sometimes denotes cancerous change.

Mumps
Mumps is an acute inflammatory condition of the salivary glands especially the parotids. The illness mainly affects children and is caused by the mumps virus, one of the parainfluenza group. Fever and headache develop and the parotid glands on one or both sides swell causing pain on swallowing. The virus is inhaled in infected droplets and in the 18–21 day incubation period the viruses multiply elsewhere in the body before spreading to the salivary glands. Serious complications are uncommon but can include pancreatitis, orchitis in males after puberty and meningitis. One attack of mumps confers lifelong immunity to the virus. A safe and effective mumps vaccine is available in combination with measles and rubella vaccines (MMR vaccine).

Nasal polyp
A nasal polyp is a growth that projects, usually on a stalk (or peduncle), from the mucous membrane lining the nose. Polyps can cause nasal obstruction and may need to be removed.

Oral candidiasis (thrush)
Thrush is the common name for an acute fungal infection of the epithelium of the mouth or vagina caused by the yeast *Candida albicans*. The organism is normally present in the mouth and vagina but it is usually kept under control by the presence of bacteria and other microorganisms. It proliferates in adults who are debilitated in some way for example, in those whose immune system is suppressed by HIV, steroids, antibiotics or cytotoxic drugs. Sore, whitish-yellow raised patches in the mouth characterize the condition.

Vincent's disease (acute gingivitis)
Acute gingivitis is an acute infection of the gums with severe necrotizing ulceration. It is caused by two commensal organisms acting together, *Borellia vincenti* and a fusiform bacillus. These organisms occur naturally in the mouth but because of poor dental hygiene, malnutrition or injury may cause serious gum disease.

NOW TRY THE WORD CHECK

WORD CHECK

This self-check exercise lists all the word components used in this unit. First write down the meaning of as many word components as you can. Then check your answers using the Exercise Guide and Quick Reference box or the Glossary of Word Components (pp. 347–371).

Prefixes

a-

dys-

endo-

intra-

macro-

ortho-

peri-

poly-

post-

prosth-

sub-

Combining forms of word roots

aden/o

aer/o

angi/o

antr/o

bronch/o

bucc/o

cheil/o

dynam/o

faci/o

gingiv/o

gloss/o

gnath/o

labi/o

laryng/o

lingu/o

man/o

myc/o

nas/o

odont/o

or/o

ot/o

palat/o

phag/o

pharyng/o

ptyal/o

rhin/o

sial/o

sin/o, sinus-

stomat/o

trich/o

tympan/o

uvul/o

Suffixes

-agogue

-al

-algia

-cele

-dynia

-eal

-ectomy

-genic

-gram

-graphy

-ia

-ic

-ics

-ist

-itis

-lalia

-lith

-logy

-meter

-metry

-osis

-pathy

-phagia

-phasia

-phonia

-phyma

-plasty

-plegia

-rrhagia

-rrhoea
(Am. -rrhea)

-schisis

-scope

-scopy

-stomy

-tomy

-us

NOW TRY THE SELF-ASSESSMENT

SELF-ASSESSMENT

Test 12A

Below are some combining forms that refer to the anatomy of the nose and mouth. Indicate which part of the system they refer to by putting a number from the diagrams (Figs 66 and 67) next to each word.

(a) gloss/o

(b) stomat/o

(c) cheil/o

(d) gingiv/o

(e) uvul/o

(f) rhin/o

(g) odont/o

(h) faci/o

Score

8

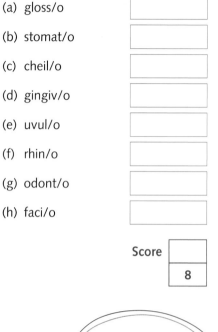

Figure 66 Section of the head showing the sinuses and salivary glands

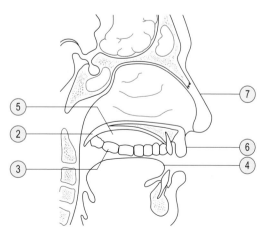

Figure 67 Sagittal section of the nasal cavity and mouth

Test 12B

Prefixes and suffixes

Match the prefixes and suffixes in Column A with a meaning in Column C by inserting an appropriate number in Column B.

Column A	Column B	Column C
(a) -agogue		1. condition of voice
(b) -cele		2. splitting
(c) -dynia		3. suturing/stitching
(d) -ectomy		4. inflammation
(e) endo-		5. condition of speech
(f) -itis		6. condition of paralysis
(g) -logy		7. straight
(h) -metry		8. measurement
(i) ortho-		9. disease
(j) -pathy		10. condition of excessive flow (of blood)
(k) peri-		11. many
(l) -phasia		12. surgical repair
(m) -phonia		13. condition of pain
(n) -plasty		14. hernia/protrusion/swelling
(o) -plegia		15. removal of
(p) poly-		16. inside/within
(q) prosth-		17. study of
(r) -rrhagia		18. around
(s) -rrhaphy		19. inducing/stimulating
(t) -schisis		20. addition of artificial part

Score

20

Test 12C

Combining forms of word roots

Match each combining form in Column A with a meaning in Column C by inserting the appropriate number in Column B.

Column A	Column B	Column C
(a) antr/o		1. gum
(b) bucc/o		2. tooth
(c) cheil/o		3. sinus
(d) dynam/o		4. pressure
(e) faci/o		5. larynx
(f) gingiv/o		6. uvula
(g) gloss/o		7. tongue
(h) gnath/o		8. nose
(i) labi/o		9. maxillary sinus/ antrum of Highmore
(j) laryng/o		10. hair
(k) man/o		11. mouth
(l) odont/o		12. jaw
(m) palat/o		13. cheek/inside mouth
(n) ptyal/o		14. palate
(o) rhin/o		15. lip (i)
(p) sial/o		16. lip (ii)
(q) sin/o		17. force
(r) stomat/o		18. face
(s) trich/o		19. saliva (i)
(t) uvul/o		20. saliva (ii)

Score [ ] 20

Test 12D

Write the meaning of:

(a) glossodynamometer [ ]

(b) sialometry [ ]

(c) stomatoglossitis [ ]

(d) gnathopalatoschisis [ ]

(e) odontogenic [ ]

Score [ ] 5

Test 12E

Build words that mean:

(a) incision into a salivary gland (use sial/o) [ ]

(b) suturing of the palate [ ]

(c) condition of fungi in the nose [ ]

(d) pertaining to the lips [ ]

(e) surgical repair of the palate [ ]

Score [ ] 5

Check answers to Self-Assessment Tests on page 325.

UNIT 13
THE MUSCULAR SYSTEM

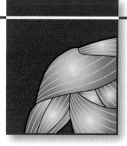

OBJECTIVES

Once you have completed Unit 13 you should be able to:

- understand the meaning of medical words relating to the muscular system

- build medical words relating to the muscular system

- associate medical terms with their anatomical position

- understand medical abbreviations relating to the muscular system.

EXERCISE GUIDE

Use this list of word components and their meanings to complete the word exercises in this unit.

Prefixes

dys-	difficult/disordered/painful
hyper-	above normal/excessive

Roots/Combining forms

aesthesi/o	sensation (Am. esthesi/o)
cardi/o	heart
electr/o	electrical
esthesi/o (Am.)	sensation
fibr/o	fibre
neur/o	nerve
paed/o	child (Am. ped/o)
ped/o (Am.)	child
phren/o	diaphragm

Suffixes

-al	pertaining to
-algia	condition of pain
-ar	pertaining to
-genic	pertaining to formation/originating in
-globin	protein
-gram	X-ray/tracing/recording
-graph	usually an instrument that records
-graphy	technique of recording/making an X-ray
-ia	condition of
-ic	pertaining to
-itis	inflammation of
-kymia	condition of involuntary twitching of muscle
-logy	study of
-lysis	breakdown/disintegration
-malacia	condition of softening
-meter	measuring instrument
-oma	tumour (Am. tumor)/swelling
-osis	abnormal condition/disease/abnormal increase
-paresis	slight paralysis
-pathy	disease of
-plasty	surgical repair/reconstruction
-rrhaphy	stitching/suturing
-rrhexis	break/rupture
-sclerosis	condition of hardening
-spasm	involuntary muscle contraction
-tome	cutting instrument
-tomy	incision into
-tonia	condition of tension/tone
-trophy	nourishment/development
-tropic	pertaining to affinity for/stimulating

ANATOMY EXERCISE

When you have finished Word Exercises 1–7, look at the word components listed below. Complete Figure 68 by writing the appropriate combining form on each line – more than one component may relate to the same position. (You can check their meanings in the Quick Reference box on p. 174.)

Muscul/o   Tendin/o
My/o   Ten/o

The muscular system

Muscles compose 40–50% of the body's weight. The function of muscle is to effect the movement of the body as a whole and to move internal organs involved in the vital processes required to keep the body alive. There are three types of muscles tissue:

- Skeletal muscle – moves the vocal chords, diaphragm and limbs.
- Cardiac muscle – moves the heart.
- Smooth muscle – moves the internal organs, bringing about movement of food through the intestines and urine through the urinary tract. It is also found in the walls of blood vessels where it acts to maintain blood pressure.

Use the Exercise Guide at the beginning of this unit to complete Word Exercises 1–7 unless you are asked to work without it.

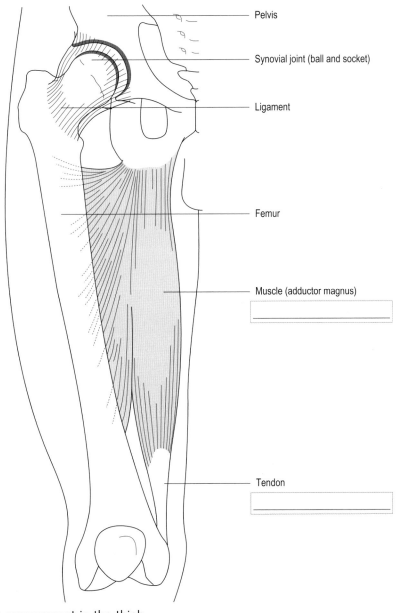

Figure 68 A muscle arrangement in the thigh

ROOT

My
*(From a Greek word **mys**, meaning muscle.)*

Combining forms   My/o, myos

WORD EXERCISE 1

Using your Exercise Guide, find the meaning of:

(a) **my/o**/neur/al

(b) **my/o**/cardi/o/pathy

(c) **my/o**/dys/trophy

(d) **myos**/itis

(e) **my/o**/fibr/osis

Using your Exercise Guide find the meaning of -globin, -oma, -sclerosis, and -spasm, then build words using my/o that mean:

(f) condition of hardening of a muscle

(g) tumour (Am. tumor) of a muscle

(h) muscle protein

(i) spasm of a muscle

The combining form **lei/o** (from Latin, meaning smooth) is added to myo to give **leiomy/o**, that refers to smooth muscle. A **leiomy**oma is a tumour (Am. tumor)/swelling of smooth muscle.

Using your Exercise Guide, find the meaning of:

(j) **my/o**/kymia

(k) **my/o**/tonia

(l) **my/o**/paresis

(m) **my/o**/rrhexis

(n) **my/o**/malacia

The contraction of a muscle can be measured, using an instrument known as a **myo**graph.

Using your Exercise Guide find the meaning of electr/o, -gram and -graphy, then build words that mean:

(o) the technique of recording muscle (contraction)

(p) the technique of recording the electrical currents generated in muscle (contraction)

(q) trace/recording made by a myograph

ROOT

Rhabd
*(From a Greek word **rhabdos**, meaning stripe. Here rhabd/o in combination with my/o it means striped muscle or striated muscle.)*

Combining form   Rhabdomy/o

WORD EXERCISE 2

Without using your Exercise Guide, write the meaning of:

(a) **rhabdomy**/oma

Using your Exercise Guide, find the meaning of:

(b) **rhabdomy/o**/lysis

ROOT

Muscul
*(From a Latin word **musculus**, meaning muscle.)*

Combining form   Muscul/o

WORD EXERCISE 3

Using your Exercise Guide, find the meaning of:

(a) **muscul/o**/tropic

(b) **muscul/o**/phren/ic

Without using your Exercise Guide, write the meaning of:

(c) **muscul**/ar dys/trophy

Note. Loss or impairment of muscular movement due to a lesion in a neuromuscular mechanism is known as a paralysis or palsy (an obsolete term). A paresis is a partial paralysis and a pseudoparesis, a condition simulating paralysis (*pseud/o-* meaning false). The latter is of hysterical (neurotic) origin and not due to organic disease within a muscle or nerve.

ROOT

Kine

(From a Greek word **kinein***, meaning movement/motion.)*

Combining forms Kine/s/i/o, kinet/o

WORD EXERCISE 4

Using your Exercise Guide, find the meaning of:

(a) **kine**/aesthes/ia
(Am. **kin**/esthes/ia)

(b) my/o/**kines**/i/meter

(c) **kinet/o**/genic

(d) hyper/**kines**/ia

Without using your Exercise Guide, build a word using kines/o that means:

(e) condition of difficult or painful movement

A Greek word *taxis* is sometimes used when describing an ordered movement in response to a stimulus. **Ataxia** refers to a disordered movement that is irregular and jerky (*a-* meaning without, i.e. condition of without normal movement). There are many types of ataxia, for example motor ataxia – an inability to control muscles and Friedreich's ataxia – an inherited movement disorder.

ROOT

Ten
(From a Greek word **tenon***, to stretch. Here ten/o and the combining forms derived from this root all mean tendon. Tendons are the white, fibrous, inelastic cords that attach muscle to bone.)*

Combining forms Ten/o, tenont/o *(Greek)* Tend/o, tendon/o, tendin/o *(Latin). Note that the combining forms tend/o and tendin/o are derived from Latin tendonis and tendines, meaning tendon.*

WORD EXERCISE 5

Using your Exercise Guide, find the meaning of:

(a) **ten**/algia

(b) **tend/o**/tome

Without using your Exercise Guide, write the meaning of:

(c) **tendin**/itis

(d) **tenont/o**/logy

Using your Exercise Guide, build words that mean:

(e) repair of a muscle and tendon (use ten/o)

(f) incision of a muscle and tendon (use ten/o)

A tendon is a fibrous non-elastic cord of connective tissue that is continuous with the fibres of a skeletal muscle; its function is to attach muscle to bone. Tendons must be strong in tension because they are used to pull bones and thereby move the body. If a tendon is wide and thin, it is known as an **aponeurosis**. This word is derived from *apo-* meaning detached/away from, *neuro-* tendon (also used to mean nerve) and *-osis* condition of.

Several words are used with **aponeur/o** meaning an aponeurosis.

Using your Exercise Guide, find the meaning of:

(g) **aponeur/o**/rrhaphy

Without using your Exercise Guide, write the meaning of:

(h) **aponeur**/itis

ROOT

(From a Greek word **orthos***, meaning straight.)*

Combining form Orth/o

WORD EXERCISE 6

Using your Exercise Guide, find the meaning of:

Orth
(a) **ortho**/paed/ic
(Am. **ortho**/ped/ic)

(Formerly this word applied to the correction of deformities in children. Orthopaedics is now a branch of surgery dealing with all conditions affecting the locomotor system in children and adults.)

Other common words related to this include:

Orthosis
a structure/appliance used to correct a deformity.

Orthotics
the knowledge of use of orthoses.

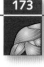

Medical equipment and clinical procedures

Revise the names of all instruments and clinical procedures mentioned in this unit before completing Exercise 7.

WORD EXERCISE 7

Match each term in Column A with a description in Column C by placing an appropriate number in Column B.

Column A	Column B	Column C
(a) myography		1. an appliance used to straighten deformities of the locomotor system
(b) electromyography		2. a recording/ trace of muscular movement
(c) myogram		3. a recording of the electrical activity of muscle
(d) myokinesiometer		4. technique of recording electrical activity of muscle
(e) orthosis		5. technique of making a recording of muscle (contraction)
(f) electromyogram		6. an instrument used for measuring movement of a muscle

ANATOMY EXERCISE

Now complete the Anatomy Exercise on page 170.

CASE HISTORY 13

The object of this exercise is to understand words associated with a patient's medical history.

To complete the exercise:

- read through the passage on Duchenne muscular dystrophy; unfamiliar words are underlined and you can find their meaning using the Word Help

- write the meaning of the medical terms shown in bold print on the lines that follow the Word Help.

Duchenne muscular dystrophy (DMD)

Miss M, a single parent, consulted her GP about her 4-year-old son R who appeared to have difficulty in climbing the stairs and running. Her son had been slow to sit up and walk and seemed less able than his peers. Her GP observed the child to have a 'waddling' gait and to stand up by 'climbing up his legs' using his hands against his ankles, knees and thighs (Gower's sign). His calf muscles appeared to be bulky and lacking strength. He was referred to the Paediatric (Am. Pediatric) Hospital with suspected muscular **dystrophy**.

Detailed examination revealed R to have proximal weakness in his limbs and **pseudohypertrophy** of his calf muscles. A muscle biopsy showed **dystrophic** changes with muscle fibre necrosis and their replacement with fat. Immunochemical staining detected an absence of dystrophin. His serum creatine phosphokinase levels were grossly elevated. **Electromyography** indicated a **myopathic** pattern with short polyphasic action potentials.

R's mother was also investigated and also found to have raised serum creatine phosphokinase levels and an abnormal **electromyogram**. R was diagnosed as having Duchenne muscular dystrophy, a fatal sex-linked condition inherited from his mother. DMD is due to a mutant gene located on the X-chromosome and as there appeared to be no previous incidence of this condition in the family, it was likely this was a spontaneous mutation. Miss M was advised by the genetics counsellor that she was a carrier of DMD and if she produced another boy there was a 50% chance that he would also have DMD.

By the age of 10 R was severely disabled and receiving daily passive physiotherapy to help prevent contractures of his muscles. At 14 he was unable to move his arms and legs and his limb bones were long and thin (disuse **atrophy**). He died at the age of 16 from **myocardial** involvement and pulmonary infection.

WORD HELP

action potential an electrochemical impulse generated by a muscle or nerve

biopsy removal and examination of living tissue

contractures abnormal shortening/contraction of muscle

dystrophin an essential structural protein found in muscle fibres

gait manner of walking

GP general practitioner (family doctor)

immunochemical pertaining to chemical basis of immunity

mutant a gene that has changed from normal form resulting in a change to the organism inheriting it

mutation a sudden change in the genetic material of cells (in this case in the mother's sex cells)

necrosis condition of localized death of tissue

passive not produced by the active effort of (the patient)

physiotherapy treatment using physical means to maintain or build physique or correct deformities due to injury or disease (Am. physical therapy)

polyphasic pertaining to many phases (here electrical potentials out of phase)

proximal near to origin/point of attachment

pulmonary pertaining to the lungs

serum a clear fluid separated from blood when it is allowed to clot

sex-linked a gene linked to a sex-chromosome (may result in increased frequency of certain disorders in one particular sex e.g. DMD affects boys only)

X-chromosome one of a pair of sex chromosomes that determine the sex of an individual

Quick Reference

Combining forms relating to the muscular system:

Aponeur/o	aponeurosis
Fibr/o	fibre
Kinesi/o	movement
Lei/o	smooth (muscle)
Muscul/o	muscle
My/o	muscle
Paed/o	child (Am. ped/o)
Ped/o (Am.)	child
Rhabd/o	striated (muscle)
Tax/o	ordered movement
Tendin/o	tendon
Tend/o	tendon
Ten/o	tendon
Tenont/o	tendon

Abbreviations

Some common abbreviations related to the muscular system are listed below. Note some are not standard and their meaning may vary from one health care setting to another. There is a more extensive list for reference on page 335.

DTR	deep tendon reflex
EMG	electromyogram/electromyography
im	intramuscular
IMHP	intramuscular high potency
MAMC	mid-arm muscle circumference
MAP	muscle action potential
MD	muscular dystrophy
MFT	muscle function test
MNJ	myoneural junction
MS	muscle shortening/strength/musculoskeletal
Ortho	orthopaedics (Am. orthopedics)
TJ	triceps jerk

Now write the meaning of the following words from the case history without using your dictionary lists:

(a) dystrophy

(b) pseudohypertrophy

(c) dystrophic

(d) electromyography

(e) myopathic

(f) electromyogram

(g) atrophy

(h) myocardial

(Answers to the case history exercise are given in the Answers to Word Exercises beginning on page 301.)

Medical Notes

Contusion

A muscle bruise caused by a minor trauma to the body such as a blow to a limb. Muscle contusions involve local internal bleeding and inflammation.

Cramp

Cramp is a painful muscle spasm (involuntary twitch) that often results from mild myositis or fibromyositis. Cramp is a symptom of irritation that may be due to an ion or water imbalance within a muscle.

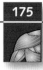

Crush injury

Severe trauma or sustained pressure to a skeletal muscle may reduce blood supply and cause ischaemia (Am. ischemia) and massive muscle necrosis. Crush injuries greatly damage the affected muscle tissue and when the circulation is restored the muscle pigment myoglobin and other necrotic products are released from the damaged area into the blood. This material is highly toxic to the kidneys and life-threatening acute renal failure may develop.

Fasciculation

A condition in which there are small, local, involuntary contractions of muscle fibres that are visible under the skin. The contractions may occur regularly and are not associated with movement of the affected muscle.

Fibrillation

A small, local involuntary muscle contraction due to activation of single muscle fibres.

Hernia

Weakness of abdominal muscles can lead to protrusion of an abdominal organ (commonly the small intestine) through an opening in the abdominal wall; this is called a hernia. There are several types, the most common *inguinal hernia*, occurs when the intestine extends through the inguinal canal into the scrotum or labia. Males experience this most often and it can occur at any age. Some women may experience *femoral hernia* because of changes during pregnancy. Hernia is referred to as reducible when the organ is manipulated back into the abdominal cavity either naturally by lying down or by manual reduction through a surgical opening into the abdomen. A *strangulated hernia* occurs when the mass is not reducible and blood flow to the affected organ is stopped. When this occurs, pain and vomiting are usually experienced and emergency surgical intervention is required.

Muscular dystrophy

Muscular dystrophy is not a single disorder but a group of genetic diseases characterized by atrophy (wasting of skeletal muscle tissues). Some but not all forms of muscular dystrophy can be fatal.

The common form of muscular dystrophy is Duchenne muscular dystrophy (DMD) in which formation of excessive amounts of fat and fibrous tissue (pseudohypertrophy) masks the atrophy of muscle. DMD is characterized by mild leg muscle weakness that progresses rapidly to the shoulder muscles. The first signs are apparent at about three years of age and the stricken child is usually severely affected within five to ten years. Death from respiratory or cardiac muscle weakness often occurs before the age of twenty-one. DMD is caused by a mutation in the X-chromosome and as boys have only one X-chromosome inherited from their mother they are affected with the disease.

Myasthenia gravis

Myasthenia gravis is a chronic disease characterized by muscle weakness, especially in the face and throat. Most forms of the disease begin with mild weakness and chronic muscle fatigue in the face, then progress to wider muscle involvement with severe weakness. When severe muscle weakness causes immobility in all four limbs, a myasthenic crisis is said to have occurred; a person in this condition is in danger of dying from respiratory failure because of weakness in the respiratory muscles. Myasthenia gravis is an autoimmune disease in which the immune system attacks muscle cells at the neuromuscular junction. Nerve impulses are then unable to fully stimulate the affected muscle.

Paralysis

Loss or impairment of muscle function resulting from a lesion of nervous or muscular origin.

Spasm

A spasm is a sudden, violent, involuntary contraction of a large group of muscles.

Tic

A spasmodic, compulsive, repetitive and involuntary movement made by muscles that are usually under voluntary control. Tics are often seen in the face and shoulders.

Tremor

A tremor is a rhythmic, involuntary, purposeless contraction of antagonistic muscles.

Torticollis

A spasmodic contraction of several superficial and deep muscles of the neck that produces twisting of the neck and an unnatural position of the head (also called wryneck).

Trichinosis

A myositis caused by infection with the parasitic nematode worm *Trichinella spiralis* that encysts in the muscles of humans, pigs and rats. Infection results from eating inadequately cooked pork; symptoms include nausea, diarrhoea (Am. diarrhea) and fever that lead to painful swelling of the muscles and oedema (Am. edema).

NOW TRY THE WORD CHECK

WORD CHECK

This self-check exercise lists all the word components used in this unit. First write down the meaning of as many word components as you can. Then check your answers using the Exercise Guide and Quick Reference box or the Glossary of Word Components (pp. 347–371).

Prefixes

a-

dys-

hyper-

Combining forms of word roots

aesthesi/o
(Am. esthesi/o)

aponeur/o

cardi/o

electr/o

fibr/o

kinesi/o

lei/o

muscul/o

my/o

neur/o

ortho-

paed/o
(Am. ped/o)

phren/o

pseud/o

rhabd/o

tax/o

tendin/o

tend/o

ten/o

tenont/o

Suffixes

-al

-algia

-genic

-globin

-gram

-graph

-graphy

-ic

-itis

-kymia

-logy

-lysis

-meter

-oma

-osis

-paresis

-pathy

-rrhaphy

-rrhexis

-sclerosis

-spasm

-taxia

-tome

-tonia

-trophy

-tropic

NOW TRY THE SELF-ASSESSMENT

SELF-ASSESSMENT

Test 13A

Prefixes, suffixes and combining forms of word roots

Match each word component from Column A with a meaning in Column C by inserting the appropriate number in Column B.

Column A	Column B	Column C
(a) aesthesi/o (Am. esthesi/o)		1. child
(b) cardi/o		2. movement
(c) electr/o		3. tumour (Am. tumor)/ swelling
(d) fibr/o		4. diaphragm
(e) -globin		5. slight paralysis/ weakness
(f) kinesi/o		6. rupture/break
(g) muscul/o		7. condition of hardening
(h) my/o		8. electrical
(i) -oma		9. protein
(j) ortho-		10. involuntary contraction of muscle
(k) paed/o (Am. ped/o)		11. condition of continuous slight contraction of muscle
(l) -paresis		12. nourishment
(m) phren/o		13. fibre
(n) -rrhexis		14. pertaining to affinity for/acting on
(o) -sclerosis		15. heart
(p) -spasm		16. muscle (i)
(q) ten/o		17. muscle (ii)
(r) -tonia		18. sensation
(s) -trophy		19. straight
(t) -tropic		20. tendon

Score [ ] 20

Test 13B

Write the meaning of:

(a) electromyograph [ ]

(b) kinesiology [ ]

(c) myotenotomy [ ]

(d) myoatrophy [ ]

(e) musculoaponeurotic [ ]

Score [ ] 5

Test 13C

Build words that mean:

(a) condition of softening of muscle [ ]

(b) pertaining to originating in muscle [ ]

(c) disease of muscle [ ]

(d) suturing of a tendon (use ten/o) [ ]

(e) cutting of a tendon (use ten/o) [ ]

Score [ ] 5

Check answers to Self-Assessment Tests on page 325.

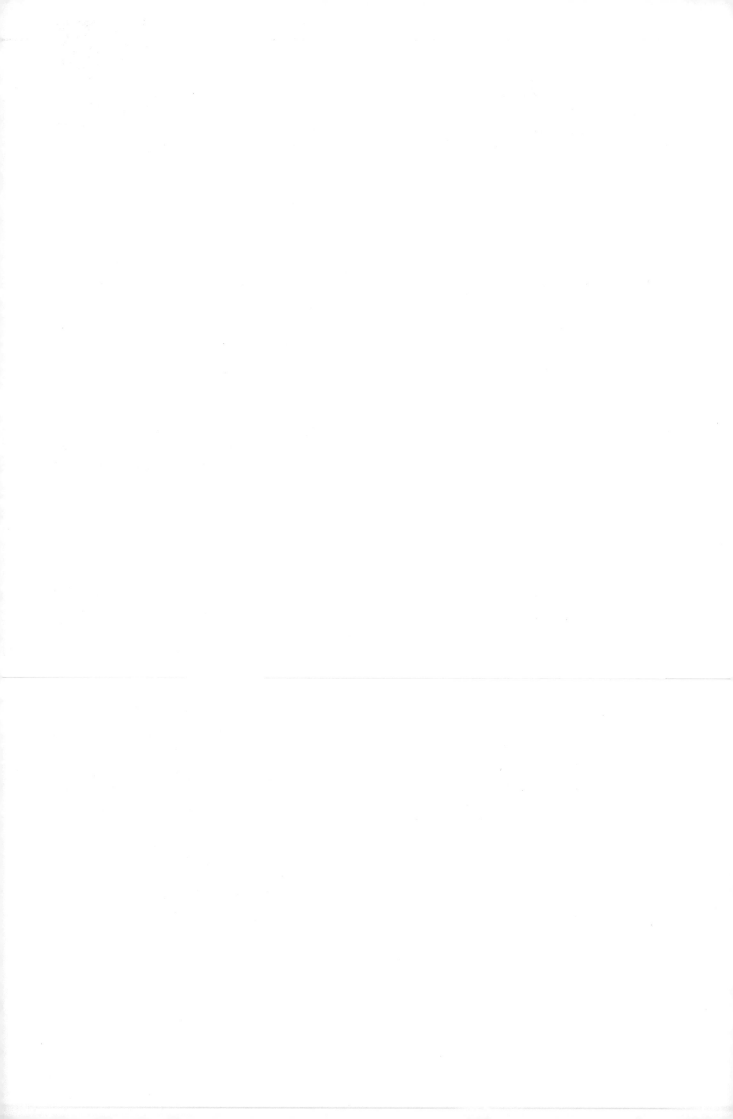

UNIT 14
THE SKELETAL SYSTEM

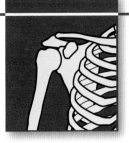

OBJECTIVES

Once you have completed Unit 14 you should be able to:

- understand the meaning of medical words relating to the skeletal system

- build medical words relating to the skeletal system

- associate medical terms with their anatomical position

- understand medical abbreviations relating to the skeletal system.

EXERCISE GUIDE

Use this list of word components and their meanings to complete the word exercises in this unit.

Prefixes

dys-	bad/difficult/painful
endo-	within/inside
poly-	many

Roots/Combining forms

calcin/o	calcium
cost/o	rib
fibr/o	fibre
my/o	muscle
petr/o	stone/rock (brittle)
por/o	pore
py/o	pus

Suffixes

-al	pertaining to
-algia	condition of pain
-blast	cell that forms . . ./immature germ cell
-centesis	puncture to remove fluid
-clasis	breaking
-clast	a cell that breaks
-desis	fixation/bind together by surgery
-eal	pertaining to
-ectomy	removal of
-genesis	capable of causing/forming
-genic	pertaining to formation/originating in
-gram	X-ray/tracing/recording
-graphy	technique of recording/making an X-ray
-ic	pertaining to
-itis	inflammation of
-lith	stone
-logist	specialist who studies . . .
-lysis	breakdown/disintegration
-lytic	pertaining to breakdown/disintegration
-malacia	condition of softening
-oid	resembling
-olisthesis	slipping
-oma	tumour (Am. tumor)/swelling
-osis	abnormal condition/disease/abnormal increase
-ous	pertaining to/of the nature of
-pathy	disease of
-phyte	plant/plant-like growth
-plasty	surgical repair/reconstruction
-scope	viewing instrument
-scopy	visual examination
-tome	cutting instrument
-trophy	nourishment/development

ANATOMY EXERCISE

When you have finished Word Exercises 1–10, look at the word components listed below. Complete Figure 69 by writing the appropriate combining form on each line. (You can check their meanings in the Quick Reference box on p. 186.)

Arthr/o	Myel/o	Spondyl/o
Chondr/o	Oste/o	Synovi/o
Disc/o		

The skeletal system

The supporting structure of the body consisting of 206 bones is known as the skeletal system. This system has five main functions:

- it supports all tissues
- it protects vital organs and soft tissues
- it manufactures blood cells
- it stores minerals that can be released into the blood
- it assists in movement.

Cartilage is found at the ends of bones and functions to form a smooth surface for the movement of one bone over another at a joint. In joints, bones are held together by tough fibrous connective tissues called ligaments. (The function of ligaments is to connect bone to bone.)

Use the Exercise Guide at the beginning of this unit to complete Word Exercises 1–10 unless you are asked to work without it.

ROOT

Oste
(From a Greek word **osteon**, *meaning bone.)*

Combining form   Oste/o

WORD EXERCISE 1

Using your Exercise Guide, find the meaning of:

(a) **oste/o/phyte**
(refers to a bony outgrowth at joint surface)

(b) **oste/o/por/osis**
(refers to loss of calcium/ phosphorus/bone density)

(c) **oste/o/malacia**
(a condition caused by lack of vitamin D in adults)

(d) **oste/o/petr/osis**
(refers to spotty calcification of bone, which becomes brittle)

(e) **oste/o/clasis**

(f) **oste/o/clast**
(a type of cell, compare with osteoblast)

(g) **oste/o/dys/trophy**

Using your Exercise Guide look up the meaning of -blast, -logist, -lytic, and -tome, then build words that mean:

(h) a cell that forms bone

(i) pertaining to breaking down of bone

(j) instrument to cut bone

(k) specialist who studies bones

(*Osseus* is a Latin word meaning of bone. The combining form oss/e/o is used in **osse**ous, meaning pertaining to bone or of the nature of bone, and **oss**ification, means to form bone.)

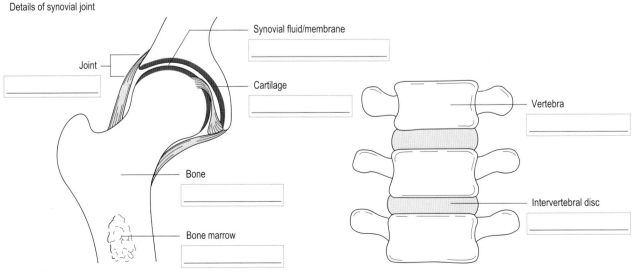

Figure 69   Joints

ROOT

Arthr

(From a Greek word **arthron**, *meaning joint or articulation, i.e. the point where two or more bones meet.)*

Combining form   Arthr/o

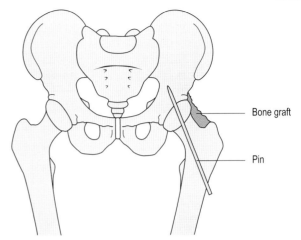

Bone graft

Pin

Figure 70   Arthrodesis of the hip

WORD EXERCISE 2

Using your Exercise Guide, find the meaning of:

(a) **arthr/o**/endo/scope

(b) **arthr/o**/py/osis

(c) **arthr/o**/graphy

(d) poly/**arthr**/itis

Rheumatoid arthritis refers to a polyarthritis accompanied by general ill health and varying degrees of crippling joint deformities, pain and stiffness (*rheumat/o* refers to rheumatism, a condition marked by inflammation, degeneration and metabolic disturbance of connective tissues especially those associated with joints). See the medical notes on page 186.

(e) **arthr/o**/desis

(Also known as an artificial **ankylosis** (from Greek *agkyloun* meaning to stiffen). An arthrodesis is achieved by surgery; see Fig. 70.)

Without using your Exercise Guide, write the meaning of:

(f) **arthr/o**/clasis

Using your Exercise Guide look up the meaning of -centesis, -gram, -lith, -pathy, -plasty and -scopy, then build words that mean:

(g) technique of viewing a joint

(h) puncture of a joint

(i) X-ray picture of a joint

(j) disease of a joint

(k) stony material in a joint

(l) surgical repair of a joint

(This operation includes the formation of artificial joints, e.g. in a hip replacement where the natural joint is replaced with a metallic prosthesis; Fig. 71.)

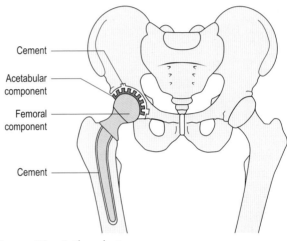

Cement

Acetabular component

Femoral component

Cement

Figure 71   Arthroplasty

ROOT

Synovi

(From a New Latin word **synovia**, *meaning the fluid secreted by the synovial membrane that lines the cavity of a joint. Here synovi/o means synovial membrane.)*

Combining forms   Synov/i/o

WORD EXERCISE 3

Without using your Exercise Guide, write the meaning of:

(a) arthr/o/**synov**/itis

Using your Exercise Guide, find the meaning of:

(b) **synov**/ectomy

(c) **synov/i**/oma

Bursae are sacs of synovial fluid surrounded by a synovial membrane; they are found between tendons, ligaments and bones. Inflammation due to pressure, injury or infection results in **burs**itis (from Latin *bursa*, meaning purse).

ROOT

Chondr

*(From a Greek word **chondros**, meaning cartilage, the plastic-like connective tissue found at the ends of bones, e.g. in joints where it forms a smooth surface for movement of a joint.)*

Combining form **Chondr/o**

WORD EXERCISE 4

Without using your Exercise Guide, write the meaning of:

(a) **chondr/o**/phyte
    (actually a cartilaginous
    growth)

(b) **chondr**/osse/ous

(d) **chondr/o**/dys/trophy

(e) **chondr/o**/malacia

Using your Exercise Guide, find the meaning of:

(f) **chondr/o**/cost/al

(g) endo/**chondr**/al

Using your Exercise Guide find the meaning of -algia, -genesis and -lysis, then build words that mean:

(h) condition of pain in a cartilage

(i) formation of cartilage

(j) breakdown of cartilage

Using your Exercise Guide, find the meaning of:

(k) **chondr/o**/calcin/osis

A cartilage that is often damaged and removed is the crescent-shaped cartilage in the knee joint. The operation to remove this is known as **menisc**ectomy (from Latin *meniscus*, meaning crescent; combining form **menisc/o**).

ROOT

Spondyl

*(From Greek word **spondylos**, meaning vertebra, one of the irregular bones that make up the vertebral column or backbone.)*

Combining form **Spondyl/o**

WORD EXERCISE 5

Without using your Exercise Guide, write the meaning of:

(a) **spondyl**/algia

(b) **spondyl/o**/py/osis

Without using your Exercise Guide, build words that mean:

(c) breakdown/disintegration of vertebrae

(d) any disease of vertebrae

Using your Exercise Guide, find the meaning of:

(e) **spondyl**/olisthesis
    (this applies to lumbar
    vertebrae)

Here we need to mention three other conditions of the vertebrae:

Kyphosis
A condition of having an abnormally curved spine (as viewed from the side), commonly called hunchback or dowager's hump. (**Kyph/o** is from Greek *kyphos*, meaning crooked/hump.) See Figure 72(a).

Scoliosis
A condition of lateral curvature of the vertebral column. (**Scoli/o** is from a Greek word *scoli*, meaning crooked/twisted.) See Figure 72(b).

Lordosis
A condition of forward curvature of the spine in the lumbar region (**Lord-** is from a Greek word *lordos* meaning to bend the body forward).

Two of these words can be combined as in:

Scoliokyphosis ⊢ both meaning lateral and

Kyphoscoliosis ⊢ posterior curvature of the spine

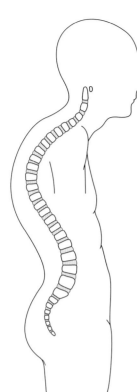

Figure 72 (a) Kyphosis

WORD EXERCISE 6

Using your Exercise Guide, find the meaning of:

(a) **disc**/oid

(b) **disc**/o/genic

Without using your Exercise Guide, build words that mean:

(c) technique of making an X-ray of an intervertebral disc

(d) removal of an intervertebral disc

The excision of degenerated intervertebral discs requires the removal of a thin layer of bone from the vertebral arch. This operation is termed a **lamin**ectomy (from Latin *lamina*, meaning thin plate; combining form **lamin/o**).

ROOT

Myel
*(From a Greek word **myelos**, meaning marrow. Here myel/o means bone marrow but it is also used to mean spinal cord and myelocyte, a type of blood cell that forms in bone marrow.)*

Combining form   Myel/o

WORD EXERCISE 7

Without using your Exercise Guide, write the meaning of:

(a) osteo/**myel**/itis

(b) **myel**/o/fibr/osis

Medical equipment and clinical procedures

Revise the names of all instruments and clinical procedures mentioned in this unit and then try Exercise 8.

WORD EXERCISE 8

Match each term in Column A with a description from Column C by placing an appropriate number in Column B.

Column A	Column B	Column C
(a) osteotome		1. puncture of a joint to withdraw synovial fluid

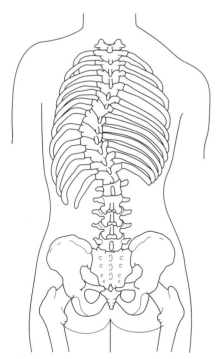

Figure 72 (b) Scoliosis

ROOT

Disc
*(From a Latin word **diskus**, meaning disc. Here disc/o means an intervertebral disc, a pad of connective tissue that acts as a shock absorber between vertebrae.)*

Combining forms   Disc/o, disk/o (Am.)

(b) arthrodesis		2.	technique of making an X-ray of a joint
(c) replacement arthroplasty		3.	fixation of a joint by surgery
(d) arthrocentesis		4.	a chisel-like instrument used to cut bone
(e) arthrography		5.	insertion of a metallic prosthesis to replace a joint

The skeleton

There are many terms that refer to specific bones within the skeleton. Look at the diagram (Fig. 73) and then complete Exercises 9 and 10.

WORD EXERCISE 9

Without using your Exercise Guide, build words that mean:

(a) surgical repair/reconstruction of the clavicle (collar bone)

(b) condition of softening of the cranium

(c) pertaining to between the ribs

(d) removal of a finger bone

(e) pertaining to the pelvis

(f) inflammation of an elbow joint

(g) pertaining to the femur and tibia

(h) surgical fixation of the scapula

(i) condition of pain in the metatarsal region

(j) surgical operation to reconstruct the hip socket

Use the boxes on Fig. 73 to practise writing the name of each bone or combining form.

WORD EXERCISE 10

Using your Exercise Guide and Fig. 73, find the meaning of:

(a) inter/**phalang**/eal

(b) **metatars**/algia

(c) tarso/**metatars**/al

(d) **metacarp**/al

ANATOMY EXERCISE

Now complete the Anatomy Exercise on page 180.

CASE HISTORY 14

The object of this exercise is to understand words associated with a patient's medical history.

To complete the exercise:

- read through the passage on rheumatoid arthritis; unfamiliar words are underlined and you can find their meaning using the Word Help

- write the meaning of the medical terms shown in bold print on the lines that follow the Word Help.

Rheumatoid arthritis

Mrs N, a 58-year-old female, was referred to the **rheumatologist** by her GP with a generalized **arthralgia** and aggravating symptoms in her left shoulder. Her GP prescribed NSAIDs for 7 weeks bringing some relief. Five years previously she had a **bursitis** in the same shoulder that had been successfully treated. There was no history of rheumatoid arthritis in her family.

Examination revealed a widespread symmetrical **polyarthritis** with swelling and tenderness in her **metacarpophalangeal** joints, proximal **interphalangeal** joints and **metatarsophalangeal** joints. Both wrists were swollen and tender, and all metatarsal heads were painful on compression. There were signs of small muscle wasting in both hands. Her back was not affected and those joints that were seemed to be stiff in the mornings for several hours. She complained of recurrent fatigue.

Mrs N had diminished movement of the chest with dullness on percussion; breath sounds were absent at the right base.

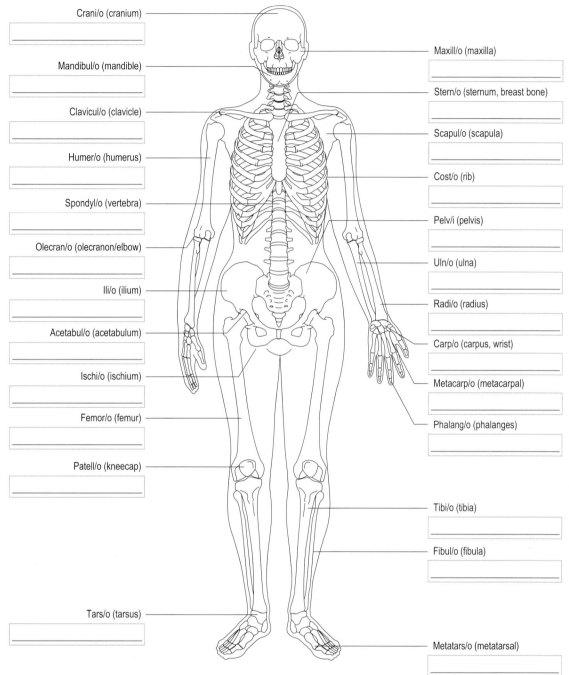

Crani/o (cranium)

Mandibul/o (mandible)

Clavicul/o (clavicle)

Humer/o (humerus)

Spondyl/o (vertebra)

Olecran/o (olecranon/elbow)

Ili/o (ilium)

Acetabul/o (acetabulum)

Ischi/o (ischium)

Femor/o (femur)

Patell/o (kneecap)

Tars/o (tarsus)

Maxill/o (maxilla)

Stern/o (sternum, breast bone)

Scapul/o (scapula)

Cost/o (rib)

Pelv/i (pelvis)

Uln/o (ulna)

Radi/o (radius)

Carp/o (carpus, wrist)

Metacarp/o (metacarpal)

Phalang/o (phalanges)

Tibi/o (tibia)

Fibul/o (fibula)

Metatars/o (metatarsal)

Figure 73   The skeleton

Joint <u>radiography</u> indicated an <u>erosion</u> in the 3rd metatarsophalangeal joint and a <u>CXR</u> confirmed a right sided <u>pleural</u> effusion. <u>Haematology</u> (Am. hematology) reported a high <u>rheumatoid factor</u>. A diagnosis of erosive rheumatoid arthritis with pleural effusion was made. Initial treatment of her inflammatory **arthropathy** was <u>enteric</u> coated aspirin 4 g/day; she was advised of possible side effects.

WORD HELP

aggravating making worse

base here it refers to the base/lower part of the right lung

compression pressing

CXR chest X-ray

effusion a fluid discharge into a part/escape of fluid into an enclosed space

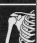
enteric pertaining to the intestine, here refers to a coating on a pill or tablet that allows it to pass to the intestine without being affected in the stomach

erosion destruction (here of a piece of bone)

GP general practitioner (family doctor)

haematology the study of blood, here refers to the department that analyses blood (Am. hematology)

NSAID a non-steroidal anti-inflammatory drug

percussion striking the body to produce a sound (here striking the thoracic wall)

pleural pertaining to the pleura (membranes that surround the lungs)

proximal near to origin/point of attachment

radiography technique of making an X-ray/ recording

rheumatoid resembling rheumatism (a painful condition marked by inflammation and degeneration of connective tissues especially around joints)

rheumatoid factor type of antibody found in the sera of patients with rheumatoid arthritis

symmetrical correspondence on opposite sides of the body/equality of parts on either side of the midline of the body

Quick Reference

Combining forms relating to the skeletal system:

Ankyl/o	fusion/adhesion/bent
Arthro	joint
Burs/o	bursa
Calcin/o	calcium
Chondr/o	cartilage
Cost/o	rib
Disc/o	intervertebral disc
Fibr/o	fibre
Kyph/o	crooked/humped
Lamin/o	lamina/part of vertebral arch
Lord/o	bend forward
Menisc/o	meniscus
Myel/o	bone marrow
Osse/o	bone
Oste/o	bone
Petr/o	stone/rock
Por/o	passage/pore
Scoli/o	crooked/twisted
Spondyl/o	vertebra
Synovi/o	synovial fluid/synovial membrane

Abbreviations

Some common abbreviations related to the skeletal system are listed below. Note some are not standard and their meaning may vary from one health care setting to another. There is a more extensive list for reference on page 335.

BM(T)	bone marrow trephine
C 1–7	cervical vertebrae 1–7
CDH	congenital dislocation of the hip
Fx	fracture
L 1–5	lumbar vertebrae 1–5
OA	osteoarthritis
Osteo	osteomyelitis
PID	prolapsed intervertebral disc
RA	rheumatoid arthritis
RF (RhF)	rheumatoid factor
T 1–12	thoracic vertebrae 1–12
THR	total hip replacement

Now write the meaning of the following words from the case history without using your dictionary lists:

(a) rheumatologist

(b) arthralgia

(c) bursitis

(d) polyarthritis

(e) metacarpophalangeal

(f) interphalangeal

(g) metatarsophalangeal

(h) arthropathy

(Answers to the case history exercise are given in the Answers to Word Exercises beginning on page 301.)

Medical Notes

Bone fracture

A bone fracture is defined as a partial or complete break in the continuity of a bone that occurs under mechanical stress. The most common cause of a fracture is traumatic injury. Bone cancer or metabolic bone disorders can also cause fractures by weakening a bone to the point that it fractures under very little stress. An *open fracture* also known as a *compound fracture*, is one in which the broken bone projects through surrounding tissue and skin, inviting the possibility of infection. A *closed fracture*, also known as a *simple fracture*, does not produce a break in the skin and therefore does not pose an immediate danger of bone infection. Fractures are also classified as 'complete' or 'incomplete'. A complete fracture involves a break across an entire section of bone, whereas an incomplete fracture involves only a partial break in which bone fragments are still partially joined. Treatment usually involves reduction (realignment) of the bone, immobilization and restoring function through rehabilitation.

Dislocation

Dislocation is the displacement of a joint as a result of trauma, it can be an emergency because of associated damage to important blood vessels and nerves. In a dislocation the articular surfaces of bones forming the joints are no longer in proper contact. The displacement can tear surrounding ligaments, alter the normal contour of the joint and cause pain and soft tissue swelling. Effective treatment involves early reduction (realignment) of the bones into their natural position.

Gout

Gout is a type of inflammatory arthritis more prevalent in males than females. It is a metabolic disorder in which blood levels of uric acid are raised leading to the deposition of sodium urate crystals in the synovial fluid of joints. The crystals are also deposited in soft tissues around joints where they form hard swellings called tophi; these trigger the chronic inflammation and tissue damage seen with the disease. In many cases only one joint is involved (monoarthritis) and is typically swollen, hot and painful. The sites most commonly affected are the metatarsophalangeal joint of the big toe and the joints at the wrists, elbows, ankles and knees. A drug for the treatment of gout called allopurinol acts to inhibit the formation of uric acid.

Osteoarthritis (OA)

Osteoarthritis also known as degenerative joint disease (DJD), is the most common non-inflammatory disorder of moveable joints. It is characterized by 'wear and tear' deterioration, atrophy of articular cartilage, formation of new bone at joint surfaces and calcification of ligaments. Osteoarthritis occurs most often in the weight-bearing joints, such as the hips, lumbar spine and knees. Symptoms include stiffness, pain on movement and limited joint motion; there is also frequent involvement of the joints in the fingers. The cause of osteoarthritis is unknown and no treatment is available to stop degeneration of the joints. Non-steroidal anti-inflammatory drugs (NSAIDs) are used to alleviate symptoms of pain and inflammation.

Osteoporosis

Osteoporosis is an age-related disorder characterized by a reduced mass of bone tissue. The condition develops when bone deposition does not keep pace with bone absorption. Peak bone mass occurs around the age of thirty-five years and then gradually declines in both sexes. Lowered levels of oestrogen after the menopause are associated with a period of accelerated bone loss in women. Common features of the condition include skeletal deformity, gradual loss of height with age due to compression of vertebrae and a hunched back. Fractures of the wrist, vertebrae and hip at the neck of the femur are frequent.

A range of environmental factors and diseases are implicated in the development of osteoporosis. These include a diet low in calcium and vitamin D, lack of exercise, smoking, early menopause and thin bodybuild in females.

Paget's disease

A chronic disease of the skeleton in which osteoclasts reabsorb excess bone softening the tissue. Overactive osteoblasts then deposit abnormal amounts of new bone that is thickened and structurally weak. This predisposes to deformities and fractures commonly of the pelvis, femur, tibia and skull. Most cases occur after forty years of age and the cause is unknown.

Rickets

A condition caused by lack of vitamin D in childhood that results in a failure to absorb calcium and phosphorus from the small intestine. As a consequence there is poor calcification of bone and when the child walks, the weight of the body causes the legs to bow. The condition may develop because of lack of vitamin D in the diet, lack of exposure of the skin to UV light, malabsorption of vitamin D or intake of drugs and other agents that result in the breakdown of vitamin D.

Rheumatism

Rheumatism is a term that refers to any painful state of the supporting structures of the body including bones, ligaments, joints, tendons and muscles. It is characterized by inflammation, degeneration and metabolic derangement of connective tissues accompanied by pain, stiffness and limited motion around joints.

Rheumatoid arthritis (RA)

Rheumatoid arthritis is a chronic progressive autoimmune disease of unknown cause. It is a systemic disease affecting not only joints but organs such as the blood vessels, eyes, lungs and heart. RA is often more severe than other forms of arthritis and is characterized by inflammation of synovial membranes, destruction of cartilage, erosion of bone and progressive crippling deformity. Common signs and symptoms include reduction in joint mobility, pain, nodular swelling and generalized aching and stiffness. As it is a systemic disease, fever, anaemia (Am. anemia) weight loss and profound fatigue are common.

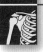
Sprain

A sprain is an acute musculoskeletal injury to the ligamentous structures surrounding a joint that disrupts the continuity of the synovial membrane. A common cause is a twisting or wrenching movement in which blood vessels may be ruptured leading to bruising and swelling around the joint. Limitation of joint motion is common in all sprain injuries.

NOW TRY THE WORD CHECK

WORD CHECK

This self-check exercise lists all the word components used in this unit. First write down the meaning of as many word components as you can. Then check your answers using the Exercise Guide and Quick Reference box or the Glossary of Word Components (pp. 347–371).

Prefixes

dys-

endo-

inter-

poly-

Combining forms of word roots

ankyl/o

arthro

burs/o

calcin/o

chondr/o

cost/o

disc/o

fibr/o

kyph/o

lamin/o

lord/o

menisc/o

myel/o

osse/o

oste/o

petr/o

phyt/o

por/o

py/o

rheumat/o

scoli/o

spondyl/o

synovi/o

Suffixes

-al

-algia

-blast

-centesis

-clasis

-clast

-desis

-eal

-ectomy

-genesis

-genic

-gram

-graphy

-ic

-itis

-lith

-logist

-lysis

-lytic

-malacia

-oid

-olisthesis

-oma

-osis

-pathy

-plasty

-scope

-scopy

-tome

-trophy

Combining forms referring to specific parts of the skeleton

acetabul/o

carp/o

clavicul/o

cost/o

crani/o

femor/o

fibul/o

humer/o

ili/o

ischi/o

mandibul/o

maxill/o

metacarp/o

metatars/o

olecran/o

patell/o

pelv/i

phalang/o

radi/o

scapul/o

spondyl/o

stern/o

tars/o

tarsometars/o

tibi/o

uln/o

NOW TRY THE SELF-ASSESSMENT

SELF-ASSESSMENT

Test 14A

Below are some combining forms that refer to the anatomy of the skeletal system and its movement. Indicate which part of the system they refer to by putting a number from the diagram (Fig. 74) next to each word.

(a) synovi/o [　　　　　]

(b) tendin/o [　　　　　]

(c) my/o [　　　　　]

(d) arthr/o [　　　　　]

(e) oste/o [　　　　　]

(f) chondr/o [　　　　　]

Score [　　]
6

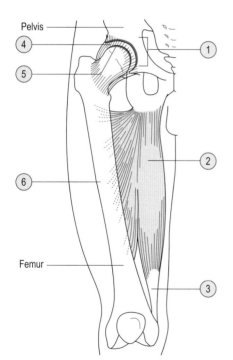

Figure 74 A muscle and skeletal arrangement in the thigh

Test 14B

Prefixes and suffixes

Match each prefix or suffix in Column A with a meaning in Column C by inserting the appropriate number in Column B.

Column A	Column B	Column C
(a) -al	[　　]	1. resembling
(b) -algia	[　　]	2. tumour (Am. tumor)/ swelling
(c) -blast	[　　]	3. slipping/dislocation
(d) -centesis	[　　]	4. condition of pain
(e) -clast	[　　]	5. technique of viewing
(f) -desis	[　　]	6. surgical repair
(g) dys-	[　　]	7. cell that breaks down a matrix
(h) -genesis	[　　]	8. pertaining to destruction/breaking down
(i) -ic	[　　]	9. condition of softening
(j) inter-	[　　]	10. instrument to cut
(k) -itis	[　　]	11. inflammation of
(l) -lytic	[　　]	12. puncture to remove fluid
(m) -malacia	[　　]	13. producing/forming
(n) -oid	[　　]	14. pertaining to (i)
(o) -olisthesis	[　　]	15. pertaining to (ii)
(p) -oma	[　　]	16. instrument to view
(q) -plasty	[　　]	17. difficult/painful/bad
(r) -scope	[　　]	18. germ cell
(s) -scopy	[　　]	19. to bind together
(t) -tome	[　　]	20. between

Score [　　]
20

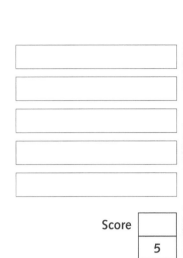

Test 14C

Combining forms of word roots

Match each combining form in Column A with a meaning in Column C by inserting the appropriate number in Column B.

Column A	Column B	Column C
(a) arthr/o		1. bone
(b) burs/o		2. marrow (of bone)
(c) calcin/o		3. synovia/synovial membrane
(d) chondr/o		4. pus
(e) cost/o		5. joint
(f) disc/o		6. vertebrae
(g) fibr/o		7. bursa/sac of fluid
(h) kyph/o		8. stone/rock
(i) lamin/o		9. calcium
(j) lord/o		10. meniscus/crescent-shaped
(k) menisc/o		11. bend forward
(l) myel/o		12. cartilage
(m) oste/o		13. crooked
(n) petr/o		14. fibre
(o) phyt/o		15. hunchback
(p) por/o		16. thin plate/lamina of vertebra
(q) py/o		17. rib
(r) scoli/o		18. passage/pore
(s) spondyl/o		19. plant-like growth
(t) synovi/o		20. intervertebral disc

Score ☐
20

Test 14D

Write the meaning of:

(a) arthrochondritis ☐

(b) bursolith ☐

(c) spondylodesis ☐

(d) chondroclast ☐

(e) kyphotic ☐

Score ☐
5

Test 14E

Build words that mean:

(a) condition of pain in a joint ☐

(b) inflammation of synovia and adjacent bones ☐

(c) condition of softening of vertebrae ☐

(d) disease of joints and bones ☐

(e) pertaining to synovia/ synovial membrane ☐

Score ☐
5

Check answers to Self-Assessment Tests on page 325.

UNIT 15
THE MALE REPRODUCTIVE SYSTEM

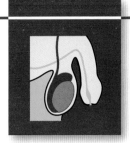

OBJECTIVES

Once you have completed Unit 15 you should be able to:

- understand the meaning of medical words relating to the male reproductive system

- build medical words relating to the male reproductive system

- associate medical terms with their anatomical position

- understand medical abbreviations relating to the male reproductive system.

EXERCISE GUIDE

Use this list of word components and their meanings to complete the word exercises in this unit.

Prefixes

a-	without
crypt-	hidden
oligo-	deficiency/few
trans-	across/through

Roots/Combining forms

cyst/o	bladder
fer/o	to carry
posth/o	prepuce/foreskin
phren/o	diaphragm

Suffixes

-al	pertaining to
-algia	condition of pain
-cele	swelling/protrusion/hernia
-cide	something that kills/killing
-ectomy	removal of
-genesis	forming/capable of causing
-graphy	technique of recording/making an X-ray

-ia	condition of
-ic	pertaining to
-ism	process of
-itis	inflammation of
-lysis	breakdown/disintegration
-megaly	enlargement
-meter	measuring instrument
-oma	tumour (Am. tumor)/swelling
-ous	pertaining to/of the nature of
-pathia	condition of disease
-pathy	disease of
-pexy	surgical fixation/fix in place
-plasty	surgical repair/reconstruction
-rrhagia	condition of bursting forth/discharge of blood
-rrhaphy	stitching/suturing
-rrhea (Am.)	excessive flow/discharge
-rrhoea	excessive flow/discharge (Am. rrhea)
-sect(ion)	cut/cutting/excision
-stomy	opening into
-tomy	incision into
-uria	condition of urine

ANATOMY EXERCISE

When you have finished Word Exercises 1–11, look at the word components listed below. Complete Figure 75 by writing the appropriate combining form on each line. (You can check their meanings in the Quick Reference box on p. 200.)

Balan/o	Phall/o	Vas/o
Epididym/o	Prostat/o	Vesicul/o
Orchi/o	Scrot/o	

The male reproductive system

The male possesses paired reproductive organs known as the testes (synonymous with testicles). These are held in position outside the main cavities of the body by a sac known as the scrotum. Each testis produces millions of sperm cells (spermatozoa) that carry the male's genetic information. Once mature, sperms are mixed with glandular secretions to form a liquid known as semen. Semen containing active swimming sperms is ejaculated from the penis during sexual intercourse. Sperms swim along the reproductive tract of the female to the oviducts where a single sperm may fuse with an egg in the process of fertilization.

Use the Exercise Guide at the beginning of this unit to complete Word Exercises 1–11 unless you are asked to work without it.

ROOT

Orch
(From a Greek word **orchi***, meaning testis (or testicle). The testis is the male reproductive organ that produces the male sex cells called spermatozoa and the hormone testosterone.)*

Combining forms Orch/i/o, orchid/o

WORD EXERCISE 1

Using your Exercise Guide, find the meaning of:

(a) **orchid/o**/pathy

(b) **orchi/o**/cele

(synonymous with scrotal hernia/scrotocele)

(c) crypt/**orch**/ism

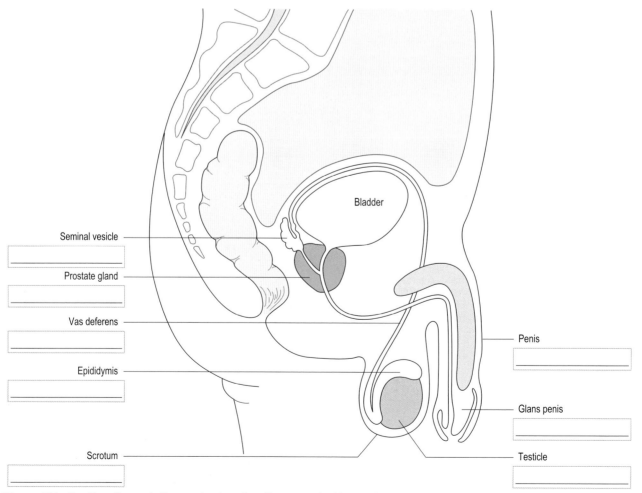

Figure 75 Section through the male showing the reproductive system

Early in fetal life the testes are located in the abdominal cavity near the kidneys but normally descend into the scrotum about two months before birth. Occasionally a baby is born with undescended testes, a condition called cryptorchism which is readily observed by palpation of the scrotum at delivery. Failure of the testes to descend may be caused by hormonal imbalances in the developing fetus or by a physical deficiency or obstruction. As the higher temperature inside the body inhibits spermatogenesis (sperm formation), measures must be taken to bring the testes down into the scrotum to prevent permanent sterility. Early treatment of this condition by surgery (orchidopexy/orchiopexy) or injection of testosterone to stimulate the testes to descend, results in normal testicular and sexual development.

(d) **orchi/o**/pexy (**orchid/o/** pexy)

Using your Exercise Guide find the meaning of -algia, -ectomy, -plasty and -tomy, then build words (using either **orch/i/o** or **orchid/o**) that mean:

(e) incision into a testicle

(f) surgical repair of a testicle

(g) removal of a testicle

(h) condition of pain in a testicle

Without using your Exercise Guide, write the meaning of:

(i) crypt/**orchid**/o/pexy

(synonymous with **orchid**/o/pexy)

Note. The word testicle comes from the Latin *testiculus* meaning testis or male gonad (reproductive organ). The combining form **test/icul/o** is used in several common medical terms for example, **testo**sterone (-sterone meaning steroid hormone) and intra/**testicul**/ar (intra- meaning within, -ar meaning pertaining to).

ROOT

Scrot
(From a Latin word meaning scrotum, the pouch containing the testicles.)

Combining form   **Scrot/o**

WORD EXERCISE 2

Without using your Exercise Guide, build words that mean:

(a) removal of the scrotum

(b) plastic surgery/repair of the scrotum

(c) hernia/protrusion of the scrotum (synonymous with **orchiocele**)

Using your Exercise Guide, find the meaning of:

(d) trans/-**scrot**/al

Two other conditions can result in a swelling of the testis:

Hydrocele
a swelling/protrusion/hernia due to an accumulation of fluid within the testis.

Varicocele
a swelling/protrusion/hernia of veins of the spermatic cords within the testis (from Latin *varicosus*, meaning varicose vein). Varicoceles need to be removed as they lead to pain and infertility.

ROOT

Phall
*(From a Greek word **phallo**, meaning penis, the male copulatory organ. Here phall/o means the penis, the male organ through which urine leaves the body via the urethra. When erect the penis transfers semen into the female reproductive system at orgasm.)*

Combining form   **Phall/o**

WORD EXERCISE 3

Using your Exercise Guide find the meaning of -ic, and -itis, then build words that mean:

(a) inflammation of the penis

(b) pertaining to the penis

Without using your Exercise Guide, build a word that means:

(c) removal of the penis

Penis is a Latin word referring to the male organ of copulation. **Pen**itis and **pen**ile are synonymous with (a) and (b) above. An abnormally enlarged penis is known as a megalo**pen**is or megalo**phall**us.

Several abnormalities of the penis have been noted at birth. The urethra sometimes opens on to the dorsal (upper) surface of the penis. This is known as an **epispadia** (*epi-* meaning above, and *-spadia* condition of drawing out). Sometimes the urethra opens on to the posterior (lower) surface. This is a **hypospadia** (condition of drawing out below).

The swelling of the penis during erotic stimulation is known as **tumescence** (from Latin *tumescere*, meaning to swell). The subsidence of the swelling is known as **detumescence** (*de* meaning lack of). Once erect the penis can be inserted into the vagina in the act of sex. Words used synonymously with sex include:

Coitus

from Latin *coire*, meaning to come together.

Intercourse

from Latin *intercurrere*, meaning to run between.

Copulation

from Latin *copulare*, meaning to bind together.

The failure to produce an erection and perform the sexual act is known as **impotence** (from Latin *impotentia*, meaning inability). This condition is often due to psychological problems, but it can arise from lesions within the reproductive tract or nervous system.

The prepuce is removed in the process of circumcision (i.e. cutting around). This is often performed for religious rather than medical reasons.

ROOT

Epididym

(Derived from Greek words **epi** *– on,* **didymos** *– twins (the testicles). Here epididym/o means the epididymis, a coiled tube that forms the first part of the duct system of each testis. The epididymes store sperm.)*

Combining form   Epididym/o

WORD EXERCISE 5

Without using your Exercise Guide, build words that mean:

(a) inflammation of the epididymis

(b) removal of the epididymis

Without using your Exercise Guide, write the meaning of:

(c) **epididym/o/-orch/itis**

ROOT

Balan

(From a Greek word **balanos**, *meaning acorn. Here balan/o means the glans penis, the sensitive, swollen end of the penis that is covered with the prepuce or foreskin.)*

Combining form   Balan/o

ROOT

Vas

(A Latin word meaning vessel or duct. Here vas/o means the vas deferens, the main secretory duct of each testis along which mature sperms move towards the penis.)

Combining form   Vas/o

WORD EXERCISE 4

Without using your Exercise Guide, build a word that means:

(a) inflammation of the glans penis

Using your Exercise Guide, find the meaning of:

(b) **balan/o/rrhagia**

(c) **balan/o/posth/itis**

The **prepuce**, or covering foreskin of the glans penis, sometimes needs to be cut, a process known as **preputio**tomy. This is performed to relieve **phimosis**, a condition in which the foreskin is too tight and cannot retract.

WORD EXERCISE 6

Without using your Exercise Guide, write the meaning of:

(a) **vas/ectomy**

(This operation (Fig. 76) is performed to sterilize the male, i.e. to make him incapable of reproduction. The cut ends of a section of the vas are tied off, a procedure known as bilateral ligation (from Latin *ligare*, meaning to bind). Following vasectomy, a reduced volume of semen is produced containing no sperm.)

Using your Exercise Guide, find the meaning of:

(b) **vas/o/epididym/o/stomy**

(c) **vas/o**/epididym/o/graphy

(d) **vas/o**/section

(e) **vas/o**/rrhaphy

Without using your Exercise Guide, write the meaning of:

(f) **vas/o**/-orchid/o/stomy

(g) **vas/o**/**vas/o**/stomy

(h) **vas/o**/tomy

ROOT

Vesicul
(From a Latin word **vesicula**, *meaning vesicle/little bladder. Here vesicul/o means the seminal vesicles, small pouches lying near the base of the bladder which secrete a nutrient fluid that becomes a component of semen.)*

Combining form **Vesicul/o**

WORD EXERCISE 7

Without using your Exercise Guide, build words that mean:

(a) technique of making an X-ray of the seminal vesicles

(b) incision into a seminal vesicle

Without using your Exercise Guide, write the meaning of:

(c) vas/o/**vesicul**/ectomy

ROOT

Prostat
(From Greek **prostates**, *meaning one who stands before. Here prostat/o means the prostate gland that surrounds the neck of the bladder and urethra in males. Secretions from the prostate gland are added to the semen during intercourse.)*

Combining form **Prostat/o**

WORD EXERCISE 8

Using your Exercise Guide, find the meaning of:

(a) **prostat/o**/cyst/o/tomy

(b) **prostat/o**/megaly

Without using your Exercise Guide, write the meaning of:

(c) **prostat**/ectomy

Benign prostatic hyperplasia (BPH) occurs in seventy-five percent of men over the age of fifty. An enlargement or hypertrophy of the prostate gland tissue characterizes the condition. As the prostate enlarges, it squeezes the urethra frequently closing it so completely that urination becomes very difficult or even impossible. In such cases surgical removal (prostatectomy) of the entire gland or part of it may become necessary. The cause of BPH is not clear but it may be associated with a decline in androgen secretion in later life that changes the androgen/oestrogen balance.

To alleviate this condition, part or the entire gland can be removed by transurethral resection of the prostate (TURP (*trans*, meaning across and *resection*, meaning removal/excision). TURP involves inserting a resectoscope, a type of endoscope into the urethra and using it to view and cut out pieces of prostate gland.)

(d) **prostat/o**/vesicul/ectomy

ROOT

Semin
(From a Latin word **seminis**, *meaning seed. Here semin/i means semen, the liquid secretion of the testicles. Note, in a few words, semin- means testicle.)*

Combining form **Semin/i**

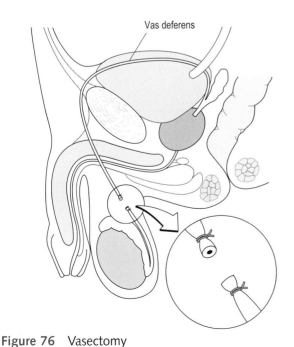
Figure 76 Vasectomy

WORD EXERCISE 9

Using your Exercise Guide, find the meaning of:

(a) **semin/i**/fer/ous

(Spermatozoa flow along seminiferous tubules of the testis.)

(b) **semin**/uria

(c) **semin**/oma

(A malignancy of the testis. A change in size and shape of the testes is a symptom of this condition; their size can be measured with an **orchidometer**. When a testis is removed it can be replaced with a prosthesis.)

In**semina**tion refers to the deposition of semen in the female reproductive tract (from Latin *seminare*, meaning to sow). Artificial insemination (AI) refers to the insertion of semen into the uterus via a cannula (tube) instead of by coitus. The sperm used in this procedure can be from two sources:

- AI by husband (AIH). In this procedure semen from the patient's husband is inseminated into the wife. It is used when there is difficulty in conceiving because of physical and/or psychological problems.
- AI by donor (AID). In this procedure semen from a male other than the female's partner is used. AID is used when the partner is sterile.

ROOT

Sperm
(From a Greek word **sperma**, meaning seed. Here sperm/o means sperm cells or spermatozoa (sing. spermatozoon). Sperm are ejaculated from the male during the peak of sexual excitement known as orgasm.)

Combining forms   **Sperm/o, spermat/o**, also **sperm/i** (from New Latin spermium)

WORD EXERCISE 10

Using your Exercise Guide, find the meaning of:

(a) a/**sperm**/ia

(b) oligo/**sperm**/ia

(c) **sperm/i**/cide

(often used as a cream in conjunction with condoms and other contraceptives)

Using your Exercise Guide, build words using spermat/o that mean:

(d) condition of disease of sperm (abnormal sperm)

(e) formation of sperm

(f) breakdown/disintegration of sperm

(g) flow of sperm (abnormal, without orgasm)

Sperm counts are performed to estimate the number of sperms, the percentage of abnormal sperms and their mobility. The actual number of sperms is important in determining the fertility of the male. A sperm count of less than 60 million sperms per cm^3 of semen results in decreased fertility, even though only one sperm is required to fertilize an egg!

Oligospermia results from reduced sperm production by the seminiferous tubules of the testes. If the *sperm count* is too low, infertility may result. A large number of sperm is needed to ensure that sufficient will reach the ovum and one will bring about fertilization. Oligospermia can result from factors such as infection, fever, radiation, malnutrition and the high temperature of undescended testes. The condition can be temporary, as in some acute infections or permanent as in untreated cryptorchism. Total absence of sperm production (*aspermia*) always results in *sterility*.

Semen containing sperms can be preserved at very low temperatures in a cryostat. Once thawed, the sperm are capable of fertilizing eggs and are used for artificial insemination.

Recently it has become possible to use sperm to fertilize eggs outside the body in laboratory glassware, a process known as in vitro fertilization (*vitro* meaning glass).

Medical equipment and clinical procedures

Revise the names of all instruments and clinical procedures mentioned in this unit and then try Exercise 11.

WORD EXERCISE 11

Match each term in Column A with a description from Column C by placing an appropriate number in Column B.

Column A	Column B	Column C
(a) sperm count		1. fusion of an egg and sperm in laboratory glassware
(b) transurethral resection		2. material used to tie a cut vas
(c) vasectomy		3. an instrument used to measure the size of a testicle
(d) orchidometer		4. removal of prostate tissue through the urethra
(e) in vitro fertilization		5. an estimate of numbers of spermatozoa in 1 cm³ semen
(f) vasoligature		6. the cutting and removal of a section of the sperm duct

ANATOMY EXERCISE

Now complete the Anatomy Exercise on page 194.

CASE HISTORY 15

The object of this exercise is to understand words associated with a patient's medical history.

To complete the exercise:

• read through the passage on seminoma; unfamiliar words are underlined and you can find their meaning using the Word Help

• write the meaning of the medical terms shown in bold print on the lines that follow the Word Help.

Seminoma

Mr O, a 32-year-old father of two children, consulted his GP about a severe back pain. Although a regular football player he could not recall any recent injury that could account for his condition. During his consultation he mentioned that several months ago he had noticed his right testicle was swollen. It felt heavy and sometimes uncomfortable but he had ignored it assuming it would resolve. When his early medical record was checked it revealed a history of **cryptorchism** of the right testicle that had been rectified by **orchidopexy** at the age of 5 years.

Palpation showed the right testicle to be hard, smooth and swollen. It was easily separated from the epididymis and did not transilluminate. Mr O had not felt any pain and otherwise appeared in good health. There was no evidence of **orchitis**, epididymitis or torsion. He was counselled by his GP who referred him to the Urology department with suspected cancer of the testis.

Ultrasonography determined the presence of an **intratesticular** mass in the right testicle. A chest X-ray was negative for lung metastases, but a CT scan of his abdominopelvic region revealed retroperitoneal and para-aortic lymphadenopathy. He had elevated levels of the serum tumour (Am. tumor) markers bHCG and lactate dehydrogenase.

Mr O was advised of the need for surgical **orchidectomy** and the consultant explained the procedure to him.

Mr O's scrotal contents were examined and his right testicle removed through an inguinal approach with early clamping of the **spermatic** cord and its vessels. (Note, **trans-scrotal** biopsy is contra-indicated as a means of evaluating scrotal masses as it causes tumour cell shedding and spread of the tumour).

Histopathological analysis confirmed the presence of a malignant **seminoma** in the right testicle; the contralateral testis was biopsied at the same time and found to be normal.

Mr O's condition was assessed as Stage IIC and he was given chemotherapy with follow up chest X-ray, abdominopelvic CT scan and serum tumour marker determination every 3 months. At 6 months the residual retroperitoneal mass has shrunk and calcified, and he remains progression free.

WORD HELP

bHCG a serum tumour marker (Am. tumor)

calcified referring to deposition of calcium salts into a tissue

chemotherapy treatment using drugs (here cytotoxic drugs that destroy cancer cells)

contralateral pertaining to the opposite side

CT computed tomography

AN INTRODUCTION TO MEDICAL TERMINOLOGY FOR HEALTH CARE

epididymis the first part of the duct system that leaves the testis and stores maturing sperm

epididymitis inflammation of the epididymis

GP general practitioner (family doctor)

histopathological pertaining to disease of a tissue

inguinal pertaining to the groin

lactate dehydrogenase a serum tumour marker (Am. tumor)

lymphadenopathy disease of lymph nodes (lymph glands)

malignant dangerous, capable of spreading

metastases parts of a tumour that have spread from one site to another

palpation act of feeling with the fingers using light pressure

para-aortic pertaining to beside the aorta

progression advancing, moving forward of a disease

retroperitoneal pertaining to behind the peritoneum

serum tumour marker certain chemicals are elevated to higher than normal levels in blood serum when tumours are present, they act as signs or markers of the presence of disease

Stage IIC staging is a system of classifying malignant disease that will influence its treatment; this patient is at Stage IIC

torsion act of twisting/rotation

transilluminate shine a bright light through (note, a solid tumour will prevent transmission of light)

ultrasonography technique of recording (an image) using high frequency sound waves

urology study of the urinary tract (here department that diagnoses and treats disease and disorders of the urinary tract)

Now write the meaning of the following words from the case history without using your dictionary lists:

(a) cryptorchism

(b) orchidopexy

(c) orchitis

(d) intratesticular

(e) orchidectomy

(f) spermatic

(g) trans-scrotal

(h) seminoma

(Answers to the case history exercise are given in the Answers to Word Exercises beginning on page 301.)

Quick Reference

Combining forms relating to the male reproductive system:

Balan/o	glans penis
Cyst/o	bladder
Epididym/o	epididymis
Orchi/o	testis
Phall/o	penis
Posth/o	prepuce/foreskin
Prostat/o	prostate
Scrot/o	scrotum
Semin/i	semen/testis
Sperm/i	spermatozoa/sperm
Varic/o	varicose vein
Vas/o	vas deferens/vessel
Vesicul/o	seminal vesicle

Abbreviations

Some common abbreviations related to the male reproductive system are listed below. Note some are not standard and their meaning may vary from one health care setting to another. There is a more extensive list for reference on page 335.

AI	artificial insemination
AID	artificial insemination by donor
ICSH	interstitial cell stimulating hormone
pros	prostate
PSA	prostate specific antigen
SPP	suprapubic prostatectomy
STD	sexually transmitted disease
Syph	syphilis
TUR	transurethral resection
TURP	transurethral resection of the prostate gland
VD	venereal disease
WR	Wasserman reaction test for syphilis

Medical Notes

Castration

Castration is the surgical removal of the testis. When performed before puberty, the male becomes a eunuch. The eunuch's reproductive system remains infantile and he does not develop secondary sexual characteristics.

Erectile dysfunction (impotence)

Failure to achieve an erection of the penis is called erectile dysfunction or impotence. Although impotence does not affect sperm production, it may cause infertility because normal intercourse may not be possible. Anxiety and psychological stress are often cited as causes of this condition. Impotence may also result from an abnormality in the erectile tissues of the penis or a failure of the nerve reflexes that control erection. Drugs and alcohol can cause temporary impotence by interfering with the nerves and blood vessels involved in erection.

Hydrocele

A common cause of scrotal swelling is an accumulation of fluid called a hydrocele. Hydroceles may be congenital, resulting from structural abnormalities present at birth. In adults the condition often occurs when fluid produced by the serous membrane (tunica vaginalis) lining the scrotum is not absorbed properly. The onset may be acute and painful or chronic; in some cases the cause of hydrocele can be linked to trauma or infection.

Infections of the penis and urethra

Inflammation of the glans penis and prepuce (foreskin) may be caused by specific or non-specific infection. In non-specific infection (*balanitis*), lack of personal hygiene is an important predisposing factor especially if *phimosis* is present.

Gonococcal urethritis (*gonorrhoea (Am. gonorrhea)*) is the most common specific infection. Non-specific infection may be spread from the bladder or be introduced by surgical procedures such as catheterization. Both types may spread throughout the system to the prostate gland, seminal vesicles epididymes and testes. If infection becomes chronic, it may cause urethral stricture or obstruction leading to retention of urine.

Inguinal hernia

An inguinal hernia forms when the intestines push through the weak area of the abdominal wall that separates the abdominopelvic cavity from the scrotum. If the intestines push into the scrotum, the digestive tract may become obstructed resulting in death. Inguinal hernia may be congenital but more often occurs when lifting a heavy object. Small hernias may be treated with external supports that prevent organs from protruding into the scrotum but more serious hernias must be repaired surgically.

Phimosis

Phimosis is a structural abnormality in which the foreskin fits so tightly over the glans that it cannot retract. The usual treatment for this condition is circumcision, a procedure in which the foreskin is cut along the base of the glans and removed. Severe phimosis can obstruct the flow of urine, possibly causing the death of an infant born with this condition. Milder phimosis can result in accumulation of dirt and organic matter under the foreskin causing severe infection.

Prostate tumours

Prostate tumour (Am. tumor)s are a relatively common cause of death in men over fifty. The cause is unknown but changes in the androgen/oestrogen balance are thought to be significant and in some cases viral infection may be involved. Invasion of local tissues is widespread before lymph-spread metastases develop in pelvic and abdominal lymph nodes. Blood-spread metastases in bone are common and bone formation rather than bone destruction is a common feature. In many cases metastases in lumbar vertebrae are the first indication of this condition.

Testicular torsion

The spermatic cord carries blood vessels, nerves, lymphatics and a sperm duct to the testis. When this becomes twisted (torsion) the blood supply to the testis is cut off leading to acute swelling and severe pain. Emergency surgery is required within 6–10 hours to restore the blood circulation and function of the testis.

Testicular tumours

Most testicular tumours (Am. tumors) arise from the sperm-producing cells of the seminiferous tubules. Malignancies of the testes are most common among men twenty to thirty-five years old. A testicular tumour tends to remain localised for a considerable time but eventually spreads in lymph to pelvic and abdominal nodes, and more widely in the blood. Besides age, this type of cancer is associated with genetic predisposition, trauma or infection of the testis and cryptorchism. Treatment of testicular cancer is most effective when diagnosis is made early in the development of the tumour.

Varicocele

A swelling of the testicular vein within the spermatic cord near the testis; the condition is associated with oligospermia and scrotal pain.

NOW TRY THE WORD CHECK

WORD CHECK

This self-check exercise lists all the word components used in this unit. First write down the meaning of as many word components as you can. Then check your answers using the Exercise Guide and Quick Reference box or the Glossary of Word Components (pp. 347–371).

Prefixes

a-

crypt-

epi-hypo-

intra-

oligo-

trans-

Combining forms of word roots

balan/o

cyst/o

epididym/o

fer/o

hydr/o

megal/o

orchi/o

phall/o

posth/o

prostat/o

scrot/o

semin/i

sperm/i

varic/o

vas/o

vesicul/o

Suffixes

-al

-algia

-ar

-cele

-cide

-ectomy

-genesis

-graphy

-ia

-ic

-ism

-itis

-ligation

-lysis

-oma

-ous

-pathia

-pexy

-plasty

-rrhagia

-rrhaphy

-rrhoea
(Am. -rrhea)

-sect(ion)

-spadia

-stomy

-tomy

-uria

NOW TRY THE SELF-ASSESSMENT

SELF-ASSESSMENT

Test 15A

Below are some combining forms that refer to the anatomy of the male reproductive system. Indicate which part of the system they refer to by putting a number from the diagram (Fig. 77) next to each word.

(a) scrot/o

(b) orchid/o

(c) phall/o

(d) balan/o

(e) vas/o

(f) prostat/o

(g) vesicul/o

(h) epididym/o

Score

8

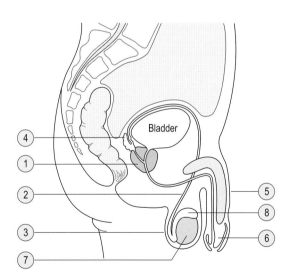

Figure 77 Section through the male showing the reproductive system

Test 15B

Prefixes and suffixes

Match each prefix or suffix in Column A with a meaning in Column C by inserting the appropriate number in Column B.

Column A	Column B	Column C
(a) -cele		1. fixation
(b) -cide		2. condition of drawing out
(c) crypt-		3. hidden
(d) epi-		4. condition of urine/ urination
(e) -genesis		5. opening into
(f) -ia		6. across
(g) -ic		7. back
(h) -ism		8. suturing
(i) oligo-		9. on/above/upon
(j) -ous		10. condition of bursting forth (of blood)
(k) -pexy		11. pertaining to (i)
(l) re-		12. pertaining to (ii)
(m) -rrhagia		13. process of
(n) -rrhaphy		14. excessive flow/ discharge
(o) -rrhoea (Am. -rrhea)		15. producing/forming
(p) -sect		16. hernia/protrusion/ swelling
(q) -spadia		17. condition of
(r) -stomy		18. to kill
(s) trans-		19. cut
(t) -uria		20. little/scanty/few

Score

20

Test 15C

Combining forms of word roots

Match each combining form in Column A with a meaning in Column C by inserting the appropriate number in Column B.

Column A	Column B	Column C
(a) balan/o		1. to carry
(b) cyst/o		2. testis
(c) epididym/o		3. penis
(d) fer/o		4. glans penis
(e) hydr/o		5. prostate gland
(f) megal/o		6. prepuce
(g) orchid/o		7. semen
(h) phall/o		8. epididymis
(i) posth/o		9. varicose vein
(j) prostat/o		10. vessel
(k) scrot/o		11. vesicle (seminal)
(l) semin/i		12. water
(m) varic/o		13. scrotum
(n) vas/o		14. bladder
(o) vesicul/o		15. abnormal enlargement

Score

15

Test 15D

Write the meaning of:

(a) orchidoepididymectomy

(b) phallorrhoea
   (Am. phallorrhea)

(c) epididymovasectomy

(d) vasoligation

(e) spermaturia

Score

5

Test 15E

Build words that mean:

(a) stitching/suturing of the testis

(b) condition of pain in the prostate

(c) formation of an opening between the vas and epididymis

(d) inflammation of the scrotum

(e) excessive flow/discharge from the prostate

Score

5

Check answers to Self-Assessment Tests on page 325.

Test your recall of the meanings of word components in Units 11–15 by completing the appropriate self-assessment tests in Unit 22 on page 296.

UNIT 16
THE FEMALE REPRODUCTIVE SYSTEM

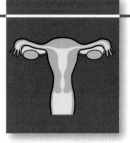

EXERCISE GUIDE

Use this list of word components and their meanings to complete the word exercises in this unit.

Prefixes

a-	without
ante-	before
dys-	difficult/painful
endo-	within/inside
eu-	good
micro-	small
multi-	many
neo-	new
nulli-	none
oligo-	deficiency/little/few
peri-	around
pre-	before/in front of
primi-	first
pro-	before
secundi-	second

Roots/Combining forms

cyst/o	bladder (cyst)
cyt/e	cell
fer/o	to carry
haem/o	blood (Am. hem/o)
hem/o (Am.)	blood
myc/o	fungus
perine/o	perineum
periton/e/o	peritoneum
phleb/o	vein
placent/o	placenta
rect/o	rectum
trachel/o	neck
vesic/o	bladder

Suffixes

-a	noun ending/a name e.g. of a condition
-agogue	agent that induces/promotes
-al	pertaining to
-algia	condition of pain
-arche	beginning
-blast	cell that forms . . . /immature germ cell
-cele	swelling/protrusion/hernia
-centesis	puncture
-dynia	condition of pain
-ectomy	removal of
-fuge	agent that suppresses/removes
-genesis	formation of
-genic	pertaining to formation
-gram	X-ray/tracing/recording
-graphy	making an X-ray/technique of recording
-ia	condition of
-ic	pertaining to
-ischia	condition of reducing/holding back
-itis	inflammation of
-lithiasis	condition of stones
-logy	study of
-malacia	condition of softening
-meter	measuring instrument
-metry	process of measuring
-oma	tumour (Am. tumor)/swelling
-osis	abnormal condition/disease of
-ous	pertaining to/of the nature of
-pathia	condition of disease

-pathy	disease of	-scope	viewing instrument
-pause	stopping	-scopy	visual examination/technique of viewing
-pexy	surgical fixation/fix in place		
-plasty	surgical repair/reconstruction	-staxis	dripping
-poiesis	formation	-stenosis	condition of narrowing
-ptosis	falling/displacement/prolapse	-stomy	formation of an opening/an opening
-rrhagic	pertaining to bursting forth (of blood)	-tic	pertaining to
-rrhaphy	suturing/stitching	-tome	cutting instrument
-rrhexis	breaking/rupturing	-tomy	incision into
-rrhea (Am.)	excessive discharge/flow	-toxic	pertaining to poisoning
-rrhoea	excessive discharge/flow (Am. -rrhea)	-trophin	hormone that stimulates/nourishes
		-tropic	pertaining to stimulating/affinity for
-sclerosis	condition of hardening	-tubal	pertaining to a tube

ANATOMY EXERCISE

When you have finished Word Exercises 1–14, look at the word components listed below. Complete Figures 78 and 79 by writing the appropriate combining form on each line – more than one component may relate to the same position. (You can check their meanings in the Quick Reference box on p. 219.)

Cervic/o	Hyster/o	Salping/o
Colp/o	Metr/o	Uter/o
Culd/o	Oophor/o	Vagin/o
Endometr/i	Ovari/o	Vulv/o

The female reproductive system

The female possesses paired reproductive organs known as ovaries; these are located in the upper pelvic cavity on either side of the uterus. The function of the ovaries is to produce reproductive cells known as ova (eggs). The ovaries pass through a regular ovarian cycle in which one egg is released (ovulation) every 28 days. The egg passes into the oviduct where it may be fertilized by sperms ejaculated into the female reproductive tract by the male. Should an egg be fertilized, it will divide and grow into a new individual after implanting into the uterus. If the egg is not fertilized, it will disintegrate and may pass out of the body at menstruation.

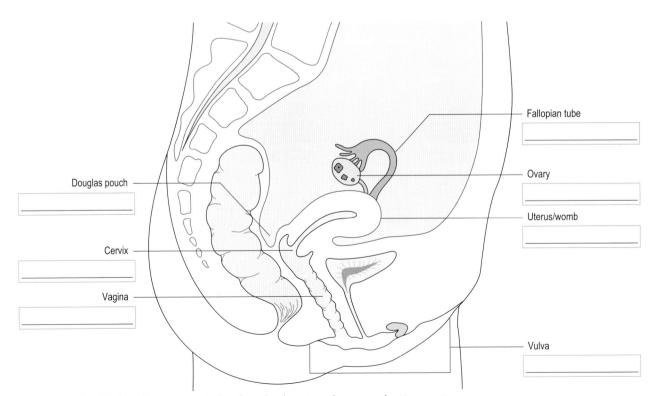

Figure 78   Sagittal section through the female showing the reproductive system

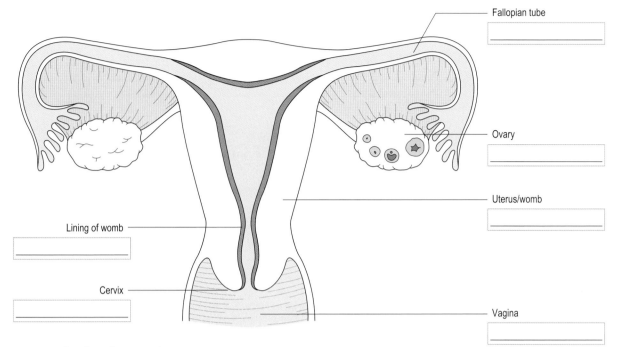

Fallopian tube

Ovary

Uterus/womb

Lining of womb

Cervix

Vagina

Figure 79 The female reproductive system

Use the Exercise Guide at the beginning of this unit to complete Word Exercises 1–26 unless you are asked to work without it.

ROOT

Oo
*(From a Greek word **oon**, meaning egg.)*

Combining form   **Oo-**

WORD EXERCISE 1

Using your Exercise Guide, find the meaning of:

(a) **oo**/blast

(b) **oo**/cyte

(c) **oo**/genesis

ROOT

Oophor
*(From a Greek word **oophoron**, derived from oion – egg, pherein – to bear. Here oophor/o means an ovary, one of the paired egg-bearing glands in the female.)*

Combining form   **Oophor/o**

WORD EXERCISE 2

Using your Exercise Guide find the meaning of -ectomy, -pexy and -tomy, then build words that mean:

(a) removal of an ovary

(b) fixation of an ovary

(c) incision of an ovary

Using your Exercise Guide, find the meaning of:

(d) **oophor/o**/cyst/ectomy
(Cyst refers to an ovarian cyst, a bladder-like growth in the ovary.)

(e) **oophor/o**/stomy

ROOT

Ovari
*(From a New Latin word **ovarium**, meaning ovary, derived from ova, meaning egg.)*

Combining form   **Ovari/o**

WORD EXERCISE 3

Without using your Exercise Guide, build words that mean:

(a) removal of an ovary (synonymous with oophorectomy)

(b) incision into an ovary
(often used to mean
the removal of an
ovarian cyst)

Using your Exercise Guide, find the meaning of:

(c) **ovari/o**/rrhexis

(d) **ovari/o**/tubal
(The tube refers to
an oviduct.)

(e) **ovari/o**/centesis

(g) condition of stones
in an oviduct

(h) surgical repair of an
oviduct

Approximately every 28 days an egg (or ovum) is
released from one of the ovaries. This process is known
as **ovulation**. Once released, the oviduct picks up the
egg and it moves towards the uterus. An ovary that fails
to release eggs is described as **anovular** meaning pertaining to without eggs.

ROOT

Salping
*(From Greek **salpigos**, meaning trumpet tube. Here
salping/o means Fallopian tube (after Gabriele
Fallopio Italian anatomist b. 1523), a structure also
known as the oviduct or uterine tube. There are two
trumpet-shaped uterine tubes, their function is to
collect eggs ovulated from the ovaries and transport
them to the uterus.)*

Combining form   Salping/o

WORD EXERCISE 4

Without using your Exercise Guide, write the
meaning of:

(a) **salping/o**/-oophor/ectomy

(b) ovari/o/**salping**/ectomy

(c) **salping/o**/pexy

Using your Exercise Guide, find the meaning of:

(d) **salping/o**/cele

(e) **salping/o**/-oophor/itis

Using your Exercise Guide find the meaning of
-graphy, -lithiais and -plasty, then build words that
mean:

(f) technique of making an
X-ray of the oviduct
(follows an injection of
opaque dye)

ROOT

Uter
*(From a Latin word **uterus**, meaning womb. Here
uter/o means the uterus, the chamber in which a
fertilized egg develops into a fetus.)*

Combining form   Uter/o

WORD EXERCISE 5

Using your Exercise Guide find the meaning of
-algia and -sclerosis, then build words that mean:

(a) condition of pain in the
uterus

(b) hardening of the uterus

Without using your Exercise Guide, write the
meaning of:

(c) **uter/o**/tubal

(d) **uter/o**/salping/o/graphy

Using your Exercise Guide, find the meaning of:

(e) **uter/o**/vesic/al

(f) **uter/o**/rect/al

(g) **uter/o**/placent/al
(The placenta is a
disc-shaped structure
that attaches the fetus
to the lining of the uterus.)

ROOT

Hyster
*(From Greek word **hystera**, meaning womb. Here
hyster/o means the uterus, the chamber in which a
fertilized egg develops into a fetus.)*

Combining form   Hyster/o

WORD EXERCISE 6

Using your Exercise Guide find the meaning of -gram, -ptosis and -scope, then build words that mean:

(a) instrument to view the uterus

(b) condition of a falling/ displaced uterus (also known as a prolapse)

(c) X-ray picture of the uterus

Without using your Exercise Guide, write the meaning of:

(d) **hyster**/o/salping/o/graphy

(e) **hyster**/o/salping/o/stomy

(f) **hyster**/o/salping/o/ -oophor/ectomy

Using your Exercise Guide, find the meaning of:

(g) **hyster**/o/trachel/o/rrhaphy

(h) **hyster**/o/trachel/o/tomy

(g) condition of narrowed uterus

(h) condition of softening of uterus

The endo**metri**um (meaning part within the uterus) refers to the lining of the uterus. The endometrium grows during the 28-day menstrual cycle and disintegrates when it ends, producing the menstrual flow.

Using your Exercise Guide, find the meaning of:

(i) endo/**metr**/itis

(j) endo/**metr**/i/oma

Without using your Exercise Guide, write the meaning of:

(k) endo/**metr**/i/osis (refers to the endometrial tissue in abnormal locations outside the uterus)

ROOT

Metr
*(From a Greek word **metra**, meaning womb. Here metr/o means the uterus, the chamber in which a fertilized egg develops into a fetus.)*

Combining form   Metr/a/i/o

WORD EXERCISE 7

Using your Exercise Guide, find the meaning of:

(a) **metr**/o/staxis

(b) **metr**/o/path/ia haemo/rrhag/ic/a (Am. **metr**/o/path/ia hemo/rrhag/ic/a)

(c) **metr**/o/periton/itis

(d) **metr**/o/phleb/itis

(e) **metr**/o/cyst/osis

(f) **metr**/o/ptosis

Using your Exercise Guide find the meaning of -malacia and -stenosis, then build words that mean:

Fibroids (**leiomyoma, myoma**) are common, often multiple, benign tumours (Am. tumors) of the myometrium (the smooth muscle layer of the uterus). They are firm masses of smooth muscle encapsulated in compressed muscle fibres and they vary greatly in size. They develop during the reproductive period and may be hormone dependent, enlarging during pregnancy and when oral contraceptives are used. Fibroids tend to regress after the menopause and malignant change is rare. Large tumours cause pelvic discomfort, frequency of micturition, menorrhagia, irregular bleeding, dysmenorrhoea and reduced fertility. The procedure of **fibroid**ectomy or **myom**ectomy (**myom-** is from myoma, meaning a muscle tumour) removes fibroids.

ROOT

Men
*(From a Latin word **mensis**, meaning month. Here men/o means menstruation, the monthly bleeding from the womb. The bleeding arises from the disintegration of the lining of the uterus known as the endometrium.)*

Combining form   Men/o

WORD EXERCISE 8

Without using your Exercise Guide, write the meaning of:

(a) **men/o**/staxis

Using your Exercise Guide, find the meaning of:

(b) **men**/arche

(c) **men/o**/pause

(d) a/**men/o**/rrhoea
(Am. a/**men/o**/rrhea)

(e) dys/**men/o**/rrhoea
(Am. dys/**men/o**/rrhea)

(f) oligo/**men/o**/rrhoea
(Am. oligo/**men/o**/rrhea)

(g) pre/**menstru**/al

Hysteroscopy and biopsy

In this procedure, a narrow endoscope known as a **hysteroscope** is inserted through the cervix to examine the uterus. Modern hysteroscopes are thin telescopes that fit through the cervix with minimal or no dilatation. The standard 4 mm hysteroscope gives a panoramic view of the cervical canal and uterine cavity and is suitable for most purposes. A diagnostic sheath around the main viewing telescope of the instrument allows saline or carbon dioxide to be pumped in, thereby inflating the uterus and improving the field of view.

Hysteroscopy is a simple, inexpensive diagnostic technique used to investigate women with abnormal uterine bleeding. It has been particularly valuable in the investigation of post-menopausal bleeding to exclude endometrial cancer. Once positioned, the hysteroscope is used to observe fibroids, polyps and adhesions, and to biopsy the endometrium (i.e. remove living suspicious tissue for examination). Benign polyps are usually removed and examined as they are difficult to differentiate from malignant lesions.

A more complex instrument the **microcolpohysteroscope** has different levels of magnification (1–150X) as well as diagnostic and operative sheaths. It can produce a panoramic view of the endocervix and uterine cavity or be used at close range to examine the cellular and vascular structure of the endometrium. During **operative hysteroscopy** various instruments including biopsy or grasping forceps, scissors, diathermy probes and laser fibres are passed into the body through the operative sheath. The surgeon controls the instruments whilst viewing the uterine cavity through the telescope component of the device.

Another instrument called a **resectoscope** used over many years for prostate and bladder surgery, has been modified for use as an operative hysteroscope. It has a built in wire loop that uses a high frequency electric current to cut and coagulate the tissues of the endometrium. The resectoscope is used for transcervical resection of the endometrium (TCRE), a technique of ablating (cutting away) the endometrium in women with dysfunctional uterine bleeding (menorrhagia). It can also remove small to medium submucous fibroids and provide biopsy specimens for histological analysis.

Flexible endoscopy using a 3–5 mm directional endoscope with an insufflating channel (to blow in gas or fluid) is also proving useful in hysteroscopy and salpingoscopy. The larger endoscopes also have a channel wide enough to accommodate surgical instruments.

Biopsy specimens removed by any of these instruments are sent to the pathology laboratory for processing and histological analysis. (The word biopsy is formed from *bio-* meaning life and *-opsy* meaning process of viewing. A biopsy is the removal and examination of tissue from a living body.)

ROOT

Cervic
*(From a Latin word **cervix**, meaning the neck. Here cervic/o means the cervix or cervix uteri, the neck of the uterus.)*

Combining form **Cervic/o**

WORD EXERCISE 9

Without using your Exercise Guide, build words that mean:

(a) inflammation of the cervix

(b) removal of the cervix

Cervical cancer or carcinoma of the cervix occurs most frequently in women between the ages of thirty and fifty and they are therefore advised to have periodic cervical smears. The procedure involves taking a sample of cells from the cervix and subjecting them to cytological examination called a **Pap test**, named after cytologist G. Papanicolaou. Neoplastic cells can be removed in their early stages of growth, thereby preventing the condition. The cancer begins with *cervical intraepithelial neoplasia* (CIN), a change in the shape, growth and number of cells in the deepest layer of the cervical epithelium. CIN may progress to the full thickness of the epithelium and is then called carcinoma-in-situ. The cancer may develop further and spread locally into the vagina, uterine body and other pelvic structures; more widespread metastases occur late in the disease. In a significant proportion of cases, the risk of developing cervical cancer is related to the number of sexual partners and is the result of transmission of the human papilloma viruses HPV-6 and HPV-7 that cause genital warts on the penis.

ROOT

Colp

*(From a Greek word **colpos**, meaning hollow. Here colp/o means the vagina, a hollow musculo-membranous passage extending from the cervix uteri to the vulva. The vagina receives the penis during copulation and allows the passage of a baby during the birth process.)*

Combining form   Colp/o

WORD EXERCISE 10

Using your Exercise Guide, find the meaning of:

(a) **colp/o**/scopy

(b) **colp/o**/micro/scope
(used in situ, i.e. to examine the vagina directly)

Without using your Exercise Guide, write the meaning of:

(c) **colp/o**/gram

(d) **colp/o**/perine/o/rrhaphy

The perineum is the region between the thighs bounded by the anus and vulva in the female. Perineotomy is used synonymously with episi/o/tomy (*episi* – meaning pubic region). This incision is made during the birth of a child when the vaginal orifice does not stretch sufficiently to allow an easy birth.

(e) **colp/o**/hyster/ectomy

(f) metr/o/**colp/o**/cele

(g) cervic/o/**colp**/itis

Without using your Exercise Guide, build words that mean:

(h) surgical repair of the perineum and vagina

(i) surgical fixation of the vagina

ROOT

Vagin

*(From a Latin word **vagina**, meaning sheath. Here vagin/o means the vagina, a hollow musculo-membranous passage extending from the cervix uteri to the vulva. The vagina receives the penis during copulation and allows the passage of a baby during the birth process.)*

Combining form   Vagin/o

WORD EXERCISE 11

Without using your Exercise Guide, write the meaning of:

(a) **vagin/o**/perine/o/tomy

(b) **vagin/o**/perine/o/rrhaphy

(c) **vagin/o**/vesic/al

Using your Exercise Guide find the meaning of -mycosis and -pathy, then build words that mean:

(d) condition of fungal infection of the vagina

(e) disease of the vagina

Investigations of disorders of the vagina and cervix usually require the use of a vaginal speculum to hold the walls of the vagina apart. There are many types of vaginal specula, one of which is shown in Figure 80.

Two small glands situated on either side of the external orifice of the vagina are known as the **greater vestibular glands** or **Bartholin's glands** (after C. Bartholin, a Danish anatomist b.1655); they produce mucus to lubricate the vagina. A condition called **bartholin**itis develops when the glands become inflamed.

ROOT

Vulv

*(From a Latin word **vulva**, meaning womb. Here vulv/o means the vulva, also known as the, pudendum femina or external genitalia.)*

Combining form   Vulv/o

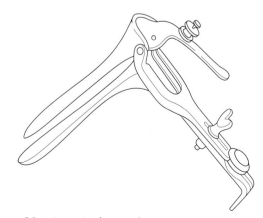

Figure 80   A vaginal speculum

WORD EXERCISE 12

Without using your Exercise Guide, write the meaning of:

(a) **vulv/o**/vagin/itis

(b) **vulv/o**/vagin/o/plasty

ROOT

Culd

(From a French word **cul-de-sac**, *meaning bottom of the bag or sack. Here culd/o means the Douglas cavity or rectouterine pouch, a blindly ending pouch that lies above the posterior vaginal fornix.)*

Combining form **Culd/o**

WORD EXERCISE 13

Without using your Exercise Guide, write the meaning of:

(a) **culd/o**/scope
(This allows examination of the uterus, oviducts, ovaries and peritoneal cavity; Fig. 81)

(b) **culd/o**/scopy

(c) **culd/o**/centesis

ROOT

Gynaec

(From a Greek word **gyne**, *meaning woman. Here gynaec/o means the female reproductive system.)*

Combining forms **Gynaec/o, (Am. Gynec/o)**

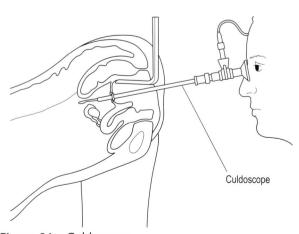

Figure 81 Culdoscopy

WORD EXERCISE 14

Using your Exercise Guide, find the meaning of:

(a) **gynaec/o**/logy
(Am. **gynec/o**/logy; refers to diseases peculiar to women, i.e. of the female reproductive tract)

(b) **gynaec/o**/genic
(Am. **gynec/o**/genic)

ANATOMY EXERCISE

Now complete the Anatomy Exercise on page 206.

Abbreviations

You should learn common abbreviations related to the female reproductive system. Note, however, some are not standard and their meaning may vary from one health care setting to another. There is a more extensive list for reference on page 335.

CACX	cancer of the cervix
DUB	dysfunctional uterine bleeding
Gyn	gynaecology (Am. gynecology)
in utero	within the uterus
IUCD	intrauterine contraceptive device
IUFB	intrauterine foreign body
LMP	last menstrual period
Pap	Papanicolaou smear test
PMB	post-menopausal bleeding
PMS	premenstrual syndrome
PV	per vagina
VE	vaginal examination

Medical Notes

Endometriosis

Endometriosis is a growth of endometrial tissue outside the uterus, most commonly in the ovaries, uterine tubes and other pelvic structures. The ectopic tissue, like the uterine endometrium is responsive to the fluctuations in sex hormone levels of the menstrual cycle, causing menstrual type bleeding in the lower abdomen and the formation of chocolate coloured cysts in the ovaries. There is intermittent pain due to swelling, and recurrent haemorrhage (Am. hemorrhage) causes fibrous tissue formation. Ovarian endometriosis may lead to pelvic inflammation, infertility and extensive pelvic adhesions, involving the ovaries, uterus, uterine ligaments and the bowel. The cause is not clear but may be due to abnormal cell differentiation during fetal development or spread of endometrial cells through the uterine tubes, blood or lymph.

Ovarian cancer

The majority of ovarian tumours (Am. tumors) are benign and usually occur in patients between twenty and forty-five years of age. The remainder occur mostly between the ages of forty-five and sixty-five years and are divided between borderline malignancy and malignancy. Three main types of cell form ovarian tumours, epithelial cells, germ cells and hormone secreting cells.

Epithelial cell tumours are borderline malignant or malignant tumours that vary in size from small to large and some may be cystic. Large tumours cause pressure on other organs leading to gastrointestinal disturbances, dysuria and formation of ascites. The principle methods of spread are invasion of local and peritoneal structures and through the lymph and blood. The prevalence of this type of cancer is higher in developed societies and in higher socio-economic groups.

Germ cell ovarian tumours occur in children and young adults and only a few are malignant.

Sex-cord stroma cell tumours develop from cells lining the ovarian follicles, luteal cells or fibrous supporting cells. Mixed tumours can also develop, some of which secrete sex hormones causing precocious sexual development in children.

Ovarian cysts

Ovarian cysts are fluid-filled sacs that are retained within the ovary. They may be benign or malignant and often originate in the ovarian follicles (follicular cysts) or corpus luteum (luteal cysts). If untreated ovarian cysts can swell to a large size creating an acute surgical emergency.

Pelvic inflammatory disease (PID)

Pelvic inflammatory disease is an acute inflammatory condition caused by bacterial infection, it can involve the uterus, uterine tubes or ovaries. PID is most commonly caused by gonorrhoea (Am. gonorrhea) and chlamydial infections that spread upward from the vagina. The condition may be accompanied by pain and fever or there may be no symptoms at all. Early treatment of PID with antibiotics can stop its spread but delay can lead to serious complications, including infertility resulting from obstruction or other damage to the reproductive tract. The infection may also spread to other tissues including the blood where it may cause septic shock and death.

Sexually transmitted disease (STD)

Sexually transmitted diseases or venereal diseases are infections caused by communicable pathogens such as viruses, bacteria, fungi and protozoa. The factor that links all these diseases and gives this disease category is the fact that they can all be transmitted by sexual contact. The term sexual contact refers to sexual intercourse in addition to any contact between the genitals of one person and the body of another. Diseases classified as STDs are not always transmitted sexually, for example HIV can also be transmitted by blood transfusion or by contact with contaminated needles and syringes. Other common STDs include gonorrhoea (Am. gonorrhea), syphylis, genital herpes and chlamydia.

Medical terms relating to pregnancy, birth and lactation

The successful entry of a sperm into an egg at fertilization is known as **conception** and it is this event that creates a new individual. The fertilized egg then divides and forms into a ball of cells (the blastocyst) that must implant into the lining (endometrium) of the uterus to complete its development. **Pregnancy** begins when implantation is complete.

Occasionally a blastocyst implants and grows outside the uterus (extrauterine development). When this occurs it is known as an **ectopic** pregnancy. The most common site is the Fallopian tube and a pregnancy here is life threatening to the mother as the tube cannot stretch to accommodate the developing fetus. Eventually the tube ruptures causing severe haemorrhage (Am. hemorrhage) and a surgical emergency.

Following implantation in a normal pregnancy a structure known as the **placenta** (from Latin meaning cake) forms. This is a vascular structure, developed about the third month of gestation and is attached to the wall of the uterus. Through the placenta the fetus is supplied with oxygen and nutrients and wastes are removed. The placenta is expelled as the afterbirth usually within 1 hour of delivery.

After approximately 9 months (**the period of gestation**) a baby is expelled from the mother's body by muscular contractions of the uterus. The onset of uterine contractions is termed labour (Am. labor) or **parturition**. The period immediately following birth is known as the **puerperium**, in which time the reproductive organs tend to revert to their original state. The terms **antepartum** and **postpartum** are also used to indicate the periods before and after birth. Antepartum is usually used to mean up to 3 months before birth.

The mammary glands become active in late pregnancy and following the birth of a baby when they produce milk. The process of secreting milk and the period in which milk is produced is called **lactation**.

ROOT

Gravida
*(From a Latin word **gravidus** meaning heavy or pregnant. Here, -gravida is used to describe a woman in relation to her pregnancies, e.g. gravida I (GI), a woman pregnant for the first time.)*

Combining form   -gravida

WORD EXERCISE 15

Using your Exercise Guide, find the meaning of:

(a) primi/**gravida**
(gravida I)

(b) secundi/**gravida**
(gravida II)

(c) multi/**gravida**
(more than twice)

ROOT

Para
(From a Latin word **parere***, meaning to bear/bring forth. Here, -para is used to describe a woman in relation to the number of her previous viable pregnancies.)*

Combining form -para

WORD EXERCISE 16

Without using your Exercise Guide, write the meaning of:

(a) primi/**para**
(Para I, primi/para can
be used synonymously
with uni/para (*uni* – one).)

(b) secundi/**para**

(c) multi/**para**

(d) nulli/**para**

Another word that refers to pregnancy is **cyesis** (from Greek *kyesis*, meaning conception). **Pseudocyesis** refers to a false pregnancy, i.e. signs and symptoms of early pregnancy, a result of an overwhelming desire to have a child.

ROOT

Fet
(From a Latin word **fetus***, meaning an unborn baby. Here fet/o means a fetus, the name given to a human embryo at 8 weeks following fertilization, i.e. when the organ systems have been laid down.)*

Combining form Fet/o

Note. Foetus is an alternative spelling of fetus. Once the usual spelling in British English, it is becoming less common.

WORD EXERCISE 17

Without using your Exercise Guide, write the meaning of:

(a) **fet/o**/logy

(b) **fet/o**/scope

(c) **fet/o**/placent/al

Using your Exercise Guide find the meaning of -toxic and -metry, then build words that mean:

(d) pertaining to poisoning
of the fetus

(e) measurement of the fetus

The part of the fetus that lies in the lower part of the uterus is known as the presenting part. In a normal birth the vertex of the skull forms the presenting part and it enters the birth canal first. If other parts enter first, e.g. the buttocks, they are known as **malpresentations**.

Various manoeuvres can be made to turn or change the position of the fetus in the uterus. The term **version** (from Latin *vertere*, meaning to turn) is used for these manoeuvres. Many types have been described, e.g.:

Cephalic version
changes the position of the fetus from breech (buttocks first) to cephalic (head first) towards the birth canal.

External version
changes the position of the fetus by manipulation through the abdominal wall.

Internal version
changes the position of the fetus by hand within the uterus.

ROOT

Amni
(From a Greek word **amnia***, meaning a bowl in which blood is caught. Here amni/o means the amnion, the fetal membrane that retains the amniotic fluid surrounding a developing fetus.)*

Combining form Amni/o

WORD EXERCISE 18

Using your Exercise Guide, find the meaning of:

(a) **amni/o**/tome

(b) feto/**amni/o**/tic

Without using your Exercise Guide, build words that mean:

(c) technique of cutting the amnion

(d) an instrument to visually examine the amnion

Without using your Exercise Guide, write the meaning of:

(e) **amni/o**/graphy

(f) **amni/o**/gram

(g) **amni/o**/centesis

Figure 82 shows the developing amnion and Figure 83 the position of the needle used to withdraw amniotic fluid during amniocentesis.

This procedure is used to remove amniotic fluid for analysis, to inject solutions that will induce abortion or infuse dyes for radiographic studies. Various fetal abnormalities can be detected by analysing the amniotic fluid, e.g. spina bifida. In this condition the vertebral arches fail to surround the spinal cord, exposing the cord and meninges which may protrude through the defective vertebrae. The disorder can be detected before birth by the presence of increased levels of alpha-fetoprotein (AFP) in the amniotic fluid. AFP is also raised when the fetus is anencephalic (without a brain).

Genetic disorders can also be identified by analysing the chromosomes present in cells sloughed off the developing fetus into the amniotic fluid, e.g. Down's syndrome (formerly known as mongolism). In this condition 47 chromosomes are present instead of the normal 46. Parents can use the information from amniocentesis to decide to continue a pregnancy or abort a defective fetus.

The outermost of the fetal membranes is known as the **chorion** (from Greek, meaning outer membrane). It develops extensions, known as villi, that become part of the placenta. The combining form **chori/o** is used to mean chorion (see Fig. 82).

Without using your Exercise Guide, write the meaning of:

(h) chori/o/**amnion**/ic

(i) chori/o/**amnion**/itis

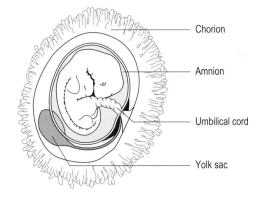

Figure 82 The amnion and related structures in a 5-week embryo

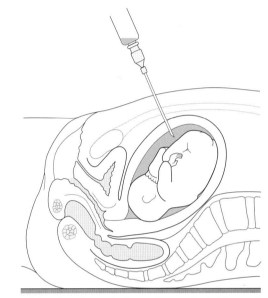

Figure 83 Amniocentesis performed at 15 weeks

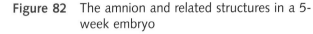

ROOT

Obstetric
(From a Latin word **obstetricare**, *meaning to assist in delivery. Here obstetr- means midwifery or obstetrics, the branch of medicine dealing with childbirth.)*

Combining forms **Obstetr-**

Obstetr- is mainly used in:

Obstetrics
The science dealing with the care of the pregnant woman during all stages of pregnancy and the period following birth.

Obstetrician
A medically qualified person who specializes in obstetrics (*-ician* meaning person associated with . . .). Often doctors specialize in obstetrics and gynaecology.

Obstetrical forceps
Large forceps consisting of two flat blades connected to a handle. They are used to pull on a fetal head or rotate it to facilitate vaginal delivery (Figs 84 and 85) (*-ical* means pertaining to).

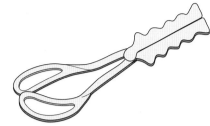

Figure 84 Obstetrical forceps

> **Adherent placenta**
> This placenta is fused to the uterine wall so that separation is slow and delivery of the placenta is delayed. When the placenta is not expelled it is known as a retained placenta.
>
> **Placenta praevia (Am. placenta previa)**
> This placenta forms abnormally in the lower part of the uterus over the internal opening of the cervix. The condition gives rise to haemorrhage (Am. hemorrhage) during pregnancy and threatens the life of the fetus.

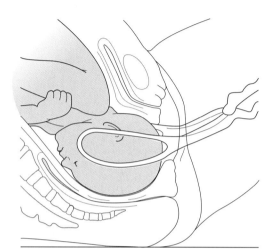

Figure 85 Obstetrical forceps in use

Another device used by obstetricians to assist delivery is the **vacuum extractor**. This suction device is attached to the head as it presents through the birth canal and is used to pull the baby out.

ROOT

Placent
*(From a Latin word **plakoenta**, meaning a flat cake. Here placent/o means the placenta, the temporary, hormone-secreting, vascular structure that facilitates the exchange of materials between the fetal and maternal blood.)*

Combining form **Placent/o**

WORD EXERCISE 19

Without using your Exercise Guide, build words that mean:

(a) technique of making an X-ray of the placenta

(b) any disease of the placenta

Many abnormalities of the placenta have been noted. Two common disorders are:

ROOT

Toc
*(From a Greek word **tokos**, meaning birth. Here toc/o means labour/childbirth (Am. labor).)*

Combining forms **Toc/o, tok/o**

WORD EXERCISE 20

Without using your Exercise Guide, write the meaning of:

(a) dys/**toc**/ia

(b) **toco**/logy
(synonymous with obstetrics)

Using your Exercise Guide, find the meaning of:

(c) eu/**toc**/ia

Labour (Am. labor) can be monitored by recording uterine contractions using a device called a **tocograph**; the procedure is known as **tocography**. When the fetal heart is monitored with the uterine contractions during delivery, it is known as **cardiotocography**.

If labour is late or slow, the uterus can be induced to produce forcible contractions by the administration of **oxytocin**, a hormone that is produced naturally by the pituitary gland. Various compounds with oxytocin-like activity are available for this purpose.

The period of 6–8 weeks following birth is known as the **puerperium** (from Latin *puerperus*, meaning childbearing). This is the time when the reproductive system involutes (reverts) to its state before pregnancy. **Puerperal** sepsis is a serious infection of the genital tract occurring within 21 days of abortion or childbirth.

Other problems can arise following birth, e.g.:

Postpartum haemorrhage
(Am. postpartum hemorrhage) excessive bleeding from the birth canal.

Eclampsia
a sudden convulsion due to pregnancy induced hypertension. The signs of pre-eclampsia include albuminuria, hypertension and oedema (Am. edema). See the medical notes on page 220.

ROOT

Nat
*(From a Latin word **natalis**, meaning birth.)*

Combining form **Nat/o**

WORD EXERCISE 21

Using your Exercise Guide, find the meaning of:

(a) neo/**nat**/al

(b) ante/**nat**/al

(c) peri/**nat**/al

Without using your Exercise Guide, write the meaning of:

(d) pre/**nat**/al

(e) neo/**nat**/o/logy
(A neonate is a newborn baby up to 1 month old.)

ROOT

Mamm
*(From a Latin word **mamma**, meaning breast. Here mamm/o means the breasts (mammary glands), the structures that secrete milk during lactation.)*

Combining form **Mamm/o**

WORD EXERCISE 22

Without using your Exercise Guide, write the meaning of:

(a) **mamm/o/graphy**

(b) **mamm/o/plasty**
(sometimes performed for cosmetic reasons to increase or decrease the size of breasts)

Using your Exercise Guide, find the meaning of:

(c) **mamm/o/tropic**

ROOT

Mast
*(From a Greek word **mastos**, meaning breast. Here mast/o means the breasts (mammary glands), the structures that secrete milk during lactation.)*

Combining form **Mast/o**

WORD EXERCISE 23

Without using your Exercise Guide, build words that mean:

(a) technique of making an X-ray of the breast

(b) surgical repair of the breast

(c) removal of the breast

There are two main forms of this operation:

- Simple mastectomy – removal of the breast and overlying skin

- Radical mastectomy – removal of the breast, overlying skin, underlying muscle and lymphatic tissue.

Some patients opt for the removal of a breast cancer (mastadenoma) by a simpler procedure known as a **lumpectomy**. In this procedure just the mass of abnormal cells is removed.

Without using your Exercise Guide, write the meaning of:

(d) **gynaec/o**/mast/ia
(Am. **gynec/o**/mast/ia; seen in males)

ROOT

Lact
*(From a Latin word **lactis**, meaning milk.)*

Combining forms **Lact/i/o**

WORD EXERCISE 24

Using your Exercise Guide, find the meaning of:

(a) **lact**/agogue

(b) **lact/i**/fer/ous

(c) **lact/o**/meter (for determining specific gravity)

(d) **lact/o**/troph/in (a hormone synonymous with prolactin)

(e) pro/**lact**/in (a hormone that acts on breasts)

(f) **lact/i**/fuge

Without using your Exercise Guide, write the meaning of:

(g) **lact/o**/genic

ROOT

Galact
(From a Greek word **gala**, meaning milk.)

Combining form   Galact/o

WORD EXERCISE 25

Without using your Exercise Guide, write the meaning of:

(a) **galact**/agogue

(b) **galact/o**/rrhoea
(Am. **galact/o**/rrhea; an abnormal condition)

(c) **galact**/ischia

(d) **galact/o**/poiesis

(d) culdoscopy
(e) fetoscope
(f) hysteroscope
(g) amniotome
(h) lactometer
(i) obstetrical forceps
(j) tocography

4. an instrument used to cut the amnion
5. an instrument used to view the vagina and cervix
6. an instrument used to measure the specific gravity of milk
7. a procedure used to examine cells from a cervical smear
8. an instrument used to assist the passage of a baby through the birth canal
9. an instrument used to hold the walls of the vagina apart
10. an instrument inserted into the amniotic cavity to visually examine a fetus

Medical equipment and clinical procedures

Revise the names of all instruments and clinical procedures mentioned in this unit before completing Exercise 26.

WORD EXERCISE 26

Match each term in Column A with a description from Column C by placing the appropriate number in Column B.

Column A	Column B	Column C
(a) vaginal speculum		1. technique of recording uterine contractions
(b) colposcope		2. an instrument used to view the uterus
(c) Pap test		3. technique of examining the peritoneal cavity via the vaginal fornix and rectouterine pouch

CASE HISTORY 16

The object of this exercise is to understand words associated with a patient's medical history.

To complete the exercise:

- read through the passage on pregnancy associated hypertension; unfamiliar words are underlined and you can find their meaning using the Word Help

- write the meaning of the medical terms shown in bold print on the lines that follow the Word Help.

Pregnancy associated hypertension

Mrs P, a **primigravida** aged 25, presented to her GP with 12 weeks of **amenorrhoea** (Am. amenorrhea); examination confirmed the dates of gestation. Her BP was at 120/80, her urine was sterile and showed no protein on dipstick testing.

Mrs P's pregnancy progressed normally until 35 weeks of gestation when her BP rose to 150/95 mmHg. She was admitted to the Obs-Gyn Unit for rest and observation. Serial ultrasound cephalometry was commenced and twice weekly 24 hour urine collection for oestrogen excretion estimation.

In addition, daily fetal **cardiotocography** was performed. All these tests were normal and her BP fell to 124/80 within 2 days of admission. After 5 days she was allowed home with instructions to rest and was seen weekly at **antenatal** clinic.

Antenatal investigations continued to be normal with evidence of good fetal growth until 3 days before term when her blood pressure increased to 155/95 and her urine was protein11. Over the next 24 hours her blood pressure was maintained and she had <u>proteinuria</u> of 3 g/24 hours. Vaginal examination showed a long cervix that was not dilated.

Mrs P had developed pregnancy associated <u>hypertension</u> or <u>pre-eclamptic toxaemia</u>, increasing the risk of **perinatal** <u>mortality</u>. The **obstetrician** considered performing a lower section Caesarean section (LSCS) since the risk becomes minimal after 24 hours of **puerperium**. Instead, the decision was taken to induce labour. Her cervix was dilated with a catheter left in place for 24 hours and partially ripened by local application of <u>prostaglandin</u>. Labour was induced by artificial rupture of the **amniotic** membranes and an infusion of <u>oxytocin</u>. After 8 hours she gave birth to a healthy male and her recovery was uneventful.

WORD HELP

BP blood pressure

dipstick testing tests using paper sticks coated with indicators that change colour when protein is present

gestation period of pregnancy

GP general practitioner (family doctor)

hypertension high blood pressure

mortality death rate

Obs-Gyn obstetrics and gynaecology (Am. gynecology)

oestrogen a female sex hormone (Am. estrogen)

oxytocin a hormone that stimulates uterine contractions (to induce birth)

pre-eclamptic condition before or leading to eclampsia, (due to toxaemia (Am. toxemia))

prostaglandin an agent that stimulates uterine contractions

proteinuria condition of protein in the urine

toxaemia the word means condition of poisoned blood, but refers to the toxic effects of eclampsia: high blood pressure, proteinuria etc. There is a risk of convulsion and toxic effects on the baby (Am. toxemia)

ultrasound cephalometry using ultrasound images to measure the size of the head

Now write the meaning of the following words from the case history without using your dictionary lists:

(a) primigravida

(b) amenorrhoea (Am. amenorrhea)

(c) cardiotocography

(d) antenatal

(e) perinatal

(f) obstetrician

(g) puerperium

(h) amniotic

(Answers to the case history exercise are given in the Answers to Word Exercises beginning on page 301)

Quick Reference

Combining forms relating to the female reproductive system:

Amni/o	amnion
Bartholin/o	greater vestibular glands/Bartholin's glands of the vagina
Cervic/o	cervix
Chori/o	chorion/outer fetal membrane
Colp/o	vagina
Culd/o	Douglas cavity/rectouterine pouch
Endometr/i	endometrium/lining of womb/uterus
Fet/o (Am.)	fetus
Galact/o	milk
-gravida	pregnancy/pregnant woman
Gynaec/o	female gynaecology
Gynec/o (Am.)	female gynaecology
Hyster/o	uterus
Lact/o/i	milk
Mamm/o	breast
Mast/o	breast
Men/o	menses/menstruation/monthly flow
Metr/o	uterus/womb
Nat/o	birth
Obstetric	pertaining to midwifery obstetrics
Oo-	egg
Oophor/o	ovary
Ovari/o	ovary
-para	to bear/bring forth offspring
Perine/o	perineum
Placent/o	placenta
Salping/o	Fallopian tube
Toc/o	labour (Am. labor)/birth
Trachel/o	neck
Uter/o	uterus
Vagin/o	vagina
Vulv/o	vulva

Abbreviations

Some common abbreviations related to obstetrics are listed below. Note some are not standard and their meaning may vary from one health care setting to another. There is a more extensive list for reference on page 335.

AB, ab, abor	abortion
AFP	alpha-fetoprotein
APH	antepartum haemorrhage (Am. hemorrhage)
BBA	born before arrival
C-Sect	caesarean section (Am. cesarean)
FDIU	fetal death in utero
GI and GII	gravida I and gravida II
IUD	intrauterine death /intrauterine device
LCCS	low cervical caesarean section (Am. cesarean)
LGA	large for gestational age
NFTD	normal full-term delivery
Obs-Gyn	obstetrics and gynaecology (Am. gynecology)

Medical Notes

Abortion

A *miscarriage* is the loss of an embryo or fetus before the twenty-fourth week of pregnancy. Technically known as a *spontaneous abortion*, the most common cause of such a loss is a structural or functional defect in the developing offspring. Other causes of spontaneous abortion include placental abnormalities, hypertension, hormonal imbalance and trauma. After twenty-four weeks delivery of a lifeless infant is termed a *stillbirth*.

Induced (non-spontaneous) abortion to intentionally terminate a pregnancy is brought on by methods such as vacuum aspiration and administration of prostaglandin preparations.

Birth defects

Birth defects, also called *congenital abnormalities*, include any structural or functional abnormality present at birth. Congenital defects may be inherited or may be acquired during gestation or delivery. Acquired defects result from agents called teratogens that disrupt normal development. Some teratogens are chemicals that can cross the placental barrier such as alcohol, antibiotics and other drugs. Viruses such as the rubella virus also cross the placenta and disrupt normal embryonic development. Exposure to ionizing radiation (X-rays etc.) and other physical factors also cause birth defects. Some teratogens damage the genetic code in the cells of the developing embryo.

Breast cancer

Approximately 90% of breast tumours (Am. tumors) are benign. Fibroadenomas are the commonest type and occur at any time after puberty; incidence peaks in the third decade. Some tumours are cystic and some solid and they usually occur in women nearing the menopause. The most common types of malignant tumour are usually painless lumps found in the upper outer quadrant of the breast. There is considerable fibrosis around the tumour that may cause retraction of the nipple and ulceration of the overlying skin.

Early spread beyond the breast is via the lymph to the axillary and internal mammary nodes. Local invasion involves the pectoral muscles and the pleura. Blood-spread metastases may occur later in many organs and bones, especially lumbar and thoracic vertebrae. The causes of breast cancer are not known but an important factor appears to be high oestrogen exposure. A genetic component is also likely, with close relatives of cancer sufferers having a significantly elevated risk of developing the disease. One per cent of all breast cancer occurs in men.

Implantation disorders

Placenta praevia (Am. previa)

In this condition the blastocyst implants in the uterine wall near the cervix or over the cervical os (opening). When this occurs, the normal dilation and softening of the cervix that occurs in the third trimester of pregnancy often causes painless bleeding as the placenta near the cervix separates from the uterine wall. The massive blood loss that may result can be life threatening for both mother and offspring.

Abruptio placentae

Separation of the placenta from the uterine wall can occur even when implantation takes place in the upper part of the uterus. When this occurs in a pregnancy of twenty weeks or more, the condition is called *abruptio placentae*. Complete separation of the placenta causes immediate death of the fetus. The severe haemorrhaging (Am. hemorrhaging) sometimes hidden in the uterus may cause circulatory shock and death of the mother within minutes. A caesarean (Am. cesarean) section and sometimes hysterectomy must be performed immediately to prevent blood loss and death.

Preeclampsia

It is not uncommon for a woman's blood pressure to rise during pregnancy and remain elevated until the end of pregnancy; this condition is called pregnancy induced hypertension (PIH) or pregnancy associated hypertension. In about six to eight percent of all pregnancies PIH may progress to a condition called preeclampsia formerly known as *toxaemia of pregnancy (Am. toxemia)*. This serious disorder is characterized by the onset of acute hypertension after the twenty-fourth week and is accompanied by proteinuria and oedema (Am. edema). The causes of PIH and preeclampsia are largely unknown but a gene that regulates salt balance may also be involved in raising blood pressure during pregnancy. Preeclampsia can result in complications such as abruptio placentae, stroke, haemorrhage (Am. hemorrhage), fetal malnutrition and low birth weight. The condition can progress to *eclampsia*, a form of PIH that causes severe convulsions, coma, kidney failure and perhaps death of the fetus and mother.

Puerperal fever

Puerperal fever or *childbed fever* is a syndrome of postpartum mothers characterized by a bacterial infection that progresses to septicaemia (Am. septicemia) and possibly death. The infection originates in the birth canal and spreads to the endometrium and other pelvic structures. Modern aseptic techniques prevent most postpartum infections and those that occur are usually successfully treated with intensive antibiotic therapy.

NOW TRY THE WORD CHECK

WORD CHECK

This self-check exercise lists all the word components used in this unit. First write down the meaning of as many word components as you can. Then check your answers using the Exercise Guide and Quick Reference box or the Glossary of Word Components (pp. 347–371).

Prefixes

a-

ante-

dys-

endo-

eu-

extra-

micro-

multi-

neo-

nulli-

oligo-

peri-

post-

pre-

primi-

pro-

pseudo-

secundi-

Combining forms of word roots

amni/o

bartholin/o

cardi/o

cervic/o

chori/o

colp/o

culd/o

cyst/o

cyt/o

fer/o

fet/o

fibr/o

galact/o

-gravida

gynaec/o
(Am. gynec/o)

haem/o
(Am. hem/o)

hyster/o

lact/o

mamm/o

mast/o

men/o

metr/o

myc/o

nat/o

obstetr-

oo-

oophor/o

ovari/o

-para

perine/o

peritone/o

phleb/o

placent/o

rect/o

salping/o

sten/o

toc/o

trachel/o

uter/o

vagin/o

vesic/o

vulv/o

Suffixes

-a

-agogue

-al

-algia

-arche

-blast

-cele

-centesis

-dynia

-ectomy

-fuge

-genesis

-genic

-gram

-graphy

-ia

-ic

-ischia

-itis

-lithiasis

-logy

-malacia

-meter

-metry

-natal

-osis

-ous

-pathia

-pathy

-pause

-pexy

-plasty

-poiesis

-ptosis

-rrhagic

-rrhaphy

-rrhexis

-rrhoea
(Am. -rrhea)

-sclerosis

-scope

-scopy

-staxis

-stenosis

-stomy

-tome

-tomy

-toxic

-trophic

-tropic

-tubal

NOW TRY THE SELF-ASSESSMENT

SELF-ASSESSMENT

Test 16A

Below are some combining forms that refer to the anatomy of the female reproductive system. Indicate which part of the system they refer to by putting a number from the diagrams (Figs 86 and 87) next to each word.

(a) oophor/o

(b) salping/o

(c) hyster/o

(d) endometr/o

(e) cervic/o

(f) colp/o

(g) vulv/o

(h) culd/o

Score 8

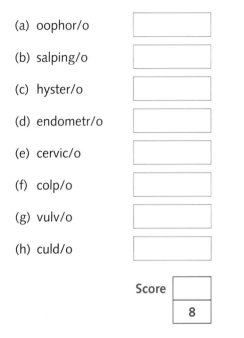

Figure 86 Sagittal section through the female showing the reproductive system

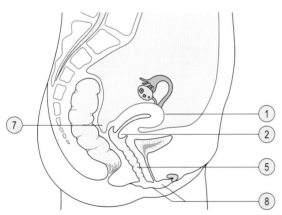

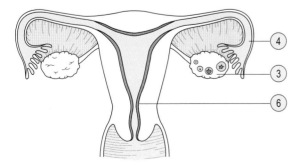

Figure 87 The female reproductive system

Test 16B

Prefixes and suffixes

Match each prefix and suffix in Column A with a meaning in Column C by inserting the appropriate number in Column B.

Column A	Column B	Column C
(a) -agogue		1. to drip (blood)
(b) ante-		2. pertaining to birth
(c) eu-		3. stop/pause
(d) -ischia		4. new
(e) multi-		5. stimulate/induce
(f) -natal		6. after
(g) neo-		7. few/little
(h) nulli-		8. condition of bursting forth (of blood)
(i) oligo-		9. pertaining to tube/oviduct
(j) -ous		10. before (i)
(k) -pause		11. before (ii)
(l) -pexy		12. good
(m) post-		13. fixation by surgery
(n) pre-		14. pertaining to stimulating
(o) primi-		15. pertaining to
(p) -rrhagia		16. second
(q) secundi-		17. none
(r) -staxis		18. first
(s) -tropic		19. condition of blocking/holding back
(t) -tubal		20. many

Score 20

Test 16C

Combining forms of word roots

Match each combining form in Column A with a meaning in Column C by inserting the appropriate number in Column B.

Column A	Column B	Column C
(a) cervic/o		1. woman
(b) colp/o		2. breast (i)
(c) culd/o		3. breast (ii)
(d) -gravida		4. menstruation/monthly
(e) gynaec/o (Am. gynec/o)		5. birth
(f) hyster/o		6. vulva (external genitalia)
(g) lact/o		7. placenta
(h) mamm/o		8. pregnant/pregnant woman
(i) mast/o		9. perineum/area between anus and vulva
(j) men/o		10. midwifery/specialty of obstetrics
(k) metr/o		11. to bear/bring forth baby
(l) nat/o		12. uterus (i)
(m) obstetr-		13. uterus (ii)
(n) oo-		14. uterus (iii)
(o) oophor/o		15. neck (of uterus)
(p) ovari/o		16. Douglas pouch/ rectouterine cavity
(q) -para		17. vagina (i)
(r) perine/o		18. vagina (ii)
(s) placent/o		19. egg
(t) salping/o		20. ovary (i)
(u) trachel/o		21. ovary (ii)
(v) uter/o		22. cervix uteri
(w) vagin/o		23. Fallopian tube

Column A	Column B	Column C
(x) vesic/o		24. milk
(y) vulv/o		25. bladder

Score [ ] / 25

Test 16D

Write the meaning of:

(a) tocometer

(b) oophorohysterectomy

(c) mastopexy

(d) hysterorrhexis

(e) metropathy

Score [ ] / 5

Test 16E

Build words that mean:

(a) surgical repair of the Douglas pouch/rectouterine pouch

(b) formation of an opening into a Fallopian tube

(c) rupture of the amnion

(d) displacement/prolapse of the vagina (use colp/o)

(e) study of cells of the vagina (use colp/o)

Score [ ] / 5

Check answers to Self-Assessment Tests on page 325.

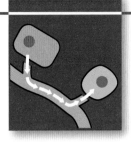

OBJECTIVES

Once you have completed Unit 17 you should be able to:

- understand the meaning of medical words relating to the endocrine system
- build medical words relating to the endocrine system

- associate medical terms with their anatomical position
- understand medical abbreviations relating to the endocrine system.

EXERCISE GUIDE

Use this list of word components and their meanings to complete the word exercises in this unit.

Prefixes

acro-	extremities/point
hyper-	above normal/excessive
hypo-	below normal/deficient
para-	beside/near

Roots/Combining forms

aden/o	gland
blast/o	germ cell/cell that forms . . .
chondr/o	cartilage
gloss/o	tongue
-gyne	woman
kal/i	potassium
natr/i	sodium

Suffixes

-aemia	condition of blood Am. -emia)
-al	pertaining to
-ectomy	removal of
-emia (Am.)	condition of blood

-genesis	formation of
-genic	pertaining to formation/ originating in
-globulin	protein
-ia	condition of
-ic	pertaining to
-ism	process of/state or condition
-itis	inflammation of
-megaly	enlargement
-micria	condition of small size
-oma	tumour (Am. tumor)/swelling
-osis	abnormal condition/disease of
-plasia	condition of growth/formation of (cells)
-ptosis	falling/displacement/prolapse
-static	pertaining to stopping/controlling
-tomy	incision into
-toxic	pertaining to poisoning
-trophic	pertaining to nourishment
-tropic	pertaining to affinity for/ stimulating
-uresis	excrete in urine/urinate
-uria	condition of urine

ANATOMY EXERCISE

When you have finished Word Exercises 1–6, look at the word components listed below. Complete Figure 88 by writing the appropriate combining form on each dotted line – more than one component may relate to the same position. (You can check their meanings in the Quick Reference box on p. 232.)

Adren/o	Orchid/o	Parathyroid/o
Adrenocortic/o	Ovari/o	Pituitar-
Hypophys-	Pancreat/o	Thyr/o
Oophor/o		

The endocrine system

The endocrine system is composed of a diverse group of glands that secrete hormones directly into the blood. Once released, the hormones travel in the blood plasma to all parts of the body and act as chemical 'messengers'. Low concentrations of hormones in the blood stimulate specific target tissues and exert a regulatory effect on their cellular processes (metabolism). They do this by attaching to receptors on the surface of target cells or within their cytoplasm and this action triggers chemical changes within the cell. To summarize their action:

The endocrine gland secretes a hormone directly into the blood → The hormone travels around the body in the blood plasma → The target tissue responds to the hormone by altering its metabolism

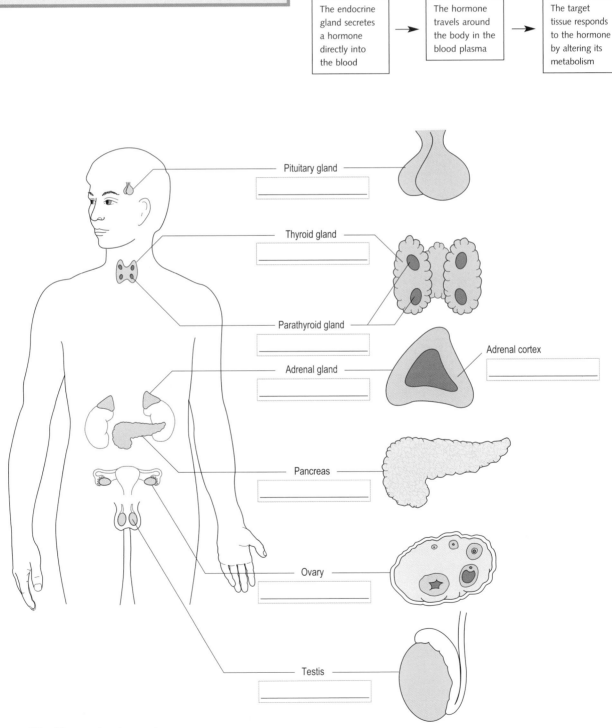

Figure 88   The endocrine system

The brain and the endocrine glands precisely regulate the concentration of hormones that circulate in the blood. Many endocrine disorders are brought about by changes in the output of hormones. Abnormal levels of hormones produce symptoms that range from minor to severely disabling disease and death.

In this unit we will examine terms associated with each endocrine gland.

Use the Exercise Guide at the beginning of this unit to complete Word Exercises 1–6 unless you are asked to work without it.

The pituitary gland

ROOT

Pituitar
(From a Latin word **pituita**, *meaning slime/phlegm. Here -pituitar- means the pituitary gland, a small structure that grows from the base of the brain on a stalk. It is commonly called the 'master' gland of the endocrine system because it releases tropic hormones that regulate other endocrine glands.)*

Combining form **-pituitar-**

(**-pituitar**ism is used when referring to the process of pituitary secretion.)

WORD EXERCISE 1

Using your Exercise Guide, find the meaning of:

(a) hypo/**pituitar**/ism

(b) hyper/**pituitar**/ism

One of the hormones produced by the pituitary gland is somatotrophin or human growth hormone (HGH). Underproduction of this results in **acromicria** and **dwarfism**. Overproduction of growth hormone produces **acromegaly** and **giantism** (see the Medical Notes on page 232).

(c) acro/micria

(d) acro/megaly

Once it was realized that the pituitary gland is not the source of spit and phlegm, scientists renamed the gland the **hypophysis** (*hypo* – below, *physis* – growth, i.e. a growth below the brain). Pituitary and hypophysis are now used synonymously. The hypophysis consists of a down-growth from the brain, known as the neurohypophysis, and attached to it a glandular part, known as the adenohypophysis.

Removal of the hypophysis is known as **hypophys/ectomy**.

The thyroid gland

ROOT

Thyr
(From a Greek word **thyreoidos**, *meaning resembling a shield. Here thyr/o and thyroid/o mean the thyroid gland, the shield-shaped gland that lies above the trachea. It secretes the thyroid hormones tri-iodothyronine (T_3) and thyroxine (T_4), that control the metabolic rate of all cells.)*

Combining forms **Thyr/o, thyroid/o**

WORD EXERCISE 2

Using your Exercise Guide, find the meaning of:

(a) **thyr**/o/gloss/al

(b) **thyr**/o/aden/itis

(c) **thyr**/o/globulin

(d) **thyr**/o/chondr/o/tomy

(e) **thyr**/o/toxic/osis
(Graves' disease, generally replaced by the term hyper/thyroid/ism)

A symptom of this disorder is **exophthalmos**, protruding eyes. The extent of this can be measured using a technique known as **exophthalmometry**.

(f) para**thyroid**

(This refers to the parathyroid glands that lie on the posterior surface of the thyroid gland (para-meaning beside or near). The parathyroid glands consist of four small glands that secrete parathyroid hormone (PTH).)

(g) **parathyroid**/ectomy

Without using your Exercise Guide, write the meaning of:

(h) hyper/**parathyroid**/ism
(leads to excess calcium in blood, hyper/calc/aemia; Am. hyper/calc/emia)

(i) **thyr**/o/megaly

Without using your Exercise Guide, build words that mean:

(j) process of secreting above normal levels of thyroid hormone

(k) process of secreting below normal levels of thyroid hormone

In infants this results in poor growth and mental retardation and is known as **congenital hypothyroidism** (formerly cretinism). It is caused by deficient secretion of thyroid hormones (T_3 and T_4) and the condition becomes evident within a few weeks or months of birth. Unless treatment begins early in life, the individual remains severely affected.

In adults the condition is known as **hypothyroidism** or **myxoedema**, (Am. myxedema), the latter term referring to the accumulation of mucopolysaccarides under the skin. Hypothyroidism is a result of below normal secretion of thyroid hormones T_3 and T_4 in adults. It gives rise to 'puffy' swollen skin, dry hair, weight-gain, bradycardia, sensitivity to cold, lethargy and loss of mental and physical vigour.

Using your Exercise Guide find the meaning of -genic, -ptosis and -tropic, then build words that mean:

(l) downward displacement of the thyroid

(m) pertaining to affinity for the thyroid gland

(n) pertaining to originating in the thyroid gland

Any enlargement of the thyroid gland is known as **goitre** (Am. **goiter**) and is a feature of several thyroid diseases. There are various types of goitre that have been grouped in different ways, three main types are:

Simple goitre (Am. goiter)
A goitre that is not producing the signs and symptoms of hyperthyroidism. Simple goitre is still common in areas of the world where the soil and water contain little iodine. As the diets in these areas are severely deficient in iodine, there is insufficient iodine for synthesis of thyroid hormones (T_3 and T_4).

Toxic goitre (Am. goiter)
A goitre that is producing the signs and symptoms of hyperthyroidism. Also known as hyperthyroiditis, exophthalmic goitre and Graves' disease.

Malignant goitre (Am. goiter)
A goitre that is the seat of new, malignant growth (carcinoma of the thyroid).

Thyroid goitre is investigated by the administration of radioactive iodine. The iodine is taken up by the thyroid gland making it slightly radioactive. The presence of radioactivity is then detected with a scanner that creates

an image of its distribution within the gland. Areas that are very active will take up more radiation and will be visible on the scan.

We will look at this in more detail in Unit 18.

The pancreas

We have already examined the role of the pancreas in digestion in Unit 2; here we examine its role as an endocrine gland. Among the cells in the pancreas that produce digestive enzymes, are small patches of tissue called the **Islets of Langerhans**. The Islets secrete the hormones **insulin** and **glucagon** directly into the blood; these play a major role in the regulation of blood glucose concentration.

ROOT

Pancreat
*(Derived from Greek **pankreas**, pan – all, kreas – flesh. Here pancreat/o means the pancreas, a large endocrine gland situated below and behind the stomach.)*

Combining form **Pancreat/o**

WORD EXERCISE 3

Without using your Exercise Guide, write the meaning of:

(a) **pancreat/o/tropic**
(Some of the pituitary hormones have such an action.)

Insulin (from Latin *insula*, meaning island) is secreted by the Islets of Langerhans. Once in the bloodstream, it stimulates the uptake of sugar (glucose) by tissue cells. Blood glucose rises following intake and digestion of carbohydrate, the overall effect of insulin is to lower blood glucose levels in the body after meals. The combining form derived from this **insulin/o** means insulin or the Islets of Langerhans.

Using your Exercise Guide, find the meaning of:

(b) **insulin/o/genesis**

(c) **insulin/oma**

Without using your Exercise Guide, write the meaning of:

(d) **insulin/itis**

(e) **hyper/insulin/ism**

If the body fails to produce insulin, blood glucose concentration rises and glucose appears in the urine; this abnormal condition is known as **diabetes mellitus**. The name diabetes is derived from two Greek words, one meaning a siphon and the other meaning to pass through. The name reflects the most obvious symptoms; excessive thirst (**polydipsia**) followed by drinking and excessive urination (**polyuria**), just like the passing of water through a siphon. The second name mellitus is a Latin word meaning honey, the substance originally used as a sweetener instead of sugar. Diabetes mellitus refers to the passing of large quantities of water containing sugar through the body.

(**Polydipsia** is formed from *poly* – meaning too much, *dips/o* – thirst and *-ia* condition of).

There are two main types of diabetes mellitus:

Type I, insulin-dependent diabetes mellitus (IDDM)
This occurs mainly in children and young adults and the onset is usually sudden. The condition is characterized by deficiency or absence of insulin due to the destruction of the β-islet cells that produce insulin in the pancreas. As insulin is required to treat this disorder throughout life, it is called insulin-dependent diabetes mellitus. It is also called *juvenile onset diabetes* because it commonly arises in those under twenty years of age. The cause is unknown but those affected have a genotype that makes them more susceptible. In many cases, an autoimmune reaction has occurred in which autoantibodies to β-islet cells are present. Without insulin treatment, IDDM is fatal.

Type II, non-insulin dependent diabetes mellitus (NIDDM)
This is the most common form of diabetes accounting for about 90% of cases. Type II is also called *maturity-onset diabetes* as it tends to develop in women over seventy-five years of age and men over sixty-five who are obese. Many type II diabetics secrete sufficient amounts of insulin into the blood but their cells are less sensitive to insulin. For this reason type II diabetes is known as non-insulin dependent diabetes and can usually be controlled by dietary changes, exercise and/or administration of antidiabetic drugs. The cause is unknown and insulin secretion may be above or below normal.

Complications of diabetes mellitus include a tendency to develop cataracts, retinopathy and neuropathy. Blood glucose estimation and glucose tolerance tests are used to diagnose the condition. The latter test involves administering a known quantity of glucose and measuring the amounts that appear in the blood and urine in a set time.

Below are terms that can be used to describe sugar (glucose) levels in blood and urine. The combining form **glyc/o/s** is used to mean sugar (from Greek *glykys*, meaning sweet).

Using your Exercise Guide, find the meaning of:

(f) hypo/**glyc**/aemia
(Am. hypo/glyc/emia)

(g) hyper/**glyc**/aemia
(Am. hyper/glyc/emia)

(h) **glycos**/uria
(Patients can estimate the state of their own blood sugar level from the amount present in their urine. Glucose oxidase papers are used to test for glucose in the urine; they change colour in the presence of glucose.)

(i) **glyc/o**/static

Untreated diabetes results in the tissue cells using fatty acids as a source of energy instead of glucose. This leads to the release of chemicals known as ketones into the blood and urine. Ketones such as acetone, have a toxic effect on the body and produces a condition known as **ketosis**. Accumulation of ketones can lead to an increase acidity of the blood (**ketoacidosis**) and this may be fatal in uncontrolled diabetes.

The adrenal gland

ROOT

Adren
*(From Latin **ad** – to/near, **renes** – kidneys. Here adren/o means the adrenal gland, a small triangle-shaped gland that lies above a kidney. The inner part of the gland called the medulla, secretes adrenalin, the outer part called the cortex, secretes steroid hormones.)*

Combining form **Adren/o**

WORD EXERCISE 4

Without using your Exercise Guide, build words that mean:

(a) an enlarged adrenal gland

(b) pertaining to poisonous to the adrenal gland

(c) pertaining to stimulating/ acting on the adrenal gland

The adrenal cortex forms the outer layer of the adrenal gland; it produces a variety of steroid hormones (**steroidogenesis**). There are three main types:

Androgens
types of male sex hormone.

Glucocorticoids
hormones that control glucose, protein and lipid metabolism.

Mineralocorticoids
hormones that regulate fluid and electrolyte balance.

Aldosterone is an example of a mineralocorticoid. It enables the body to retain sodium and excrete potassium. Abnormal aldosterone production results in the disturbances of sodium and potassium levels named in (d), (e) and (f) below.

Using your Exercise Guide, find the meaning of:

(d) hyper/natr/aemia
(Am. hyper/natr/emia)

(e) hypo/kal/aemia
(Am. hypo/kal/emia)

(f) natr/i/uresis

The combining form **adrenocortic/o** is used when referring to the adrenal cortex itself. Corticosteroid refers to the steroid hormones of the adrenal cortex.

(g) **adrenocortic/o/trophic**
(ACTH produced by the pituitary has this effect.)

(h) **adrenocortic/o/hyper/plasia**

Three major endocrine disorders caused by abnormal secretion of hormones from the adrenal cortex include:

Cushing's disease
A rare disorder mainly affecting females in which over-production of adrenocorticotrophic hormone (ACTH) by the pituitary stimulates the adrenal cortex to release steroid hormones; these raise blood pressure, increase sodium retention and bring about hyperglycaemia (Am. hyperglycemia). Other signs and symptoms include obesity, moon face, muscle wastage, acne, hirsutism and psychotic disturbances. (*Cushing's syndrome* is a clinically similar disorder caused by tumours (Am. tumors) of the adrenal cortex or secretion of ACTH by non-endocrine tumours).

Adrenogenital syndrome
This condition is also called *adrenal virilism* and is due to over-production of male sex hormones (androgens) by the adrenal gland. When present at birth, there is premature sexual development, the female develops an

enlarged clitoris and may be confused with a male. The male child may develop pubic hair and an enlarged penis. In both sexes there is rapid growth, muscularity and advanced bone age.

Adrenal tumours (Am. tumors) or adrenal hyperplasia (increase in number of cells) can cause this condition to develop in adult women. When this occurs, it is characterized by the appearance of secondary male characteristics (virilism). Symptoms include hirsutism (excessive hair growth in the male pattern on the face and body) amenorrhoea (Am. amenorrhea), acne and deepening of the voice.

Addison's disease (chronic adrenal cortex insufficiency)
A condition due to the failure of the adrenal cortex to produce sufficient glucocorticoids and mineralocorticoids. The most common cause of this condition is development of antibodies to cells of the adrenal cortex. It results in loss of sodium and water, and a fall in blood pressure. Patients will die within 4–14 days unless given specific hormone replacement therapy.

The ovary and testis

The ovary and the testis are endocrine organs as well as reproductive organs. In their endocrine role they produce sex hormones that function to control the development of the reproductive system and maintain its activity. Note that we have already used the combining forms for the ovary (oophor/o and ovari/o) and testis (orchid/o) in Units 15 and 16.

First, let's examine the endocrine role of the testis. This gland secretes male sex hormones called **androgens** that stimulate the development of the male reproductive tract and secondary sexual characteristics such as beard growth, a deep voice and the male physique. The main androgen produced by the testis is **testosterone**; it is also produced in small quantities by the adrenal cortex of both men and women. In women excess secretion leads to virilism (masculinization), one obvious effect being the growth of facial hair (hirsutism).

ROOT —————————————————

Andr
(From a Greek word **aner**, *meaning man/male.)*

Combining form **Andr/o**

WORD EXERCISE 5

Using your Exercise Guide, find the meaning of:

(a) **andr/o/gyn/ous**

(b) **andr/o/blast/oma**

The ovary is also an endocrine gland secreting several types of sex hormone, for example:

Oestrogens (Am. estrogens)
Steroid hormones that regulate the development of the female reproductive tract, menstrual cycle and secondary sexual characteristics, such as the growth of pubic hair and breasts. Compounds that have oestrogen-like actions on the body are described as **oestrogenic** (Am. estrogenic).

Progestogens
Steroid hormones that maintain the receptivity of the uterus to fertilized eggs and stimulate the growth of the uterus during pregnancy.

Medical equipment and clinical procedures

Revise the names of medical equipment and clinical procedures mentioned in this unit and then try Exercise 6. Some imaging techniques used for examining the endocrine system will be studied in Unit 18 as they are similar to those used for other systems.

WORD EXERCISE 6

Match each term in Column A with a description from Column C by placing an appropriate number in Column B.

Column A	Column B	Column C
(a) adrenal function test		1. imaging of the thyroid gland following administration of radioactive iodine
(b) glucose tolerance test		2. a test for hypothyroidism by measuring concentration of iodine in blood
(c) protein bound iodine test (PBI)		3. a test used to diagnose diabetes mellitus
(d) glucose oxidase paper strip test (Clinistix)		4. measurement of the 24-hour output of corticosteroids
(e) thyroid scan		5. a simple test that indicates the relative amount of glucose in urine

ANATOMY EXERCISE

Now complete the Anatomy Exercise on page 226.

CASE HISTORY 17

The object of this exercise is to understand words associated with a patient's medical history.

To complete the exercise:

• read through the passage on diabetes mellitus; unfamiliar words are underlined and you can find their meaning using the Word Help

• write the meaning of the medical terms shown in bold print on the lines that follow the Word Help.

Diabetes mellitus

W, a 14-year-old boy on holiday in the locality, was brought into Accident and Emergency by his worried parents. Prior to admission he had complained of tiredness and insomnia, and his mother had noticed that despite a good appetite he had become thinner. On the morning of admission he suffered abdominal pain, nausea and vomiting, his breathing had become irregular and at times he appeared semiconscious. Further questioning of the parents indicated the patient had recently developed polydipsia and **polyuria**.

On admission he was conscious and hyperventilating; he was dehydrated and his breath had the fruity odour of ketones. Blood and urine samples were analysed and quickly indicated clinically significant levels of **glycosuria**, **hyperglycaemia** and **ketonaemia**. W's condition was diagnosed as diabetic **ketoacidosis** and emergency treatment was commenced.

Vital signs on admission

Pulse	Oral temp	BP
98 per minute	36.0°C	110/70
Blood glucose 28 mmol/L	Urine 3+ ketones	Hyperventilating

He was given an initial intravenous infusion of 6 units of soluble insulin followed by 6 units hourly. His fluid and electrolyte loss were replaced by an intravenous saline infusion. His blood glucose was monitored hourly and electrolytes 2 hourly in the initial phase of treatment. When his blood glucose reached its normal value, he was given a saline infusion of 5% dextrose containing 20 mmol/L KCl. The dose of insulin was adjusted according to the hourly blood glucose results.

W's parents were informed their son was suffering from Type 1 diabetes mellitus also known as insulin-dependent diabetes mellitus (IDDM), a chronic incurable condition brought on by a failure of the **pancreatic** islets to produce insulin.

Once recovered from his acute attack he was referred to the diabetic clinician for advice on insulin therapy and his GP was informed. He responded well to advice, and now self-administers two daily injections of insulin. His <u>regimen</u> was adjusted to avoid **hypoglycaemia** and give good **glycaemic** control. Both injections consist of a mixture of short and intermediate-acting insulin, the first before breakfast and the second before his evening meal.

WORD HELP

clinician an expert on treating and advising patients

chronic lasting/lingering for a long time

electrolyte the ionized salts in the blood (e.g. sodium and potassium ions)

GP general practitioner (family doctor)

hyperventilating above normal ventilation rate of the lungs (rapid deep breathing)

insomnia condition of inability to sleep

insulin a hormone secreted by the pancreas that lowers blood sugar

islets small islands of cells that secrete insulin in the pancreas (Islets of Langerhans)

ketones ketone bodies (chemicals formed in diabetes from breakdown of fat)

polydipsia condition of too much/excessive thirst

regimen a regulated scheme (e.g. of taking drugs/medication)

Now write the meaning of the following words from the case history without using your dictionary lists:

(a) polyuria

(b) glycosuria

(c) hyperglycaemia (Am. hyperglycemia)

(d) ketonaemia (Am. ketonemia)

(e) ketoacidosis

(f) pancreatic

(g) hypoglycaemia (Am. hypoglycemia)

(h) glycaemic (Am. glycemic)

(Answers to the case history exercise are given in the Answers to Word Exercises beginning on page 401)

Quick Reference

Combining forms relating to the endocrine system:

Aden/o	gland
Adren/o	adrenal gland
Adrenocortic/o	adrenal cortex
Andr/o	male
Cortic/o	cortex
Estr/o (Am.)	estrogen
-globulin	protein
Glyc/o	sugar
Hypophys-	hypophysis/pituitary gland
Insulin/o	insulin/Islet of Langerhans
Kal/i	potassium
Ket/o	ketones
Natr/i	sodium
Oestr/o	oestrogen (Am. estr/o)
Oophor/o	ovary
Orchid/o	testis
Ovari/o	ovary
Pancreat/o	pancreas
Parathyroid/o	parathyroid gland
Pituitar-	pituitary
Progest/o	progesterone
Thyr/o	thyroid gland

Abbreviations

Some common abbreviations related to the endocrine system are listed below. Note some are not standard and their meaning may vary from one health care setting to another. There is a more extensive list for reference on page 335.

ACTH	adrenocorticotrophic hormone
BSS	blood sugar series
FSH	follicle-stimulating hormone
HGH	human growth hormone
HRT	hormone replacement therapy
IDDM	Insulin-dependent diabetes mellitus
LH	luteinizing hormone
NIDDM	non-insulin-dependent diabetes mellitus
OGTT	oral glucose tolerance test
PRL	prolactin
T_3, T_4	tri-iodothyronine, tetraiodothyronine (thyroxine)
TSH	thyroid stimulating hormone

Medical Notes

Acromegaly

Hypersecretion of human growth hormone (HGH) after skeletal fusion has occurred in adults' results in acromegaly. In this condition, excess HGH causes bones to become abnormally thick and leads to enlargement of the hands, feet, face and jaw.

Acromicria

A condition of smallness of the hands, nose, jaws and feet, probably due to deficiency of human growth hormone from the pituitary gland.

Diabetes insipidus

A condition due to under secretion of anti-diuretic hormone (ADH) caused by damage to the pituitary gland or hypothalamus. Lack of ADH results in failure of water reabsorption by the renal tubules of the kidneys leading to excessive excretion of urine, dehydration, and extreme thirst (polydipsia).

Dwarfism

Hyposecretion of human growth hormone (HGH) during growth years results in stunted body growth known as *pituitary dwarfism*. In this condition the epiphyseal plates of long bones ossify before normal height is reached and other organs fail to grow to their normal size.

Giantism

Hypersecretion of human growth hormone (HGH) while epiphyseal cartilages of long bones are still growing and before their ossification is complete results in giantism. The bones of the limbs are particularly affected and individuals may grow to heights of 2.1–2.4 metres although body proportions remain normal.

Graves' disease (exophthalmic goitre)

Graves' disease accounts for 90% of cases of hyperthyroidism or thyrotoxicosis in which body tissues are exposed excessive levels of thyroid hormones (T_3 and T_4). The main signs and symptoms are due to an increased basal metabolic rate and patients may suffer from weight loss, nervousness, increased heart rate and exophthalmos (protruding eyes). In Graves' disease, autoantibodies mimic the action of thyroid stimulating hormone (TSH) and stimulate the secretion of high levels of thyroid hormones.

Hyperparathyroidism

A condition characterized by excessive secretion of parathyroid hormone (PTH) by the parathyroid glands. Hyperparathyroidism is often caused by the presence of adenoma or by hyperplasia (increase in number of cells) in the parathyroid glands. The action of PTH brings about reabsorption of calcium from bones into the blood. The resulting increase in blood calcium results in *osteitis fibrosa cystica*, a condition characterized by decalcification of bones, bone pain, spontaneous fractures, cyst formation and kidney damage.

Hypoparathyroidism

A condition characterized by deficient secretion of parathyroid hormone (PTH) by the parathyroid glands. Lack of PTH causes reduced calcium absorption from the small intestine and reduced reabsorption from bones. Abnormally low levels of calcium in the blood result in tetany (strong, painful spasms of muscles),

psychiatric disturbances, grand mal epilepsy and paraesthesia (abnormal sensation Am. paresthesia).

Phaeochromocytoma (Am. pheochromocytoma)

Phaeochromocytoma is a tumour (Am. tumor) that develops in the adrenal medulla, it secretes excessive amounts of adrenaline and noradrenaline into the blood. The symptoms are due to excess of these hormones and include raised BP, excessive metabolic rate, headache and nervousness. The name comes from the fact that the tumour is selectively coloured when stained with chromium salts (phae/o or phe/o meaning dark).

Thyroid tumours (Am. tumors)

Thyroid tumours may be benign or malignant. Adenomas are benign tumours that sometimes secrete sufficient thyroid hormones to cause hyperthyroidism; they have a tendency to become malignant in the elderly.

Malignant cancers (carcinomas) are rare, they vary in their rate of growth and malignancy and can be anaplastic. A hard, rapidly growing lump in the gland is usually an indication of thyroid cancer.

Benign adenomas are distinguishable from thyroid carcinomas by radionuclide scanning. Adenomas take up large amounts of iodine and form 'hot' nodules. 'Cold' nodules taking up little iodine can be benign or malignant and ultimately need to undergo biopsy.

NOW TRY THE WORD CHECK

WORD CHECK

This self-check exercise lists all the word components used in this unit. First write down the meaning of as many word components as you can. Then check your answers using the Exercise Guide and Quick Reference box or the Glossary of Word Components (pp. 347–371).

Prefixes

acro-

hyper-

hypo-

para-

poly-

Combining forms of word roots

acid/o

aden/o

adren/o

andr/o

blast/o	
chondr/o	
cortic/o	
dips/o	
estr/o (Am.)	
-globulin	
gloss/o	
-gyne	
insulin/o	
kal/i	
ket/o/n	
natr/i	
oestr/o (Am. estr/o)	
pancreat/o	
-physis	
pituitar-	
progest/o	
thyr/o	

Suffixes

-aemia (Am. -emia)	
-al	
-ectomy	
-emia (Am.)	

-genesis	
-genic	
-ia	
-ic	
-ism	
-itis	
-megaly	
-micria	
-oid	
-oma	
-osis	
-plasia	
-ptosis	
-static	
-tomy	
-toxic	
-trophic	
-tropic	
-uresis	
-uria	

NOW TRY THE SELF-ASSESSMENT

SELF-ASSESSMENT

Test 17A

Below are some combining forms that refer to the anatomy of the endocrine system. Indicate which part of the system they refer to by putting a number from the diagram (Fig. 89) next to each word.

(a) adren/o ☐

(b) parathyroid/o ☐

(c) andr/o ☐

(d) thyroid/o ☐

(e) pancreat/o ☐

(f) ovari/o ☐

(g) pituitar- ☐

(h) adrenocortic/o ☐

Score ☐
8

Test 17B

Prefixes, suffixes and combining forms of word roots

Match a word component from Column A with a meaning in Column C by inserting the appropriate number in Column B.

Column A	Column B	Column C
(a) acro-	☐	1. germ cell
(b) aden/o	☐	2. small
(c) andr/o	☐	3. pancreas
(d) blast/o	☐	4. progesterone
(e) -globin	☐	5. pertaining to constant/unchanging/controlling
(f) glyc/o	☐	6. condition of growth (increase of cells)
(g) hyper-	☐	7. oestrogen (Am. estrogen)
(h) hypo-	☐	8. sugar
(i) insulin/o	☐	9. hypophysis
(j) micr/o	☐	10. below
(k) oestr/o (Am. estr/o)	☐	11. gland
(l) pancreat/o	☐	12. thyroid
(m) para-	☐	13. pertaining to affinity for/acting on
(n) -plasia	☐	14. pertaining to nourishment
(o) pituitar-	☐	15. insulin/islets of Langerhans
(p) progest/o	☐	16. extremity/point
(q) -static	☐	17. beside/near
(r) thyr/o	☐	18. above
(s) -trophic	☐	19. protein
(t) -tropic	☐	20. man/male

Score ☐
20

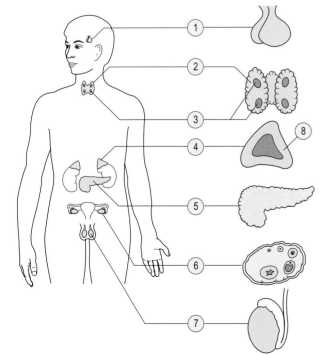

Figure 89   The endocrine system

Test 17C

Write the meaning of:

(a) thyroparathyroidectomy

(b) pituicyte

(c) adrenomegaly

(d) glycotropic

(e) hyperketonaemia
(Am. hyperketonemia)

Score

5

Test 17D

Build words that mean:

(a) process of producing too much insulin

(b) condition of too little sodium in the blood

(c) pertaining to nourishing the thyroid gland (use thyr/o)

(d) pertaining to acting on/stimulating the adrenal gland

(e) process of producing too little parathyroid hormone

Score

5

Check answers to Self-Assessment Tests on page 325.

UNIT 18
RADIOLOGY AND NUCLEAR MEDICINE

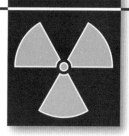

OBJECTIVES

Once you have completed Unit 18 you should be able to:

- understand the meaning of medical words relating to radiology and nuclear medicine

- build medical words relating to radiology and nuclear medicine

- understand medical abbreviations relating to radiology and nuclear medicine.

EXERCISE GUIDE

Use this list of word components and their meanings to complete the word exercises in this unit.

Prefixes

ultra-   beyond

Roots/Combining forms

angi/o	vessel
cardi/o	heart
encephal/o	brain
esophag/o (Am.)	esophagus/gullet
oesophag/o	oesophagus/gullet (Am. esophag/o)

Suffixes

-er	one who
-genic	pertaining to formation/ originating in

-gram	X-ray picture/tracing/recording
-graph	usually an instrument that records/an X-ray picture
-graphy	technique of recording/making an X-ray
-ist	specialist
-logist	specialist who studies
-logy	study of
-scope	viewing instrument
-therapist	specialist who treats (disease)
-therapy	treatment

Radiology

Radiology is the study of the diagnosis of disease by the use of radiant energy (radiation). In the past this meant the use of X-rays to make an image of the internal components of the body. Today many other forms of radiation are used to aid both diagnosis and treatment of disease. Developments in physics and technology are bringing rapid changes to this branch of medicine.

Before completing the first exercise, review the terms below:

-gram
a recording/picture/tracing/X-ray.

-graph
usually refers to an instrument that records by making a picture or tracing but it is also used here to mean a recording or X-ray picture.

-graphy
a technique of making a recording, such as a picture, X-ray, tracing or writing.

Use the Exercise Guide at the beginning of this unit to complete Word Exercises 1–10 unless you are asked to work without it.

ROOT

Radi
*(From a Latin word **radius**, meaning a ray. Here radi/o means X-rays, the invisible rays produced by an X-ray machine. This combining form is also used to mean radiation/radioactivity.)*

Combining form   **Radi/o**

WORD EXERCISE 1

Using your Exercise Guide, find the meaning of:

(a) **radi**/o/log/ist
(a physician specializing in radiology who is medically qualified)

(b) **radi**/o/graph
(here refers to an X-ray picture)

(c) **radi**/o/graphy

(d) **radi**/o/graph/er
(refers to a technician who is not medically qualified)

(e) **radi**/o/therap/ist

Some radiographic procedures require the use of a contrast medium or agent to improve the quality of the image. Contrast agents are required because there is little difference in the density of the soft parts of the body and X-rays pass through them without producing a distinct image of individual organs. The contrast medium is administered to the patient, filling a cavity such as the stomach. The X-ray is taken and the outline of the cavity recorded on the radiograph.

An example of a contrast medium is barium sulphate, a radio-opaque substance that absorbs X-rays. It shows up on X-ray film as a white area that has not allowed X-rays to pass. This property of barium sulphate makes it particularly useful for outlining the digestive tract where it is administered as:

A barium 'meal' (swallow)
To outline the upper parts of the digestive system the barium is given as a drink.

A barium enema
To outline the lower parts of the digestive system. In this procedure barium is injected via the anus into the rectum and colon. Sometimes air is also administered with the barium to increase contrast; this is known as a **double contrast radiograph**.

Iodine is another contrast agent that can be added to make various fluids radio-opaque. It is often the contrast agent used in angiocardiography, arteriography and venography.

ROOT

Roentgen
*(From the name of Wilhelm K. **Roentgen**, a German physicist (b.1845) who discovered X-rays. Here roentgen/o means X-rays/Roentgen rays.)*

Combining form   **Roentgen/o**

WORD EXERCISE 2

Without using your Exercise Guide, write the meaning of:

(a) **roentgen**/o/graphy

(b) **roentgen**/o/logist
(synonymous with radiologist)

Using your Exercise Guide, find the meaning of:

(c) **roentgen**/o/gram
(synonymous with radiograph, but as the German name is less easy to pronounce, radiograph is more commonly used)

(d) **roentgen**/o/cardio/gram

The movement of internal parts of the body can be observed using a technique known as fluoroscopy. In this procedure X-rays pass through the body on to a phosphor screen (a fluorescent screen, i.e. one from which light flows). As the X-rays strike the screen, the phosphor emits light, producing an image that is viewed as it is generated. Fluoroscopy is useful for observing movement of the oesophagus (Am. esophagus), stomach and heart. If necessary, a recording/picture can be made of the light image from the screen. (**Fluor** is from Latin *fluere*, meaning to flow. It is used to mean something that is luminous, i.e. emitting light.)

Using your Exercise Guide find the meaning of - scope and then build a word that means:

(e) instrument used for the direct X-ray examination of the body (fluoroscopy)

Without using your Exercise Guide, build a word that means:

(f) technique of recording a radiographic image produced by fluoroscopy

ROOT

Cine
*(From a Greek word **kinein**, meaning movement. Here the combining form cine/o means movement or motion. Cinemat/o means a motion picture on film, video or other recording device.)*

Combining forms   Cine/o, cinemat/o

WORD EXERCISE 3

Without using your Exercise Guide, write the meaning of:

(a) **cine**/radi/o/graph

(b) roentgen/o/**cinemat**/o/graphy

Using your Exercise Guide, find the meaning of:

(c) **cine**/angi/o/cardi/o/graphy

(d) **cine**/oesophag/o/gram (Am. **cine**-esophag/o/gram)

ROOT

Tom
*(From a Greek word **tomos**, meaning a slice or section.)*

Combining form   Tom/o

A **tomograph** is an instrument that uses X-rays to obtain images of sections through the body. It uses a thin beam of X-rays that rotates around the patient. X-ray photons emitted from the patient are detected and converted into an image by a computer. The images produced by this device show more detail than a simple X-ray.

WORD EXERCISE 4

Without using your Exercise Guide, write the meaning of:

(a) **tom**/o/gram

(b) **tom**/o/graphy (This procedure is usually called computed tomography (CT), but it is also known as CT scanning, computerized axial tomography (CAT) and CAT scanning).

Nuclear medicine

This branch of medicine uses **radioisotopes** (also called **radionuclides**) to diagnose and treat disease. In some texts it is called nuclear radiology. Terms used for diagnostic radiology include nuclear imaging and radionuclide imaging.

Radioisotopes

Radioisotopes are elements that exhibit the property of spontaneous decay, emitting radiation in the process. The radiation is in the form of high-speed particles and energy-containing rays. Elements that emit alpha, beta or gamma radiation are used as diagnostic labels to trace the route and uptake of chemicals administered into the body. The radioisotope behaves like a transmitter, passing radiation from inside to the outside of the body. Ideally, radioisotopes should give off gamma radiation as alpha and beta particles can damage cells. Many different diagnostic techniques have been devised that use radioisotopes; one procedure is described below.

First the specific isotope or tracer is given to the patient. Once in the body it continues to emit radiation and is absorbed or excluded from the tissues and organs under investigation. Next a Geigy–Muller tube or gamma camera is passed over the surface of the body to detect gamma rays emitted by the isotope; this is also known as a **radioisotope scan**. Finally an image is constructed showing the distributon of radioactivity within the tissues and organs. **Radioisotope scans** are used to image the heart, liver, biliary tract, bones, thyroid and kidney.

Here are some examples of the use of specific radioisotopes:

---

^{99M}Tc (technetium)

^{99M}Tc is administered to the patient in trace quantities. It is excluded from normal brain tissue but accumulates in some brain tumours (Am. tumors). A tumour can be detected by locating the gamma rays emitted from it.

^{123}I (Iodine)

^{123}I is rapidly taken up by the thyroid gland. A radioisotope scan of the gland will outline the now radioactive gland and information from this will aid the diagnosis of various thyroid disorders, e.g. thyrotoxicosis.

^{57}Co (cobalt)

^{57}Co is used to trace the uptake of vitamin B_{12} by the body and from this a diagnosis of megaloblastic anaemia can be made.

Scintigraphy

Scintigraphy is the technique of producing a radioisotope scan. A radioisotope with an affinity for a particular organ or tissue is injected into the body and the distribution of the radioactivity is followed using an instrument called a **scintillation counter (scintiscanner)**. This device contains a **scintillator**, a substance that emits light when in contact with ionizing radiation. There is a flash of light for each ionizing event and the number of flashes (or counts) is related to the radioactivity present in the area being scanned. Scintillation counters can be moved over the outer surface of the body to locate radioisotopes within particular organs and build an image (scintigram/scintiscan) of their distribution. The **gamma camera** mentioned earlier is a scintillation counter.

ROOT

Scint
(*From a Latin word* **scintillatio**, *meaning spark/emitting sparks/light.*)

Combining forms   Scint/i, scintill/a

WORD EXERCISE 5

Without using your Exercise Guide, write the meaning of:

(a) **scinti**/gram

(b) **scinti**/graphy

Positron emission tomography (PET)

This is another imaging technique that traces the distribution of radioisotopes within the body. **Positron emission tomography** (PET scanning) uses radioisotopes (radionuclides) that emit short-lived particles called positrons (β^+ radiation). Particular tissues take up the isotopes, which are injected intravenously, for example 11C-2-deoxy-D-glucose penetrates the blood–brain barrier and is used by brain cells as a source of energy. Once inside a brain cell the isotope decays emitting positrons; the more active the cell, the more labeled glucose is taken up and the more positrons are emitted.

The positrons immediately collide with electrons, yielding gamma ray photons that have sufficient energy to leave the body. These photons are detected by a large array of scintillation detectors that surround the patient. The position of the emerging photons is determined and used to construct a cross sectional computerized image that shows the distribution of the radioisotopes in the tissues.

PET is used to investigate physiological processes such as the blood perfusion of organs and metabolism and has found particular application in the study of the brain in patients with neurological deficits caused by strokes and epilepsy.

The half-life of radionuclides used in PET is short-lived so they cannot be stored and used when required. The technique is dependent on the immediate production of radionuclides in a complex and expensive device called a **cyclotron** and the services of **radiochemical** and **radiopharmaceutical** laboratories. These restrictions have limited its use to special centres with appropriate facilities. Recently, mini cyclotrons have been designed for on site production of radionuclides and these are leading to increased use of this imaging technique.

Radiotherapy

Radiotherapy is the treatment of disease by X-rays and other forms of radiation. In particular the radiation is used to destroy malignant cancer cells by exposing them to a lethal dose of radiation.

Teletherapy (external beam therapy)

This is the administration of radiation from an external source at a distance from the body (*tele-* meaning far away/operating at a distance). Radiotherapy machines generate the radiation used in this form of treatment and there has been a move towards ever more powerful devices. To maximize the therapeutic advantages of radiotherapy, it is necessary to give a tumouricidal (Am. tumoricidal) dose of radiation to a planned target volume and minimize the dose to surrounding tissue. (Here *tumour-* means a mass of cancer cells, *-cidal* pertaining to killing).

The first high-energy beams were produced by the decay of radioactive sources. The cobalt sixty (^{60}Co) radiotherapy machine still in use produces radiation at energies of between 1 and 4 MeV (mega-electron- volts, 1 MeV=1 million electronvolts). At its centre is a cobalt sixty high energy radiation source that emits gamma(γ)-ray photons that are directed at the patient through an opening called a collimator. This machine has been particularly useful for treating tumours of the head, neck and metastases in lymph nodes.

Cobalt sixty machines have been largely superseded by linear accelerators that generate X-ray photons or electron beams at very high energy levels (3–35 MeV) and contain no radioactive sources. In electron mode these complex machines accelerate a beam of electrons to near the speed of light and direct them on to superficial lesions near the surface of the body. In photon mode the beam of electrons is made to collide with a metal target generating high energy X-ray photons that can be used to destroy tumours deep within the body.

Brachytherapy

The term **brachytherapy** (*brachy-* meaning short) means the administration of radiation in close proximity to a tumour. It is accomplished by the implantation of radioactive sources into the body. The sealed source has been used to deliver radiation in three main ways: into the surface of the skin, into a cavity (intracavity) and directly into a tissue or tumour (interstitial).

Needles containing radium (^{226}Ra) and emitting gamma ray photons at 0.2–2.4 MeV were first used. A needle consists of a platinum or alloy tube with a sharp (trocar) point at one end and an eyelet for a thread at the other. The radioactive material is loaded into the needle in cells (this minimizes spillage if damaged) and they are sealed in with gold solder. The needle is inserted directly into a tumour and left for a fixed time before being withdrawn. Caesium (^{137}Cs) (Am. Cesium) has been used as a radium substitute for intracavity and interstitial brachytherapy.

Tubes and seeds are similar to needles, but they have no sharp points; instead they fit into an applicator for insertion into a body cavity. Radon gas seeds (^{222}Rn) were used as a substitute for radium, and gold (^{198}Au) seeds for interstitial implants have superseded these. Typically they have a length of 5mm and a diameter of 1.35mm, small enough to be inserted into a tumour and left forming harmless foreign bodies once their radioactivity has decayed to a negligible value (half-life 3.8 days).

Other sources include: Caesium (^{137}Cs) needles, Gold (^{198}Au) grains and tubes, and iridium (^{192}Ir) wires, hairpins, seeds and ribbons.

In the 1930s brachytherapy needles were inserted into the patient manually; this exposed medical and nursing staff to high doses of radiation. The afterloading technique has been developed to reduce the handling times of radioactive sources. In this procedure, non-radioactive needles, tubing and applicators are precisely positioned in the patient before the introduction of the

radioactive sources. The sources are only introduced when they can be quickly loaded into the appropriate points in the patient, thereby reducing exposure to medical staff. Improved afterloading machines are now available that further reduce unwanted exposure. This, with the development of new radionuclides, has made brachytherapy a much safer form of treatment.

Radionuclides are also administered to patients in unsealed forms, for example, Iodine (^{131}I) emits beta radiation and is used as a treatment for thyrotoxicosis. The iodine is available as an injection, drink or capsule, the latter being safer as it reduces the risk of spillage. Once absorbed, the iodine is preferentially absorbed by the thyroid gland delivering a therapeutic dose of radiation. This causes the gland to atrophy and reduce its output of thyroid hormones.

WORD EXERCISE 6

Without using your Exercise Guide, write the meaning of:

(a) **radi/o**/therapy

(b) **radi/o**/therap/ist
(a physician, medically qualified)

Ultrasonography

When high-frequency sound waves are directed at the body, internal organs and masses reflect the sound to a different extent. They are said to have different echo textures. These internal echoes are detected and converted into an image. The size and shape of easily recognized organs can be investigated using this technique and it is widely used for examining a fetus in utero.

ROOT

Son
(From a Latin word **sonus**, *meaning sound.)*

Combining form **Son/o**

Note the next exercise refers to techniques using **ultrasound**, high-frequency sounds beyond human hearing.

WORD EXERCISE 7

Using your Exercise Guide, find the meaning of:

(a) ultra/**son/o**/gram

Without using your Exercise Guide, write the meaning of:

(b) ultra/**son/o**/graphy

(c) ultra/**son/o**/graph

ROOT

Echo
(A Greek word meaning sound. Here echo- means an ultrasound echo generated by the reflection of sound waves off an obstacle.)

Combining form   **Echo-**

WORD EXERCISE 8

Using your Exercise Guide, find the meaning of:

(a) **echo**/encephalo/gram

Using your Exercise Guide find the meaning of -genic and then build a word that means:

(b) pertaining to forming/ generating an echo

Without using your Exercise Guide, build words that mean:

(c) a recording/picture of echoes (synonymous with ultrasonogram)

(d) an instrument that records echoes from the brain

(e) a recording/picture of heart echoes

(f) technique of making a picture/tracing/recording using echoes

Thermography

Thermography is the technique of recording temperature differences throughout the body on film or computer monitor.

Our bodies radiate a range of infrared waves at different frequencies. The frequency of the radiation depends on the temperature of the body. Thermography uses electronic equipment to detect infrared radiation coming from the body and displays it as an image on a screen. As tumours contain abnormally active cells, they give off more heat than surrounding areas and this enables them to be detected. Thermography has proved of great benefit in the detection of breast and testicular tumours.

ROOT

Therm
*(From a Greek word **therme** meaning heat.)*

Combining form   **Therm/o**

WORD EXERCISE 9

Without using your Exercise Guide, write the meaning of:

(a) **therm/o**/gram

(b) scrotal **therm/o**/graphy

Medical equipment and clinical procedures

Revise the names of all instruments and clinical procedures mentioned in this unit before trying Exercise 10.

WORD EXERCISE 10

Match each term in Column A with a description in Column C by placing an appropriate number in Column B.

Column A	Column B	Column C
(a) radiography		1. an instrument that detects gamma rays from radioisotopes
(b) fluoroscopy		2. technique of using ultrasound echoes to image the heart
(c) thermo-graphy		3. a chemical used to improve the detail of an X-ray
(d) ultra-sonograph		4. technique of making an X-ray
(e) computerized tomograph		5. an instrument that makes a tracing/picture using reflected sound
(f) radiotherapy		6. an instrument that uses X-rays to image a slice through the body
(g) cineradio-graphy		7. direct observation of an X-ray picture using a fluorescent screen
(h) gamma camera		8. technique of recording body heat on film
(i) echocar-diography		9. the treatment of disorders using radiation
(j) contrast medium		10. technique of using X-rays to make a moving picture

CASE HISTORY 18

The object of this exercise is to understand words associated with a patient's medical history.

To complete the exercise:

* read through the passage on cancer of the larynx; unfamiliar words are underlined and you can find their meaning using the Word Help

* write the meaning of the medical terms shown in bold print on the lines that follow the Word Help.

Cancer of the larynx

Mr R, aged 42, was referred to the ENT clinic with suspected cancer of the larynx. He had been a 15 per day cigarette smoker for 22 years. His main symptom was hoarseness (dysphonia) that had been present for about 2 months; otherwise, he seemed to be in good health. He was admitted to have his larynx formally assessed.

Direct laryngoscopy under anaesthesia confirmed the presence of a glottic tumour affecting both vocal cords. Following biopsy, histological analysis classified the tumour as a squamous cell carcinoma.

A chest **radiograph** excluded the presence of metastatic deposits and bronchial carcinoma. Computed **tomography** excluded lymph node and cartilage involvement with no spread into the hypopharynx.

Following discussion at a joint clinic, the ENT surgeon and **radiotherapist** staged Mr R's tumour at T1b N0 with no metastatic involvement. He was prescribed a course of radical **radiotherapy** to try to conserve his larynx.

Immobilization of Mr R's neck was achieved by a well-fitting perspex shell reaching from the angle of the jaw down to just below the clavicle. The radiotherapist placed him in the supine position (without a mouthbite) with his neck straight to prevent the spinal cord curving anteriorly. The tumour was localized using CT scanning and the dose distribution outlined on the **tomogram** centring on the proposed target volume.

Mr R was placed in the same perspex shell and position for radiotherapy. The aim of his treatment was to administer a **tumouricidal** (Am. **tumoricidal**) dose of radiation centred on his vocal cords. As he had a short neck, two anterior, oblique beams were used to irradiate the whole larynx. The wedged beams were angled at 90° to give a homogeneous dose to the target volume and to reduce the dose to the skin and spinal cord. He was administered 60 Gy in twenty-five fractions in 5 weeks (4–6 MeV) from a **linear accelerator**.

Mr R was advised of the possibility of side-effects such as difficulty in swallowing, exacerbated hoarseness, desquamation and rarely oedema (Am.

edema) leading to obstruction. These often peak around the twelfth treatment with resolution of the tumour in approximately 2 months.

Mr R made an uneventful recovery, his only complaints being difficulty in swallowing and a sore throat. Recent follow-up examinations by the ENT surgeon and diagnostic **ultrasonography** showed no evidence of tumour recurrence. He appears well, and his voice is showing signs of recovery.

WORD HELP

anterior front/from the front of the body

biopsy removal and examination of living tissue

carcinoma a malignant growth from epidermal cells

clavicle the collar bone

desquamation the shedding of cells from the epidermis

dysphonia condition of difficulty/pain on speaking

ENT ear, nose and throat

glottic pertaining to the glottis (vocal apparatus of the larynx)

Gy gray (SI unit of absorbed radiation dose)

histological pertaining to histology (here histological analysis for classification and signs of malignancy)

hoarseness rough, grating, discordant voice making speech difficult

homogeneous uniform quality in all parts

hypopharynx the laryngeal part of the pharynx

laryngoscopy technique of viewing the larynx

localized here refers to determination of the position of the target volume in relation to the patient's anatomy and skin reference points

metastatic pertaining to metastases (parts of a tumour that have spread from one site to another)

MeV mega-electronvolt

oblique slanting

oedema (Am. edema) accumulation of fluid in a tissue

squamous pertaining to scale-like/from squamous epithelium

supine lying on the back so the face is upward

target volume tumour volume

radical direct to the root or cause (treatment to eliminate disease) extensive

resolution abatement of a pathological process and the return of affected tissues to normal

T1b N0 staging symbols T – tumour, N – node, T1b – tumour at stage 1b and N0–no node involvement

wedge wedge-shaped devices that act as filters to absorb radiation. They are used to adjust the dose received on either side of the body

Now write the meaning of the following words from the case history without using your dictionary lists:

(a) radiograph

(b) tomography

(c) radiotherapist

(d) radiotherapy

(e) tomogram

(f) tumouricidal
(Am. tumoricidal)

(g) linear accelerator

(h) ultrasonography

(Answers to the case history exercise are given in the Answers to Word Exercises beginning on page 301.)

Quick Reference

Combining forms relating to radiology and nuclear medicine:

Cine/o	movement/motion (picture)
Ech/o	reflected sound
Fluor/o	fluorescence/fluorosopy
Radi/o	radiation/X-ray
Roentgen/o	X-ray
Scint/i	spark/flash of light
Son/o	sound
Therm/o	heat
Tom/o	slice/section
Ultrason/o	ultrasound

Abbreviations

Some common abbreviations related to radiation and nuclear medicine are listed below. Note some are not standard and their meaning may vary from one health care setting to another. There is a more extensive list for reference on page 335.

AXR	abdominal X-ray
Ba	barium
CT	computerized tomography
CXR	chest X-ray
DSA	digital subtraction angiography
DXT	deep X-ray therapy
EUA	examination under anaesthesia (Am. anesthesia)
MRI	magnetic resonance imaging
NMR	nuclear magnetic resonance
PET	positron emission tomography
US	ultrasound/ultrasonography
XR	X-ray

NOW TRY THE WORD CHECK

WORD CHECK

This self-check exercise lists all the word components used in this unit. First write down the meaning of as many word components as you can. Then check your answers using the Exercise Guide and Quick Reference box or the Glossary of Word Components (pp. 347–371).

Prefixes

ultra-

Combining forms of word roots

angi/o

cardi/o

cine/o

ech/o

encephal/o

esophag/o (Am.)

fluor/o

oesophag/o
(Am. esophag/o)

radi/o

roentgen/o

scint/i

son/o

therm/o

tom/o

Suffixes

-cidal

-er

-genic

-gram

-graph

-graphy

-ist

-logy

-scope

-scopy

-therapy

NOW TRY THE SELF-ASSESSMENT

SELF-ASSESSMENT

Test 18A

Prefixes, suffixes and combining forms of word roots

Match each word component in Column A with a meaning in Column C by inserting the appropriate number in Column B.

Column A	Column B	Column C
(a) angi/o		1. X-ray/radiation
(b) cinemat/o		2. X-rays
(c) ech/o		3. specialist
(d) -er		4. treatment
(e) fluor/o		5. beyond/excess
(f) -genic		6. slice/section/cut
(g) -gram		7. sound
(h) -graph		8. heat
(i) -graphy		9. technique of recording/making a picture X-ray
(j) -ist		10. technique of visual examination
(k) radi/o		11. vessel
(l) roentgen/o		12. picture/tracing/X-ray picture
(m) scint/i		13. movement/motion picture
(n) -scope		14. pertaining to formation/originating in
(o) -scopy		15. reflected sound
(p) son/o		16. instrument to view
(q) -therapy		17. fluoroscope/fluoroscopy
(r) -therm/o		18. spark (flash or light)
(s) tom/o		19. instrument that records or the picture/tracing/X-ray itself
(t) ultra-		20. one who

Score

20

Test 18B

Write the meaning of:

(a) roentgenotherapy

(b) sonologist

(c) thermoradiotherapy

(d) radiocinematograph

(e) ultrasonotomography

Score

5

Test 18C

Build words that mean:

(a) treatment using ultrasound

(b) pertaining to examination by a fluoroscope

(c) technique of making a picture of vessels using sparks/flashes of light

(d) an instrument used to detect and image heat from the body

(e) technique of imaging the brain using echoes (use ech/o)

Score

5

Check answers to Self-Assessment Tests on page 325.

UNIT 19
ONCOLOGY

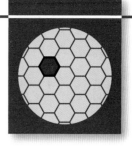

OBJECTIVES

Once you have completed Unit 19 you should be able to:

- understand the meaning of medical words relating to oncology

- build medical words relating to oncology

- understand medical abbreviations relating to oncology.

EXERCISE GUIDE

Use this list of word components and their meanings to complete the word exercises in this unit.

Roots/Combining forms

angi/o	vessel
chondr/o	cartilage
haem/o	blood (Am. hem/o)
hem/o (Am.)	blood
leiomy/o	smooth muscle
mening/i	meninges (membranes of CNS)
rhabdomy/o	striated muscle

Suffixes

-eal	pertaining to
-genesis	formation of
-genic	pertaining to formation/originating in
-ia	condition of
-ic	pertaining to
-ist	specialist
-logist	specialist who studies
-logy	study of
-lysis	breakdown/disintegration
-oma	tumour (Am. tumor)/swelling
-osis	abnormal condition/disease/abnormal increase
-static	pertaining to stopping/controlling
-tropic	pertaining to stimulating/affinity for

Oncology

This branch of medicine deals with the study and treatment of malignant tumours (Am. tumors) commonly called cancers. A tumour is a mass or swelling forming from dividing cells which appear to be out of control. Benign tumours remain localized and do not threaten life but malignant tumours spread and may lead to death. Tumours spread when they release cells into the blood and lymph; the tumour cells multiply in new sites forming secondary growths or **metastases** (from Greek *meta histanai*, *meta* meaning changed in form, *histanai* to place/set, i.e. a growth in a different position).

As tumours grow they consume nutrients, depriving normal cells of essential metabolic components. A clinical feature called **cachexia** is seen in advanced stages of disease (from Greek *kakos* meaning bad and *hexis* meaning state). The body appears to suffer from malnutrition and becomes thin and 'wastes' away.

In this unit we will examine terms that relate to common types of tumour.

Use the Exercise Guide at the beginning of this unit to complete Word Exercises 1–3 unless you are asked to work without it.

ROOT ─────────────────────

Onc
(From a Greek word **ogkos**, *meaning a swelling. Here onc/o means a tumour (Am. tumor).)*

Combining form   **Onc/o**

WORD EXERCISE 1

Using your Exercise Guide, find the meaning of:

(a) **onc**/osis

(b) **onc/o**/genesis

(c) **onc/o**/trop/ic

Using your Exercise Guide find the meaning of -genic, -logist and -lysis, then build words that mean:

(d) pertaining to formation of a tumour

(e) breakdown/disintegration of a tumour

(f) person who specializes in the study and treatment of tumours

The process of tumour formation is also known as **neoplasia** (*neo-* meaning new, *-plas-* forming/growing and *-ia* condition of) and the tumour itself as a **neoplasm**. Neoplastic, derived in the same way, is also used to mean pertaining to a new growth (synonymous with oncogenic).

Before we study the next word root, we need to examine the use of the suffix *-oma*. Used by itself in combination with a tissue type, it indicates a benign tumour, e.g. ost**oma** – a benign bone tumour.

Malignant tumours may also be designated by *-oma* but they are usually preceded by the word **malignant**, e.g. **malignant melanoma**, a malignant tumour of the pigment cells and **malignant lymphoma**, a malignant tumour of lymphatic tissue.

The suffix *-oma* is also used in **blastoma**, meaning a tumour that forms from embryonic (germ) cells of an organ. Examples include: **glioblastoma**, a tumour that contains neuroglia (a type of brain cell or gliacyte) and **retinoblastoma** a tumour that grows from embryonic cells in the retina of the eye.

(To confuse matters, *-oma* is occasionally used for a non-neoplastic condition such as **haematoma** (Am. **hematoma**), that refers to a swelling filled with blood and is not a new growth of cells.)

Two terms that are widely used when referring to malignant tumours are:

Carcinoma
a malignant tumour of epithelial origin. Remember epithelia cover organs and line cavities and form membranes and glands.

Sarcoma
a malignant tumour of supporting tissues, including all connective tissues and muscle.

These terms are studied in the exercises that follow:

ROOT

Carcin
(*From a Greek word* **karkinos**, *meaning crab. Here carcin/o means a malignant tumour/cancer.*)

Combining form **Carcin/o**

A **carcin**oma is a tumour of an epithelium and there are numerous types. They are usually named by using the word carcinoma preceded by the histological type and followed by the organ of origin, for example:

Squamous cell carcinoma of the lung
originates in non-glandular epithelium.

Adenocarcinoma of the breast
originates in a glandular epithelium within the breast.

Often carcinomas are more simply named, e.g. as carcinoma of the colon or carcinoma of the urinary bladder.

Note. A substance that stimulates the formation of a malignant tumour is known as a **carcinogen**.

WORD EXERCISE 2

Without using your Exercise Guide, write the meaning of:

(a) **carcin/o**/gen/ic

(b) **carcin/o**/lysis

Using your Exercise Guide, find the meaning of:

(c) **carcin/o**/stat/ic

Also from this root we have the word cancer, which is imprecisely used to mean carcinoma or cancer in situ. It is sometimes preceded by words that indicate the cause of a cancer, for example:

• radiologist's cancer
• smoker's cancer
• asbestos cancer.

ROOT

Sarc
(From a Greek word **sarkoma***, meaning a fleshy growth. Here sarc/o means a malignant tumour of connective tissue.)*

Combining form **Sarc/o**

Sarcomas are malignant tumours that are less common than carcinomas. They are derived from cells that have developed from the supporting tissues of the body, such as the connective tissues, i.e. bone, cartilage, blood and lymph, and from muscle tissue. The word **sarcoma** is preceded by the tissue type as in osteo**sarcoma**, a malignant bone tumour. (**Sarcomat/o** is the combining form of sarcoma.)

WORD EXERCISE 3

Using your Exercise Guide, find the meaning of:

(a) chondr/o/**sarcoma**

(b) lei/o/my/o/**sarcoma**

(c) rhabd/o/my/o/**sarcoma**

(d) mening/eal **sarcoma**

(e) haem/angi/o/**sarcoma**
   (Am. hem/angi/o/**sarcoma**)

Without using your Exercise Guide, write the meaning of:

(f) **sarcomat**/osis

Most malignant tumours arise from epithelial tissues. When malignant cells grow they sometimes resemble the cells from which they originate and are said to be **well-differentiated**. Other malignant cells may be **undifferentiated** and may change their character back to a more primitive or embryonic type. When this occurs they are described as **anaplastic** (*ana-* meaning backward, *-plast-* to mould or form and *-ic* pertaining to). A characteristic of all malignant cells within a tumour is that they have an increased capacity to divide.

Another form of malignancy is the mixed tissue tumour. This type contains cells that may resemble both epithelial and connective tissue cells.

Diagnosis of malignant tumours (cancers)

Precise classification of malignant tumours is essential for determining their likely growth characteristics. Once

a tumour has been classified, appropriate treatment can be planned and the patient can be given a prognosis (forecast of the probable course of their disease).

The classification of a tumour usually requires the microscopic examination of a sample of its cells; this procedure is called a **biopsy**. The word biopsy is formed from *bio-* meaning life and *-opsy* meaning process of viewing. A biopsy is the removal and examination of tissue from a living body.

A biopsy will determine a tumour's type, whether benign or malignant and whether it has spread to other tissues. Most biopsies are minor procedures but some require general anaesthesia (Am. anesthesia). There are several types including:

* a **needle biopsy** – removal of a small sample of cells using a fine, hollow needle
* an **incision biopsy** – removal of a small sample of skin or muscle through an incision
* an **excision** or **resection biopsy** – removal of a whole tumour which is then sent for analysis
* an **open biopsy** – removal of tissue from within the body during an operation
* an **endoscopic biopsy** – removal of tissue using forceps attached to a fibre-optic endoscope.

Cancer classification

Cancers are classified in two main ways:

* by the type of tissue in which the cancerous cells originate (histological type)
* by the location or primary site where the cancer first developed.

Histological types of cancer

Here the many different types of cancer are grouped into six main categories based on their origin:

Carcinoma

A carcinoma is a malignant tumour of epithelial origin. Epithelial tissue consists of epithelial membranes and epithelial glands that form the internal and external linings of the body. Carcinomas are divided into two major subtypes: adenocarcinoma that develops from an epithelial gland, and squamous cell carcinoma that develops from a squamous epithelium. Carcinomas often affect glands or organs covered or lined with epithelial membranes that are capable of secretion such as the breast, prostate gland, bronchus and colon.

Sarcoma

A sarcoma is a malignant tumour that originates in connective tissue such as cartilage, bone, adipose tissue or muscle tissue. Sarcomas also include tumours arising from blood forming tissue (leukaemia), lymphatic tissue (lymphoma) and connective tissue in the brain (glioma).

A solid sarcoma usually forms a painful mass in a bone or other tissue and resembles the tissue from which it originates.

Leukaemia (Am. Leukemia)

Leukaemia is a cancer of the blood-forming cells in the bone marrow. The disease affects the immature cells that produce leucocytes (Am. leukocytes), hence the term leuk/aem/ia meaning a condition of white blood or too many white cells.

Leucocytes normally protect us from disease but the leukaemic white cells lose their ability to protect us against micro-organisms leaving the patient prone to infection. Leukaemia can also affect the immature cells that produce erythrocytes, resulting in the symptoms and signs of anaemia (Am. anemia), and interference with blood clotting.

There are many types including:

- granulocytic leukaemia – a malignancy of the granulocytic series of leucocytes
- lymphocytic leukaemia – a malignancy of the lymphocytic series of blood cells
- polycythaemia vera (Am. polycythemia vera) – a malignancy of red blood cells. The condition carries an increased risk of acute leukaemia.

Myeloma

A myeloma is a tumour that originates in the plasma cells of bone marrow. The cancerous cells produce many of the proteins found in blood. For example in multiple myeloma plasma cells derived from β lymphocytes produce an abnormal amount of immunoglobulin.

Lymphoma

Lymphoma develops in the nodes and organs of the lymphatic system. A lymphoma is a solid tumour that arises in an organ such as the spleen, tonsil, thymus gland or lymph node. Extra-nodal lymphomas are also found in other organs such as the stomach or brain. Lymphomas are classified into two sub-types:

- Hodgkin's lymphoma (Hodgkin's disease)
- non-Hodgkin's lymphoma.

Mixed tumours

In mixed tumours the cells may be of different origins and they can be grouped into different categories, for example:

- carcinosarcoma – a malignant tumour composed of cells originating in epithelial and connective tissue
- adenosquamous carcinoma – a malignant tumour composed of cells that originate in squamous epithelia and glandular tissue.

Staging

Attempts to develop an international language for describing the extent of malignant disease have been made. One of these is in widespread use and is known as the **TNM** system.

T – tumour
categorizes the primary tumour and its size.

N – nodes
defines the number of lymph nodes that have been invaded.

M – metastases
indicates the presence or absence of metastases.

The extent of malignant disease defined by these categories is termed **staging**. Staging defines the size of tumour, its growth and progression at any one point.

Many different staging systems are in use for different cancers. It is not possible to study them here, but we have included a basic system that is outlined below.

T		
	T_0	no primary tumour
	T_1	primary tumour limited to site of origin
	T_{2-4}	progressive increase in size of primary tumour
	T_x	primary tumour cannot be assessed
	T_{is}	primary tumour in situ
N		
	N_0	no evidence of spread to nodes
	N_1	spread to nodes in immediate area
	N_{2-4}	increasing number of lymph nodes invaded
	N_x	lymph nodes cannot be assessed
M		
	M_0	no evidence of metastases
	M_{1-3}	ascending degrees of metastases

Using the above system, we can see the principle of how a cancer is staged. For example, a tumour classified at stage T_2 N_1 M_0, indicates the primary tumour is large and has spread to deeper structures (T_2). It has spread to one lymph node draining the area (N_1) and there is no evidence of a distant metastasis (M_0).

Staging is not an exact description of a tumour's progress but it is a useful way to estimate the course of the disease when planning treatment (therapy). A patient can be re-staged following a period of treatment and assessment of its effect.

Effective treatment can lead to the disappearance of all signs and symptoms of disease, this is known as **remission**. However if treatment does not completely eradicate the cancerous cells, symptoms of disease will return, this is known as a **relapse**. Sometimes a cancer is described as **refractory** that is resistant to treatment and the patient may never go into remission.

If treatment is deemed to be successful the patient will be asked to attend the outpatient clinic on a regular basis for assessment by the oncologist. This is known as **follow-up** and its purpose is to monitor the patient for signs of re-occurrence of the disease.

Medical equipment and clinical procedures

We have already described the main instruments and clinical procedures that are used in the diagnosis and treatment of cancers in Unit 18. Tumours can be detected using radiography, computerized tomography, thermography, magnetic resonance imaging, positron emission tomography etc.

The main types of treatments are:

- radiotherapy: the use of radiation/X-rays by medically qualified radiotherapists (-*ist* meaning specialist) to destroy tumour cells
- chemotherapy: the use of chemicals i.e. cytotoxic drugs to poison tumour cells
- excision surgery: the use of surgery to remove a tumour.

CASE HISTORY 19

The object of this exercise is to understand words associated with a patient's medical history.

To complete the exercise:

- read through the passage on glioblastoma multiforme; unfamiliar words are underlined and you can find their meaning using the Word Help
- write the meaning of the medical terms shown in bold print on the lines that follow the Word Help.

Glioblastoma multiforme

Mr. S, a 59-year-old male senior office worker noticed a loss of verbal fluency and had difficulty in recalling the names of common objects and friends. His employer reprimanded him over a decline in his previously high standard of written work. His condition worsened, and he was persuaded by his colleagues to seek medical advice. He was referred to the neurology unit by his GP.

On examination by the neurologist he appeared alert and intelligent but made several mistakes when asked to name common objects and spell simple words. He could not remember a simple name and address after 5 minutes.

His optic discs were normal, but there was no venous pulsation. Vision was restricted in the upper temporal visual field in the right eye and upper nasal field in the left eye. There was a mild lower facial weakness and a slight increase in reflexes of the right arm and leg. The right plantar reflex was extensor.

The presence of dysphasia, memory loss, right homonymous field restriction and mild pyramidal signs suggested a lesion affecting the upper temporal lobe of the left cerebral hemisphere.

A CXR excluded a bronchial **neoplasm** which is the commonest cause of cerebral **metastases** in a smoker. A CT scan demonstrated a mixed, high and low density intracranial lesion in the left temporal region and excluded **meningioma**. EEG demonstrated a wave abnormality in the left temporal region and a left carotid arteriogram indicated displacement of cerebral branches by a temporal **mass**. The commonest cause of lesions presenting in this way is malignant **glioma**.

A case conference was arranged with the **oncologist** to disclose the prognosis to Mr. S and his family and to outline the options for treatment. The **radiotherapist** required histological confirmation of the diagnosis before commencing treatment. Mr. S was administered dexamethasone to reduce the oedema (Am. edema) around the tumour and improve the symptoms of raised intracranial pressure. A brain biopsy confirmed glioblastoma multiforme.

Mr. S underwent neurosurgery, part of the temporal lobe was removed to provide an internal decompression and the tumour was sucked out. Unfortunately, malignant gliomas infiltrate into brain tissue and are difficult to remove completely. A radical course of cobalt sixty radiotherapy in combination with **chemotherapy** and small doses of steroids followed surgery. His speech defect and writing improved considerably for many months following surgery. Now, a year later, he shows signs of deterioration with a right hemiparesis, dysphasia and occasional grand mal seizures.

WORD HELP

arteriogram tracing/X-ray picture of arteries

biopsy removal and examination of living tissue

carotid the carotid artery in the neck

cerebral hemisphere a lateral half of the cerebrum

cobalt sixty (^{60}Co) isotope of cobalt that emits gamma rays that can destroy cancer cells

CT computed tomography

CXR chest X-ray

decompression relief of pressure

dysphasia condition of difficulty in speaking

EEG electroencephalogram/electroencephalography

extensor straightening (here refers to the Babinski reflex, a response in which the toes curl upwards or dorsiflex when the sole of the foot is stroked, instead of the normal plantar flexion in which the toes curl down)

glioblastoma tumour of embryonic/germ cells that contains neuroglia (types of supporting cell found in the brain)

GP general practitioner (family doctor)

grand mal seizure a form of epileptic fit in which consciousness is lost

hemiparesis partial or slight paralysis, weakness of a limb

histological pertaining to histology (here histological analysis for classification and signs of malignancy)

intracranial pertaining to within the cranium

homonymous corresponding halves

lesion a pathological change in a tissue

malignant dangerous, capable of spreading

multiforme having many forms (here referring to the fact that the tumour may be derived from different types of cells)

oedema (Am. edema) accumulation of fluid in a tissue

plantar pertaining to the sole of the foot

prognosis a forecast of the probable outcome and course of a disease

pyramidal referring to the pyramidal tract in the brain, an area that initiates voluntary skilled movements of skeletal muscles, especially the fingers

radical direct to the root or cause (treatment to eliminate disease), extensive

steroid a drug used to suppress inflammation and reduce oedema (Am. edema)

temporal pertaining to the temple/temporal bone (the temple is the flat region on either side of the head)

Now write the meaning of the following words from the case history without using your dictionary lists:

(a) neoplasm

(b) metastases

(c) meningioma

(d) mass

(e) glioma

(f) oncologist

(g) radiotherapist

(h) chemotherapy

(Answers to the case history exercise are given in the Answers to Word Exercises beginning on page 301.)

Quick Reference

Combining forms relating to oncology:

Aden/o	gland
Blast/o	embryonic/germ cell
Cancer/o	cancer
Carcin/o	cancerous/malignant tumour
Melan/o	pigment
Onc/o	tumour (Am. tumor)
Sarc/o	connective tissue/fleshy
Sarcomat/o	sarcoma/malignant tumour

Abbreviations

Some common abbreviations related to oncology are listed below. Note some are not standard and their meaning may vary from one health care setting to another. There is a more extensive list for reference on page 335.

BCC	basal cell carcinoma
BT	bone tumour (Am. tumor)
BX or Bx	biopsy
CA or Ca	cancer/carcinoma
CACX	cancer of the cervix
CF	cancer free
MEN	multiple endocrine neoplasia
Metas	metastasis
N & V	nausea and vomiting
SA	sarcoma
T	tumour (Am. tumor)
t	terminal

NOW TRY THE WORD CHECK

WORD CHECK

This self-check exercise lists all the word components used in this unit. First write down the meaning of as many word components as you can. Then check your answers using the Exercise Guide and Quick Reference box or the Glossary of Word Components (pp. 347–371).

Prefixes

ana-

meta-

neo-

Combining forms of word roots

aden/o

angi/o

blast/o

cancer/o

carcin/o

chem/o

chondr/o

cyt/o

gli/a/o

haem/o

hem/o (Am.)

leiomy/o

melan/o

meningi/o

onc/o

rhabdomy/o

sarc/o

sarcomat/o

Suffixes

-genic

-genesis

-ia

-ic

-ist

-logy

-lysis

-oma

-osis

-plasia

-plastic

-static

-therapy

-toxic

-tropic

NOW TRY THE SELF-ASSESSMENT

SELF-ASSESSMENT

Test 19A

Prefixes, suffixes and combining forms of word roots

Match each word component in Column A with a meaning in Column C by inserting the appropriate number in Column B.

Column A	Column B	Column C
(a) aden/o		1. pertaining to
(b) ana-		2. change position or form
(c) cancer/o		3. pertaining to formation/ originating in
(d) carcinoma		4. membranes of CNS
(e) chondr/o		5. striated muscle
(f) -genic		6. condition of growth (increase of cells)
(g) -ic		7. pertaining to stopping/ controlling
(h) -ist		8. pertaining to affinity for/acting on
(i) leiomy/o		9. gland
(j) melan/o		10. cancer (general term)
(k) meningi/o		11. cancer/tumour (medical term)
(l) meta-		12. cartilage
(m) neo-		13. tumour/swelling (benign or malignant)
(n) -oma		14. malignant tumour of epithelium

Column A	Column B	Column C
(o) onc/o		15. malignant tumour of supporting tissue
(p) -plasia		16. specialist
(q) rhabdomy/o		17. smooth muscle
(r) sarcomat/o		18. pigment (melanin)
(s) -static		19. new
(t) -tropic		20. backward

Score [20]

Test 19B

Write the meaning of:

(a) fibrosarcoma (fibr/o – fibre/fibrous)

(b) gastric adenocarcinoma (gastr/o – stomach)

(c) hepatocellular carcinoma (hepat/o – liver)

(d) anaplastic thyroid carcinoma (thyr/o – thyroid)

(e) bronchogenic carcinoma (bronch/o – bronchus)

Score [5]

Test 19C

Build words that mean:

(a) malignant tumour
   of lymph (use sarc/o)

(b) benign tumour
   of cartilage

(c) a malignant tumour
   originating in bone
   (use sarc/o)

(d) condition of a new
   growth of cells

(e) the treatment of
   tumours

Score

5

Check answers to Self-Assessment Tests on page 325.

UNIT 20
ANATOMICAL POSITION

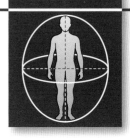

EXERCISE GUIDE

Use this list of word components and their meanings to complete the word exercises in this unit.

Prefixes

epi-	above/upon/on
hypo-	below/under

Roots/Combining forms

bucc/o	cheek
cardi/o	heart
cephal/o	head
chondr/o	cartilage
cost/o	rib
crani/o	cranium/skull
derm/o	skin
faci/o	face
-ganglion	ganglion
gastr/o	stomach
hepat/o	liver

ili/o	hip/ilium/flank
mamm/o	breast/mammary gland
nas/o	nose
or/o	mouth
ot/o	ear
placent/o	placenta
stern/o	sternum
ven/o	vein
vertebr/o	vertebra/spine

Suffixes

-ac	pertaining to
-al	pertaining to
-ary	pertaining to
-ic	pertaining to
-ous	pertaining to/of the nature of
-ver(ted)	turned

Anatomical position

In this unit we will examine a selection of terms that refer to the position of organs and tissues within the body. Many of these terms are also used to indicate the position of injuries, pain, disease and surgical operations.

The **anatomical position** of the body (Fig. 90) is a reference system that all doctors and medical texts use when describing body components. We always refer to position in the patient's body as if he/she were standing upright with arms at the sides and palms of the hands facing forward, head erect and eyes looking forward.

With the body in the anatomical position we can draw an imaginary line down the middle of the body (Fig. 90). This is called the **midline** or **median line** and it bisects the body into right and left sides. Note that right

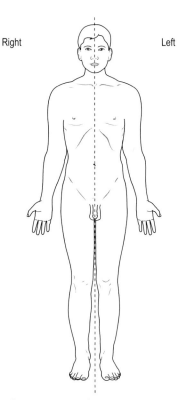

Right   Left

Figure 90   The anatomical position

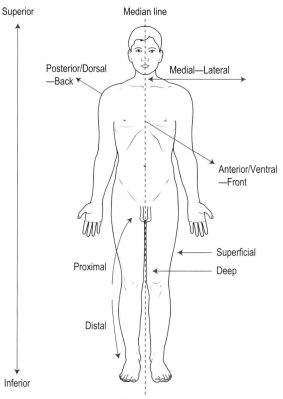

Superior   Median line

Posterior/Dorsal —Back

Medial—Lateral

Anterior/Ventral —Front

Superficial

Proximal

Deep

Distal

Inferior

Figure 91   Anatomical directions

and left refer to the sides of the patient in the anatomical position, not those of the observer.

Directions

We can now see how the imaginary midline can be used to indicate directions when a body is in the anatomical position. Parts that lie nearer to the median line of the body than other parts are described as **medial** to that part. Any part that lies further away is said to be **lateral** to the first part (Fig. 91). To summarize:

Medial   pertaining to towards the median line (or midline)

Lateral   pertaining to away from the median line (or midline)

Other directions can also be seen in Figure 91.

Superior towards the head, upper
Inferior away from the head, lower
Anterior (ventral) front
Posterior (dorsal) back
Proximal pertaining to near point of attachment or point of origin
Distal pertaining to further from point of attachment or origin
Superficial pertaining to near the surface of the body
Deep away from the surface of the body

WORD EXERCISE 1

Using the information in Figure 91, complete the following sentences by deleting the incorrect word:

(a)   The eyes are superior/inferior to the mouth.

(b)   The mouth is superior/inferior to the nose.

(c)   The ear is medial/lateral to the eye.

(d)   The nostril is medial/lateral to the eye.

(e)   The umbilicus lies on the anterior/posterior surface of the abdomen.

(f)   The vertebrae lie close to the dorsal/ventral surface of the body.

(g)   The wrist is proximal/distal to the elbow.

(h)   The ankles are proximal/distal to the toes.

(i)   The ribs are superficial/deep to the lungs.

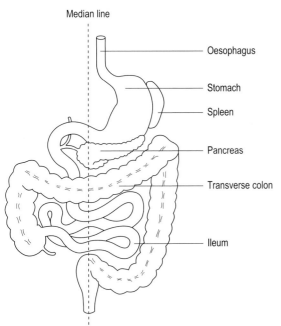

Figure 92   The digestive system in the anatomical position

These terms can also be applied to organ systems and tissues within the body. They too are described as if they are in the anatomical position, e.g. the digestive system (Fig. 92).

WORD EXERCISE 2

Using information from Figure 92, complete the following sentences by deleting the incorrect word:

(a) The pancreas is superior/inferior to the stomach.

(b) The oesophagus (Am. esophagus) is superior/inferior to the stomach.

(c) The stomach is medial/lateral to the spleen.

(d) The oesophagus (Am. esophagus) is proximal/distal to the stomach.

(e) The transverse colon is anterior/posterior to the ileum.

(f) The ileum is dorsal/ventral to the transverse colon.

Regions

With the body in the anatomical position, it can be divided into the cephalic, thoracic, abdominal and pelvic regions (Fig. 93).

Each of these regions can be subdivided; the simplest example is perhaps the division of the abdominopelvic region into quadrants (Fig. 94).

Doctors and health personnel often use this simple system to describe the position of abdominopelvic pain. Imaginary vertical and horizontal lines through the umbilicus form the quadrants. A more complex method is to divide the abdominopelvic region into nine regions (Fig. 95).

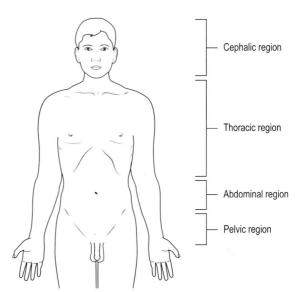

Figure 93   Regions of the trunk and head

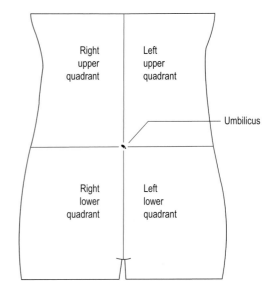

Figure 94   Abdominopelvic region (quadrants)

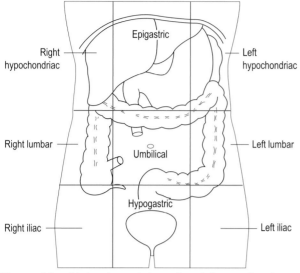

Figure 95   Abdominopelvic region (nine regions)

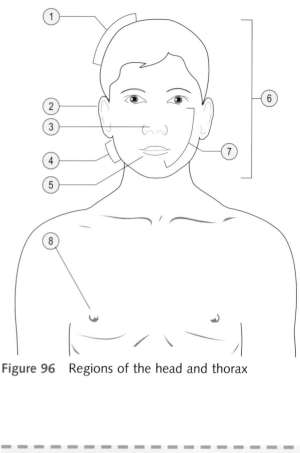

Figure 96   Regions of the head and thorax

WORD EXERCISE 3

Using your Exercise Guide, find the meaning of:

(a) hypo/chondr/i/ac region (The word refers to the cartilage of the rib-cage.)

(b) epi/gastr/ic region

(c) ili/ac region

(f) mammary region

(g) nasal region

(h) buccal region

The cephalic regions and the upper and lower extremities can also be subdivided into regions. These are examined in the next two exercises. Use your Exercise Guide to find the meaning of unfamiliar words.

WORD EXERCISE 4

Examine Figure 96 and match the regions listed in Column A with a number from the diagram:

Column A	Number
(a) cephalic region	
(b) cranial region	
(c) facial region	
(d) otic region	
(e) oral region	

WORD EXERCISE 5

Look at Figures 97 and 98 and label the regions of each limb by selecting an appropriate region from the list below. The first region has been labelled for you.

hallux region	great toe
crural region	leg
pedal region	foot
digital/phalangeal region	toes
patellar region	knee
femoral region	thigh
tarsal region	ankle bones
axillary region	armpit
palmar/volar region	palm
antebrachial region	forearm
digital/phalangeal region	fingers
brachial region	arm
pollex region	thumb
carpal region	wrist bones

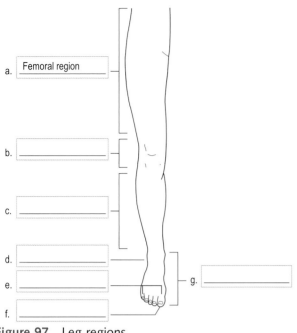

a. | Femoral region |

b. |_____|

c. |_____|

d. |_____|

e. |_____| g. |_____|

f. |_____|

Figure 97   Leg regions

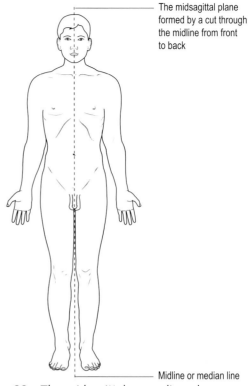

The midsagittal plane formed by a cut through the midline from front to back

Midline or median line

Figure 99   The midsagittal or median plane

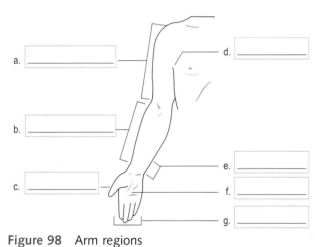

a. |_____| d. |_____|

b. |_____|

c. |_____| e. |_____|

f. |_____|

g. |_____|

Figure 98   Arm regions

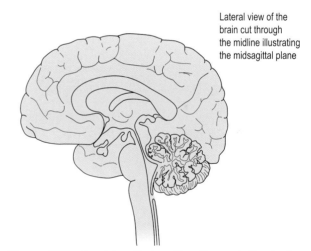

Lateral view of the brain cut through the midline illustrating the midsagittal plane

Figure 100   A midsagittal section through the brain

Planes

Planes are imaginary flat surfaces that form a reference system indicating the direction in which organs have been cut, drawn or photographed. When a body structure is studied, it is often viewed in section and the section is formed from a cut made in relation to one of the planes.

Imagine a vertical cut made along the midline from the front of the body to the back dividing it into right and left halves. The flat surfaces formed in each cut half illustrate the **median** or **midsagittal plane**. Figure 99 shows the direction of the cut that forms the midsagittal plane. Figure 100 shows a midsagittal section through the brain when cut in this plane and viewed from the side.

Any plane parallel to the midsagittal or median plane is called a **parasagittal** or **paramedian plane** (*para* meaning besides) (Fig. 101).

Two other planes are shown in Figure 102 and Figure 103. A horizontal cut illustrates the **horizontal** or **transverse plane** (Fig. 102). This is the equivalent of a cross-section through the body dividing it into superior and inferior portions.

A vertical side cut divides the body into anterior and posterior portions at right angles to the sagittal plane and illustrates the **frontal** or **coronal plane** (Fig. 103).

Figure 104 summarizes the three main planes of the body.

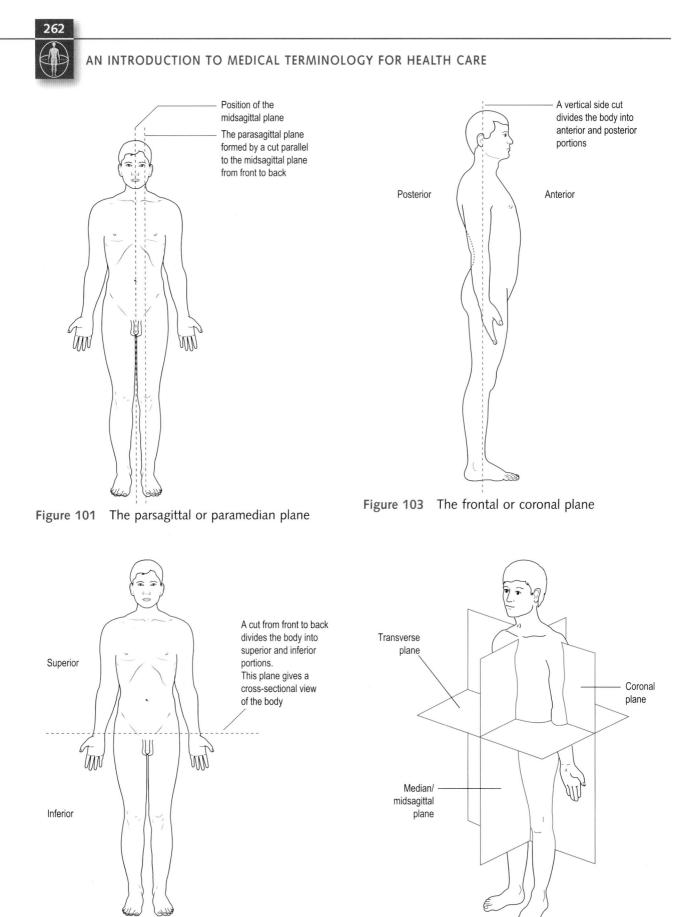

Position of the
midsagittal plane

The parasagittal plane
formed by a cut parallel
to the midsagittal plane
from front to back

Figure 101   The parsagittal or paramedian plane

A vertical side cut
divides the body into
anterior and posterior
portions

Posterior   Anterior

Figure 103   The frontal or coronal plane

Superior

A cut from front to back
divides the body into
superior and inferior
portions.
This plane gives a
cross-sectional view
of the body

Inferior

Figure 102   The horizontal or transverse plane

Transverse
plane

Coronal
plane

Median/
midsagittal
plane

Figure 104   The planes of the body

WORD EXERCISE 6

Match a description in Column A to a plane in Column C by inserting a number in Column B.

Column A	Column B	Column C
(a) divides the body into superior and inferior portions		1. midsagittal plane
(b) a plane parallel to the median plane		2. transverse plane
(c) divides the body into right and left halves		3. frontal plane
(d) divides the body into anterior and posterior portions		4. parasagittal plane

WORD EXERCISE 7

Use the locative prefix list to fill in each blank with an appropriate prefix:

Column A	Column B	Column C
(a) The region beside the nose		nasal region
(b) Disc between vertebrae		vertebral disc
(c) Region upon the stomach		gastric region
(d) Pertaining to after a ganglion		ganglionic
(e) Condition of right displacement of heart		cardia
(f) Nerve below orbit of eye		orbital nerve

Locating parts of the body

There are a large number of locative prefixes that act as prepositions when placed in front of word roots. These tell us about the position of structures within the body. Use the list of locative prefixes below to complete the next two exercises.

WORD EXERCISE 8

Use your Exercise Guide and the locative prefix list to find the meaning of:

(a) peri/cardi/al

(b) intra/ven/ous

(c) inter/cost/al

(d) retro/verted uterus

(e) supra/hepat/ic

(f) infra/stern/al

(g) pre/ganglion/ic

(h) extra/placent/al

(i) sub/epiderm/al

Locative prefixes	
Above	epi-, hyper-, super-, supra-
Across	trans-
After	meta-, post-
Against	anti, contra-
Around	circum-, peri-
Away	ab-, apo-, ef-
Back	dorsi-, dorso-, post-, re-, retro-
Backward	opistho-, retro (also means back/behind)
Before/front	ante-, pre-, pro-, ventr-
Below	hypo-, infra-, sub-
Behind/after	dorsi-, dorso-, post-
Beside	para-
Between	inter-
Down	de-
Front/in front	pro-, ventr-
In/inside	em-, en-, endo-, in-, intra-
Left	laevo- (Am. levo-)
Middle	medi-, meso-
Out/outside	ec-, ect-, ef-, exo-, extra-
Right	dextro-
Side	later-
Through	dia-, per-
To/towards/near	ad-, af-
Under	infra-, sub-
Upon	epi-
Within	intra-

Some of the locative prefixes we have listed are incorporated into words that indicate the direction of movement of parts of the body. Before noting some examples we need to describe the main actions of muscles.

Muscles that bend limbs by decreasing the angles between articulating bones are called **flexors** and those that increase the angles after they have flexed are called **extensors**. The action of flexors is known as **flexion** and that of extensors, **extension**. Examples of prefixes that indicate direction of movements at joints are shown in bold:

Abduction	the movement of a part away from the midline (*ab-* meaning away from).
Adduction	the movement of a part towards the midline (*ad-* meaning to)
Circumduction	the movement in which the distal ends of a bone move in a circle (*circum-* meaning around). Not a separate plane of movement
Protraction	the movement of a part forward/in front e.g. the jaw (*pro-* meaning in front/before)
Retraction	the movement of a protracted part back (*re-* meaning back/contrary)
Elevation	the upward movement of a body part e.g. the jaw (from Latin *elevare* meaning to raise)
Depression	the downward movement of a body part (*de-* meaning down/from)
Dorsiflexion	the movement that bends the foot back (upwards) from the anatomical position (*dorsi-* meaning back)
Plantar flexion	the movement that bends the foot downwards from the anatomical position (*plantar* meaning pertaining to the sole of the foot)
Inversion	the movement of the sole inward so the soles face each other (*in-* meaning in/inward)
Eversion	the movement of the sole in the outwards, so the soles face away from each other (*e-* meaning out from)
Pronation	the movement of the forearm that turns the palm of the hand posteriorly or inferiorly (from Latin *pronare* meaning bend forward)
Supination	the movement of the forearm that turns the palm of the hand anteriorly or superiorly (from Latin *supinare* meaning bend backward)

CASE HISTORY 20

The object of this exercise is to understand words associated with a patient's medical history.

To complete the exercise:

- read through the passage on an unusual fracture of the tibia; unfamiliar words are underlined and you can find their meaning using the Word Help

- write the meaning of the medical terms shown in bold print on the lines that follow the Word Help.

An unusual fracture of the tibia

A 13-year-old male was referred to the <u>Orthopaedic</u> Department after sustaining a <u>hyperextension</u> injury to his right knee during a school football match. He had immediate onset of pain and swelling during the first few hours following the injury. On admission he could not bear weight on the knee and <u>flexion</u> and <u>extension</u> <u>exacerbated</u> the pain. His medical record indicated no previous injury to his right <u>lower extremity</u> and he appeared to be in good health.

Examination of the right lower extremity revealed a knee <u>effusion</u> with soft tissue swelling and diffuse tenderness over the **proximal** <u>tibial</u> growth plate. There were **superficial** skin <u>lacerations</u> on the **anterior** and **medial** surface of his right thigh. He could not **dorsiflex** or <u>evert</u> his foot and sensation in the **lateral** <u>calf</u> and foot was reduced. <u>Vascular</u> insufficiency in the injured extremity was assessed; the <u>popliteal</u>, <u>dorsalis pedis</u> and <u>posterior tibial</u> pulses were <u>palpable</u> with good **distal** refilling.

Lateral and **anteroposterior** <u>radiographs</u> demonstrated a proximal tibial fracture classified as a <u>Salter-Harris</u> <u>type III</u>. The <u>intra-articular</u> fracture extended along the articular surface into the medial and lateral <u>plateaus</u>. The <u>epiphyseal</u> plate was anteriorly displaced on the <u>metaphysis</u>.

He underwent <u>open reduction</u> and internal fixation with a 3 mm Steinmann pin; recovery was uneventful and his articular surface was preserved.

WORD HELP

calf the fleshy back part of the leg below the knee

dorsalis pedis pulse the pulse on the dorsal foot (the upper part of the foot)

effusion a fluid discharge into a part/escape of fluid into an enclosed space

flexion decreasing the angle between two bones (here bending the leg)

epiphyseal pertaining to the epiphysis, the end of a long bone separated from the main shaft by a cartilage plate

evert turn the sole of the foot outward at the ankle joint

extension increasing the angle between two bones (here straightening the leg)

exacerbated increased severity of symptoms

hyperextension forcible over-extending of a limb (here extending the knee joint so far that the lower leg bends forwards)

intra-articular within a joint or inside the cavity of a joint laceration a tear in a tissue

lower extremity a leg (hip, thigh, leg, ankle and foot taken as one structure)

metaphysis the wider part at the end of the main shaft of a long bone adjacent to the epiphysis

open reduction an operation that exposes bones for restoration of displaced tissue

orthopaedic pertaining to orthopaedics (study of the locomotor/movement system)

palpable able to be felt using light pressure with the fingers

plateau a flat region (here the expanded end of the tibia that articulates with the femur)

popliteal pulse pertaining to the pulse behind the knee

posterior tibial pulse the pulse in the foot posterior to the lower end of the tibia

radiograph here meaning an X-ray picture/recording

Salter-Harris type III a classification system for growth plate injuries

tibial pertaining to the tibia

vascular pertaining to blood vessels

Quick Reference

Combining forms relating to anatomical parts and positions of the body:

Anter/o	front/anterior
Axill/o	armpit
Brachi/o	arm
Bucc/o	cheek
Carp/o	carpal/wrist bones
Cephal/o	head
Crani/o	cranium
Crur/o	leg
Digit/o	finger/toe
Faci/o	face
Femor/o	femur/thigh
Hallux	great toe
Ili/o	ilium/flank
Infer/o	towards the feet/inferior
Later/o	side
Mamm/o	breast/mammary gland
Nas/o	nose
Or/o	mouth
Ot/o	ear
Palm/o	palm
Patell/o	patella/knee cap
Ped/o	foot
Phalang/o	phalange/finger/toe
Pollex	thumb
Poster/o	back/posterior
Super/o	towards the head/superior
Tars/o	tarsus/ankle bones
Vol/o	palm

Now write the meaning of the following words from the case history without using your dictionary lists:

(a) proximal

(b) superficial

(c) anterior

(d) medial

(e) dorsiflex

(f) lateral

(g) distal

(h) anteroposterior

(Answers to the case history exercise are given in the Answers to Word Exercises beginning on page 301.)

Abbreviations

Some common abbreviations related to anatomical position are listed below. Note some are not standard and their meaning may vary from one health care setting to another. There is a more extensive list for reference on page 335.

ant	anterior
inf	inferior
lat	lateral
LLQ	left lower quadrant
LUQ	left upper quadrant
med	medial
pos	position
post	posterior
prox	proximal
RLQ	right lower quadant
RUQ	right upper quadrant
sup	superior

NOW TRY THE WORD CHECK

WORD CHECK

This self-check exercise lists all the word components used in this unit. First write down the meaning of as many word components as you can. Then check your answers using the Exercise Guide and Quick Reference box or the Glossary of Word Components (pp. 347–371).

Prefixes

ab-

ad-

af-

ante

anti-

apo-

circum-

contra-

dextro-

dia-

dorso-

ec-

ect-

ef-

em-

en-

endo-

exo-

extra-

in-

infra-

inter-

intra-

laevo-
(Am. levo-)

medi-

meso-

para-

per-

peri-

pre-

pro-

retro-

super-

supra-

trans-

ventro-

Combining forms of word roots

anter/o

axill/o

brachi/o

bucc/o

cardi/o

carp/o

cephal/o

chondr/o

cost/o

crani/o

crur/o

derm/o

digit/o

faci/o

femor/o

-ganglion

gastr/o

hallux

hepat/o

ili/o

infer/o

later/o

mamm/o

nas/o

or/o

ot/o

palm/o

patell/o

ped/o

phalang/o

placent/o

pollex

poster/o

stern/o

super/o

tars/o

ven/o

verteb/o

vol/o

Suffixes

-ac

-al

-ary

-ia

-iac

-ic

-ous

-ver(ted)

NOW TRY THE SELF-ASSESSMENT

AN INTRODUCTION TO MEDICAL TERMINOLOGY FOR HEALTH CARE

SELF-ASSESSMENT

Test 20A

Combining forms relating to parts of body

Match each combining form in Column A with a meaning in Column C by inserting the appropriate number in Column B.

Column A	Column B	Column C
(a) abdomin/o		1. head
(b) axill/o		2. leg
(c) brachi/o		3. great toe
(d) carp/o		4. ankle bones/tarsus
(e) cephal/o		5. palm (i)
(f) crani/o		6. palm (ii)
(g) crur/o		7. knee
(h) digit/o		8. finger/toe (i)
(i) femor/o		9. finger/toe (ii)
(j) hallux		10. pelvis
(k) ili/o		11. thumb
(l) palm/o		12. thigh/femur
(m) patell/o		13. abdomen
(n) ped/o		14. skull/cranium
(o) pelv/i		15. thorax
(p) phalang/o		16. foot
(q) pollex		17. arm
(r) tars/o		18. armpit
(s) thorac/o		19. ilium/flank
(t) vol/o		20. wrist bones

Score ☐
20

Test 20B

Locative prefixes

Match each locative prefix from Column A with a meaning in Column C by inserting the appropriate number in Column B.

Column A	Column B	Column C
(a) ab-		1. through (i)
(b) ad-		2. through (ii)
(c) circum-		3. backward/behind
(d) dextro-		4. across
(e) dia-		5. between
(f) ec-		6. side
(g) en-		7. around (i)
(h) epi-		8. around (ii)
(i) infra-		9. away
(j) inter-		10. before/in front of
(k) laevo- (Am. levo-)		11. beside
(l) later-		12. towards
(m) para-		13. after/behind
(n) per-		14. right
(o) peri-		15. upon
(p) post-		16. in
(q) pre-		17. above
(r) retro-		18. left
(s) supra-		19. below
(t) trans-		20. out

Score ☐
20

Test 20C

Write the meaning of:

(a) interphalangeal

(b) dextroversion

(c) retrobuccal

(d) supracostal

(e) intranasal

Score

5

Test 20D

Build words that mean:

(a) pertaining to the side

(b) a turning towards the left

(c) pertaining to after a ganglion

(d) pertaining to below the liver

(e) pertaining to across the skin

Score

5

Check answers to Self-Assessment Tests on page 325.

UNIT 21
PHARMACOLOGY AND MICROBIOLOGY

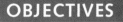

OBJECTIVES

Once you have completed Unit 21 you should be able to:

- understand the meaning of medical words relating to pharmacology and microbiology
- deduce the use or action of drugs from their classification

- understand medical abbreviations associated with pharmacology and microbiology.

EXERCISE GUIDE

Use this list of word components and their meanings to complete the word exercises in this unit.

Prefixes

a-	without
an-	without
anti-	against
dia-	through
neo-	new
oxy-	quick
retro-	back/backward

Roots/Combining forms

acid/o	acid
aem-	blood (Am, -em)
aesthet/o	sensation/sensitivity (Am. esthet/o)
anxi/o	anxiety
alges/i/o	sense of pain
bacill/o	bacillus/bacilli
bacteri/o	bacterium/bacteria
bio-	life/living
bronch/i/o	bronchus/bronchial tubes
cocc/o	coccus/cocci
cycl/o	ciliary body
cyt/o	cell
dynam/o	force/power (of movement)
em- (Am.)	blood
epilept/o	epilepsy
esthet/o (Am.)	sensation/sensitivity
estr/o (Am.)	estrogen/estrus

fibrin/o	fibrin (a protein that forms the fibres of blood clots)
fung/i/o	fungus
gonad/o	gonads/reproductive organs
haem/o	blood (Am. hem/o)
hem/o (Am.)	blood
helmint/h/o	worms
hypn/o	sleep
immun/o	immune/immunity
kerat/o	epidermis/cornea
kinet/o	motion/movement
lact/i/o	milk
muc/o	mucus
oestr/o	oestrogen /oestrus (Am. estr/o)
pharmac/o	drug
plas/m/o	growth
prurit/o	itching
psych/o	mind
(r)rhythm/o	rhythm
septic/o	sepsis/infection
staphylococc/o	staphylococcus/staphylococci
spasm/o/d	spasm
spirill/o	spirillum/spirilla
streptococc/o	streptococcus/streptococci
thyroid/o	thyroid
toc/o	labour/birth
tox/ic/o	poison/poisonous to
troph/o	nourish/stimulate
tuss/i	cough
ur/o	urine
vir/o	virus/virion

Suffixes

-aemia	condition of blood (Am. -emia)
-al	pertaining to/type of drug
-ase	an enzyme
-cidal	pertaining to killing
-cide	agent that kills/killing
-emia (Am.)	condition of blood
-form	having the form/structure of
-gen	precursor/agent that produces
-genic	pertaining to formation
-gnosy	process of judgment/knowledge
-ia	condition of
-ic	type of drug/pertaining to
-in	non-specific suffix indicating a chemical
-ine	substance thought to be derived from ammonia
-ist	specialist
-ite	end-product
-ity	state/condition
-ive	pertaining to/type of drug
-logist	specialist who studies
-logy	study of
-lytic	drug that breaks down . . . / pertaining to breakdown
-oid	resembling
-ose	carbohydrate/sugar/starch
-osis	abnormal condition/disease of
-plegic	drug that paralyses/condition of paralysis
-rrhea (Am.)	excessive discharge/flow
-rrhoea	excessive discharge/flow (Am. -rrhea)
-static	pertaining to stopping/agent that stops
-uria	condition of urine
-y	process/condition

Pharmacology

Pharmacology is the science that deals with the study of drugs. By drugs we mean medicinal substances that can be used to treat, prevent or diagnose disease and illness. Research into the properties and potential use of substances showing physiological activity has enabled the pharmaceutical industry to market new and more effective drugs.

ROOT

Pharmac
(From a Greek word **pharmakon** *meaning drug.)*

Combining form   **Pharmac/o**

WORD EXERCISE 1

Without using your Exercise Guide write the meaning of:

(a) **pharmac/o/logy**

(b) **pharmac/o/log/ist**

(c) **pharmac/o/psych/osis**

There are several specialisms related to pharmacology that are not completely understood from their name:

Pharmacognosy
the study of (*gnos-* knowledge of) crude drugs of vegetable and animal origin.

Pharmacokinetics
the study of the way drugs are absorbed, metabolized and excreted, i.e. what the body does to the drug and how it moves through the body.

Pharmacodynamics
the study of the action of drugs, i.e. what the drug does to the body.

Pharmacy
the study of the process of preparing and dispensing medicinal drugs or a place where drugs are compounded or dispensed.

Therapeutics
the branch of medicine that deals with the treatment of disease. Treatment can be **palliative** i.e. alleviates symptoms or **curative**. In common usage, therapeutics refers mainly to the use of drugs to treat disease.

Chemotherapy
the treatment of disease using chemical agents (a main type of treatment for cancer).

Toxicology
the study of poisons and other toxic substances and their effect on the body.

Naming drugs

Drugs are known by several different names.

1. **The brand, trade or proprietary name**
    Following extensive research and development, pharmaceutical companies assign brand names to their products for marketing purposes. Each drug and its name are the exclusive property of the

company with patent rights to its manufacture. The patent will expire after a fixed time (usually 17 years) allowing time for development costs to be recouped. When the patent expires, other companies may manufacture the drug under different brand names or under the drug's generic name.

2. **The generic name**

Each drug has an official non-proprietary or generic name. This name is assigned to it in its early stage of development and is often a description of its chemical composition or class. Once the patent expires, any number of companies may manufacture a generic drug under different brand names.

A recent EEC directive requires the use of a recommended International Non-proprietary Name (rINN) for medicinal substances. Many British Approved Names (BANs) have been changed or modified to comply with the rINN directive.

3. **The chemical name**

This name indicates a drug formula. A manufacturer or pharmacist uses the name when making up a formulation.

Authoritative information about the use, structure, manufacture and the dosage of medicinal drugs is documented in large reference texts known as a *pharmacopoeia*.

WORD EXERCISE 2

In pharmacology certain suffixes are used to denote types of substance:

Suffix	Meaning	Examples
-ase	indicates an enzyme	amy**lase**/suc**rase**
-gen	a precursor or agent that produces something	trypsino**gen**
-ic	denotes a type of medicinal drug	mucoly**tic**
-in	a non-specific suffix denoting a chemical agent	triste**rin**
-ine	a substance derived from ammonia	am**ine**/alan**ine**
-ite	an end product	metabo**lite**
-ose	a type of sugar	glu**cose**/mal**tose**

Match a biochemical name from Column A with a description in Column C by inserting the appropriate number in Column B.

Column A	Column B	Column C
(a) lip/ase		1. a sugar
(b) rib/ose		2. a chemical that produces an action
(c) ser/ine		3. an enzyme

(d) progesto/gen		4. a medicinal agent
(e) mydria/t/ic		5. a chemical related to ammonia

Drug classification

Drugs can be classified by their therapeutic use or action. Exercises 3–14 list the classifications of drugs used to treat disorders associated with the body systems we have studied in this book.

Note. The suffixes -al, -ant, -ent, -ic, and -ive are used to mean *pertaining to* but they are also used in pharmacology to indicate a type of drug.

The action of a drug can often be deduced from its classification. To do this we split the word classification into its components, find their meaning and then try to deduce an action or use. The technique can be practised in Word Exercises 3–14.

WORD EXERCISE 3

Many classifications have the prefix **anti-** meaning against. Using your Exercise Guide write the meaning of:

(a) **anti**/bacter/i/al

(b) **anti**/bio/t/ic

(c) **anti**/fung/al

(d) **anti**/vir/al

(e) **anti**/prurit/ic

In the following examples the *i* of the prefix ***anti-*** is dropped for roots beginning with a vowel or the letter h.

(f) **ant**/acid

(g) **ant**/helmint/ic

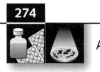
WORD EXERCISE 4

Several drug classifications have the prefix **an-** meaning without. Using your Exercise Guide write the meaning of:

(a) **an**/alges/ic

(b) **an**/aesthe/t/ic
    (Am. an/esthe/t/ic)

Word Exercises 5–14 list common types of drug associated with the systems studied in this book.

Drug classifications associated with the digestive system

WORD EXERCISE 5

Without using your Exercise Guide write the meaning of:

(a) anti/diarrhoe/al
    (Am. antidiarrheal)

(b) anti/spasmod/ic
    (acts on intestines)

Others include:

Laxative
promotes evacuation of the bowels

H$_2$–receptor antagonist
prevents the secretion of acid by the gastric mucosa (lining of the stomach) and promotes the healing of ulcers

Drug classifications associated with the respiratory system

WORD EXERCISE 6

Using your Exercise Guide write the meaning of:

(a) muc/o/lyt/ic

(b) anti/tuss/ive

(c) bronch/o/dilat/or (dilate means to widen, not listed in the Exercise Guide)

Others include:

Antihistamine
a type of drug that counteracts the effects of histamine, a chemical that is released during allergic reactions such as asthma.

Corticosteroid
a type of drug that reduces inflammation. Corticosteroids are used for prophylaxis in the treatment of asthma by reducing inflammation in the bronchial mucosa (lining).

Decongestant
a type of drug that reduces the feeling of congestion in the nose.

Drug classifications associated with the cardiovascular system and blood

WORD EXERCISE 7

Using your Exercise Guide write the meaning of:

(a) fibrin/o/lyt/ic

(b) anti/fibrin/o/lyt/ic

(c) anti-/a/rrhythm/ic

(d) haem/o/stat/ic
    (Am. hem/o/stat/ic)

Others include:

Anticoagulant
a type of drug that prevents clotting/coagulation of blood.

Antiplatelet drug
a type of drug that decreases platelet aggregation in arteries, thereby inhibiting clot formation.

Antihypertensive
a type of drug that reduces high blood pressure. Antihypertensives are used to treat hypertension (high blood pressure).

Diuretic
a type of drug that promotes the excretion of urine, thereby relieving the oedema (Am. edema) of heart failure.

Inotropic
a type of drug used to increase or decrease the force of contraction of heart muscle (myocardium).

Sympathomimetic
a type of drug that mimics the action of the sympathetic nervous system, sympathomimetics are used to raise blood pressure.

Drug classifications associated with the urinary system

Anti-diruretic hormone
a hormone that acts on the kidney stimulating reabsorption of water thereby reducing the formation of urine.

Diuretic
a type of drug that promotes the excretion of urine.

Uricosuric
a type of drug that increases the excretion of uric acid in urine thereby relieving the symptoms of gout.

Xanthine-oxidase inhibitor
a type of drug used for the palliative treatment of gout.

Drug classifications associated with the nervous system

WORD EXERCISE 8

Using your Exercise Guide write the meaning of:

(a) hypn/o/t/ic

(b) anxi/o/lyt/ic

(c) anti/epilep/t/ic

(d) anti/psych/o/t/ic

Others include:

Antidepressant
a type of drug that prevents or relieves depression.

CNS stimulant
a type of drug that has limited use for treating narcolepsy (a recurrent, uncontrollable desire to sleep).

Anti-emetic
a type of drug that prevents vomiting (emesis).

Opioid analgesic
a type of drug that relieves moderate to severe pain particularly of visceral origin (opioid – refers to a synthetic narcotic resembling but not derived from opium).

Drug classifications associated with the eye

WORD EXERCISE 9

Using your Exercise Guide write the meaning of:

(a) cycl/o/pleg/ic

Others include:

Eye lotion
a solution used for irrigating the eye.

Topical anti-infective preparation
an antibacterial, antifungal or antiviral agent that is applied directly to the eye.

Topical corticosteroid
an anti-inflammatory steroid that is applied directly to the eye.

Mydriatic
a type of drug that dilates the pupil for eye examination.

Local anaesthetic (Am. anesthetic)
a type of drug that reduces sensation in the eye.

Miotic
a type of drug used to treat glaucoma that narrows the pupil.

Drug classifications associated with the ear

Topical astringent
a type of drug used to treat inflammation that dries the tissue.

Topical anti-infective preparation
an antibacterial or antifungal applied directly to the external ear for treatment of otitis externa.

Drug classifications associated with the mouth and nose

Oral antihistamine
a type of drug that reduces the symptoms of histamine, it is used for treatment of nasal allergy.

Systemic nasal decongestant
a type of drug used for symptomatic relief in chronic nasal congestion.

Topical decongestant
a type of drug applied directly to the nose as drops or spray to relieve congestion.

Drug classifications associated with the skin

WORD EXERCISE 10

Using your Exercise Guide write the meaning of:

(a) anti/prurit/ic

(b) kerat/o/lyt/ic

Others include:

> **Vehicle**
> an inert substance added to a drug that gives it a suitable consistency for transfer into the body; vehicles do not possess therapeutic properties.
>
> **Emollient**
> an agent that softens or soothes the skin.
>
> **Desloughing agent**
> an agent that removes dead tissue from a wound.

Drug classifications associated with the musculoskeletal system

> **Non-steroidal anti-inflammatory drug (NSAID)**
> a type of drug that in full dose has analgesic and anti-inflammatory effects. NSAIDs are used to treat painful inflammatory conditions such as rheumatic disease; aspirin is a familiar example.
>
> **Relaxant**
> a type of drug that blocks the neuromuscular junction and produces relaxation of muscles, they are widely used in anaesthesia.
>
> **Uricosuric**
> a type of drug that promotes the excretion of uric acid in the urine thereby relieving the symptoms of gout.

Drug classifications associated with the reproductive system

WORD EXERCISE 11

Using your Exercise Guide write the meaning of:

(a) oxy/toc/ic

(b) gonad/o/troph/in

Without using your Exercise Guide write the meaning of:

(c) anti-/oestr/o/gen
   (Am. anti-/estr/o/gen)

Others include:

> **Oral contraceptive**
> a type of drug that prevents conception i.e. the fertilization of an egg by a sperm. Family planning pills contain sex hormones that inhibit the release of eggs from the ovary thereby preventing a pregnancy.
>
> **Prostaglandin**
> a type of drug used to induce abortion, augment labour and minimize blood loss from the placental site.

> **Sex hormone**
> a type of hormone used for hormone replacement therapy (HRT). In women small doses of the female sex hormone oestrogen are used to relieve menopausal symptoms. In castrated males sex hormones called androgens are used for replacement therapy.

Drug classifications associated with the endocrine system

(This section deals with examples of drug classifications other than those that act on the reproductive system.)

WORD EXERCISE 12

Without using your Exercise Guide write the meaning of:

(a) anti/thyroid

Others include:

> **Antidiabetic**
> a drug that is used to treat non-insulin dependent diabetes, it acts against diabetes by increasing insulin secretion.
>
> **Insulin**
> insulin is a hormone that lowers blood glucose in patients with diabetes mellitus. Many different forms of insulin e.g. short, intermediate and long-acting are available for injection.
>
> **Corticosteroid**
> a steroid produced by the adrenal cortex or its synthetic equivalent used for replacement therapy. Corticosteroids are used when secretion by the adrenal glands is insufficient.
>
> **Human growth hormone**
> a growth hormone of human origin (somatotrophin) used to stimulate growth in patients of short stature. This has been replaced by somatotropin, a biosynthetic human growth hormone that has a similar effect.

Drug classifications associated with oncology

Drugs used in oncology aim to prevent the replication of cancer cells and destroy them by interfering with their metabolism. The process of using drugs in this way to destroy tumours is called **chemotherapy**.

WORD EXERCISE 13

Using your Exercise Guide write the meaning of:

(a) cyt/o/tox/ic

(b) anti/neo/plas/t/ic

Others include:

Alkylating drugs
drugs that damage DNA (genes) and interfere with the replication of cancer cells.

Antimetabolite
a drug that combines with and inhibits vital cell enzymes.

Vinca alkaloids
drugs originally derived from the plant species *Vinca* that have the ability to directly interrupt the process of cell division.

Drug classifications associated with the immune system

These drugs are used to suppress rejection of transplanted organs in their recipients and treat autoimmune diseases (*auto-* meaning self, **autoimmunity** is an abnormal response of the immune system to the body's own tissues).

WORD EXERCISE 14

Without using your Exercise Guide write the meaning of:

(a) immun/o/suppress/ant (suppress means prevent/stop)

_____

(b) cyt/o/toxic/ immun/o/suppress/ant

_____

Abbreviations

Some common abbreviations related to drug administration are listed below. Note some are not standard and their meaning may vary from one health care setting to another. There is a more extensive list for reference on page 335.

bid	twice a day (bis in die)
cap	capsule
disp	dispense
im	intramuscular
iv	intravenous
od	every day
OTC	over the counter (non-prescription drugs)
po	per os, by mouth, orally
prn	when required
qid	four times a day (quater in die)
tab	tablet
tid	three times a day (ter in die)

Microbiology

Microbiology is the study of small organisms (*micro* – small, *bio* – life, *logy* – study of). In the field of health, pathogenic microorganisms such as bacteria, protozoa, fungi and viruses are responsible for infectious disease. Swabs, fluids and tissues taken from patients suspected of having an infection are sent to the microbiology laboratories for analysis. The microbiology laboratory is often part of the pathology department in a large hospital. This section examines words associated with microorganisms.

Microbiology is divided into the following specialities:

Bacteriology	study of bacteria
Mycology	study of fungi
Virology	study of viruses
Protozoology	the study of protozoa

Naming microorganisms

Species of microorganisms are given Latin names according to the binomial (two name) system. The first name denotes the group or **genus** to which the organism belongs and always begins with a capital letter. The second name is the **species** or specific name and this begins with a lower case letter for example:

Salmonella typhi Salmonella is the genus, typhi the species

Clostridium tetani Clostridium is the genus, tetani the species

---

Often the name of the genus is abbreviated if it is widely used, as in *E. coli* for *Escherichia coli* and *Staph. aureus* for *Staphylococcus aureus*.

The species name of microorganisms is sometimes formed from words that indicate:

---

their colour	e.g. *Staphylococcus aureus* (from aurum, meaning gold)
the place where they are found	e.g. *Staphylococcus epidermidis* (in the epidermis of the skin)
the disease they cause	e.g. *Bacillus anthracis* (causes anthrax)
the scientist who studied or named them	e.g. *Escherichia coli* (after Dr Theodor Escherich, German physician, b.1857)

Bacteriology

Bacteria are small single-celled organisms that can only be seen with an optical microscope. There are thousands of different types classified according to their shape, group arrangement, colony characteristics, structure and chemical characteristics. The combining form **bacteri/o** is used to mean bacteria (from Greek *bakterion* meaning staff).

Classification of bacteria using the Gram staining reaction

For more than a century bacteria have been classified using the **Gram** staining reaction named after Christian Gram who devised it in 1884. His method is based upon the ability of bacteria to retain the purple crystal violet-iodine complex when stained and treated with organic solvents:

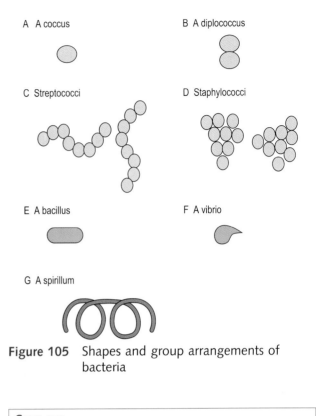

Figure 105 Shapes and group arrangements of bacteria

Gram-positive bacteria (Gram +ve) retain the stain and appear purple.

Gram-negative bacteria (gram –ve) cannot retain the purple dye complex and need to be stained with a red dye before they can be seen with an optical microscope.

Classification by shape and grouping

Individual bacteria have one of three basic shapes: they are either spherical, cylindrical or spiral. Spherical cells are called **cocci** (singular **coccus**), cylindrical cells **bacilli** (singular **bacillus**) and helical or spiral cells **spirilla** (singular **spirillum**).

The coccus (plural – cocci)

The word coccus comes from a Greek word *kokkos* meaning berry. They are usually round but can be ovoid or flattened on one side when adhering to another cell. Cocci can grow in several different arrangements or groups depending on the plane of cell division and whether the new cells remain together. Each arrangement is typical of a species and contributes to an organism's classification. When a coccus divides in one plane and the two new cells remain together the arrangement is called a **diplococcus**.

When cocci divide repeatedly in one plane and remain together to form a twisted row of cells they are called **streptococci** (*strepto-* from a Greek word meaning twisted, singular streptococcus). Others divide in three planes and remain together in irregular, grape-like patterns; these are called **staphylococci** (*staphylo-* from a Greek word meaning grapes, singular staphylococcus). See Figure 105 for examples:

Some cocci are of great medical importance, for example:

Gram +ve
Streptococcus pneumoniae causes pneumonia and meningitis.

Staphylococcus aureus causes serious infection in hospitals (MRSA – methicillin resistant *Staphylococcus aureus*).

Gram –ve
Neisseria gonorrhoeae causes gonorrhoea.

Neisseria meningitidis causes meningitis.

(*Neisseria* are sometimes seen in pairs and are grouped as diplococci.)

The bacillus (plural – bacilli)

These are rod-shaped bacteria (*bacillus* is a Latin word meaning a stick or rod); they are also classified using the Gram staining procedure (see Fig. 105E). There are large differences in the length and width of bacilli and their ends can be square, rounded or tapered.

Some bacilli are of medical importance, for example:

Gram +ve
Bacillus anthracis causes anthrax. It produces highly resistant spores that are difficult to destroy except at high temperatures.

Clostridium tetani found in soil, causes tetanus.

Gram –ve
Escherichia coli found in the human gut, certain strains are pathogenic.

Salmonella typhi causes typhoid.

Gram-negative bacilli that appear curved in shape (like a comma) are called vibrios (see Fig. 105F), for example:

Vibrio cholerae causes cholera, a water-borne infection.

The spirillum (plural – spirilla)

The spirilla are spiral or helical-shaped bacteria that look like tiny corkscrews (see Fig. 105G). Those that belong to the genus *Spirillum* consist of Gram –ve, non-flexous (non-flexible) spiral-shaped filaments. Another group distinguished by their flexibility belongs to the genus *Spirochaeta*. (Note: the use of this group is becoming obsolete and most of the bacteria assigned to this group have been transferred to other genera.) Examples are:

Spirillum minus causes rat-bite fever in man. *Treponema pallidum* a spirochaete (Am. spirochete) that belongs to the order Spirochaetales and causes syphilis.

It should be noted that the cells of a given species are rarely arranged in exactly the same pattern. It is the predominant arrangement that is important when studying bacteria.

Some terms denoting shape, for example bacillus, may be used as generic names as in *Bacillus anthracis*.

Culture and sensitivity testing

Infected swabs, fluids and tissues are sent to microbiology laboratories for **culture and sensitivity testing**. To culture an organism, it is placed at an optimum temperature in a special culture medium (broth or agar jelly) that contains all the nutrients required for growth. In ideal conditions the microorganism multiplies rapidly producing a huge clone of identical cells. Samples from the culture are then exposed to a range of different antibiotics. If an organism is sensitive to a particular antibiotic, it will be destroyed or its growth inhibited. Antibiotics that are found to destroy the cultured organisms are administered to the patient to try and rid them of the infection.

WORD EXERCISE 15

Match a description in Column A with a bacterium in Column C by inserting a number in Column B.

Column A	Column B	Column C
(a) A bacterium that appears rod-shaped		1. diplococci
and purple following staining with the Gram staining procedure		
(b) A rod that appears comma-shaped and pink following staining with the Gram staining procedure		2. *Staphylococcus aureus*
(c) Cocci arranged into a twisted chain that infects the lungs		3. Gram –ve *Vibrio cholerae*
(d) Gold coloured cocci arranged into irregular grape-like groups that cause serious suppurative infections, sometimes resistant to common antibiotics		4. Gram –ve *E. coli*
(e) Cocci belonging to the genus Neisseria that arrange themselves into pairs		5. Gram +ve *Bacillus anthracis*
(f) A helical bacterium that causes syphilis		6. *Streptococcus pneumoniae*
(g) A bacterium that appears rod-shaped and pink following staining with the Gram procedure		7. *Treponema pallidum* (a spirochaete)

WORD EXERCISE 16

Using your Exercise Guide write the meaning of:

(a) **bacteri/o/log/ist**

(b) **streptococc/al**

(c) **bacteri/ur/ia**

(d) **bacteri/cid/al**

(e) **bacteri/o/stat/ic**

(f) **bacteri/o/lyt/ic**

(g) **bacill/aem/ia**
(Am. **bacill/em/ia**)

(h) **bacill/o/gen/ic**

(i) **streptococc/i/cide**

(j) **strept/o/septic/aem/ia**
(Am. **strept/o/septic/em/ia**)

(k) **spirill/osis**

Mycology

Fungi are non-green plants that act as decomposers in the environment, breaking down the dead bodies of plants and animals. The group includes the familiar mushrooms and toadstools and microscopic moulds and yeasts.

Certain types of moulds and yeasts are pathogenic and infect the body causing disease. When they infect the skin they are called **dermatophytes** (*dermat/o* meaning skin, *-phyte* meaning plant). A common condition is Athlete's foot caused by several species of fungi (e.g. *Trichophyton rubrum*) that infect skin between the toes. In warm, moist conditions the fungi grow and digest the skin causing it to itch and split. The fungal spores that generate the infection are usually picked up on changing room floors so the condition is common among sports enthusiasts. Athlete's foot is easily treated and harmless, unlike some fungal infections found in tropical climates.

When round, red patches of skin infected with fungi begin to heal in the centre first, they often take on a ring-like appearance and because of this the infection became inaccurately known as 'ringworm'. The medical name for Athlete's foot is **Tinea pedis** or ringworm of the foot (*Tinea* is a Latin word meaning gnawing worm, and *-pedis* means the foot). Other superficial fungal infections of the skin are named in a similar way: **Tinea capitis** (ringworm of the head), **Tinea corporis** (ringworm of the body).

Fungal infections are life-threatening in patients whose immune system is compromised; for example, *Candida albicans* can cause serious infections of the mouth, digestive system and reproductive systems in AIDS patients. This type of infection is known as **candidiasis** (from Latin *candidus* meaning white and *-iasis* meaning abnormal condition).

Fungi are named according to the binomial system with a generic and specific name as in *Candida albicans*.

ROOT

Myc
(From a Greek word **mykes**, *meaning fungus.)*

Combining forms **Myc/o**

WORD EXERCISE 17

Without using your Exercise Guide, write the meaning of:

(a) **myc/osis**

(b) **mycot/ic**

(c) **myc/o/tox/in**

(d) **myc/o/toxic/osis**

ROOT

Fung
(From a Greek word **fungus**, *meaning mushroom. Here fung/i/o means fungus or fungal infection.)*

Combining forms **Fung/i/o**

WORD EXERCISE 18

Without using your Exercise Guide, write the meaning of:

(a) **fung/i/form**

(b) **fung/i/tox/ic**

(c) **fung/i/cide**

(d) **fung/i/stat/ic**

Using your Exercise Guide, find the meaning of:

(e) **fung/oid**

(f) **fungos/ity**

Virology

A virus (virion) is an extremely small infectious particle that does not show the usual characteristics of life; for example, it does not move, respire, feed or respond to stimuli.

Viruses do reproduce but only within a specific host cell. (Note: a host is an organism that harbours a parasite.) When a virus comes into contact with a host cell, it inserts its genes into the cell. Once inside the viral genes alter the metabolism of the host cell and instruct it to make new viruses. The host cell fills with copies of the original virus and may burst, releasing the new infectious particles into the surrounding environment.

Viruses have characteristic shapes, different chemical structures and different methods of replication. They can only be seen in an electron microscope that produces a large magnification and has the ability to resolve their fine detail. Characteristics of viruses and the conditions they cause are incorporated into their names. In the examples given below the words have been split to show their meaning.

Onco/rna/virus
type of virus that causes cancer (onc/o) and contains ribonucleic acid (-rna-).

Papo/va/virus
type of virus that causes vacuoles (va) inside host cells and the formation of papillomas/tumours (papo – papilloma).

Pico/rna/virus
type of virus that is very small (pico-) and contains ribonucleic acid (-rna-).

Retro/virus
type of virus that carries the enzyme reverse transcriptase (retro – back, the enzyme converts viral RNA back to DNA).

Rhino/virus
type of virus that infects the nose (rhin/o – nose).

Entero/virus
type of virus that infects the intestines.

Bacterio/phage
type of virus that uses a bacterium as a host.

The modern convention for naming viruses is to use the host name followed by the major effect e.g. human immunodeficiency virus.

ROOT

Vir

(From a Greek word **virus***, meaning poison. Here vir/o means virus, a minute infectious particle that replicates only within a living host cell. Each particle consists of viral genes enclosed in a protein coat.)*

Combining forms **Vir/o/u**

Protozoology

This is a branch of medicine concerned with single-celled animals called protozoa. Some of these organisms are pathogenic and responsible for serious disease. Infection with protozoa is generally referred to as a **protozo**iasis (*-iasis* meaning abnormal condition of). Examples are given below:

Plasmodium falciparum
(a type of sporozoan) that causes malaria

Trypanosoma gambiense
(a type of flagellate) that causes African sleeping sickness

Entamoeba histolytica
(a type of amoeba) that causes amoebic (Am. amebic) dysentery

---

CASE HISTORY 21

The object of this exercise is to understand words associated with a patient's medical history. To complete the exercise:

• read through the passage on HIV infection; unfamiliar words are underlined and you can find their meaning using the Word Help

• write the meaning of the medical terms shown in bold print on the lines that follow the Word Help.

HIV infection

Mr U, a 38-year-old homosexual man, presented to the Accident and Emergency Department with a fever, non-productive cough and dyspnoea (Am. dyspnea). During the previous 7 days he had become increasingly short of breath and complained of an inability to sleep because he was hot and sweating profusely. He was a non-smoker and had no haemoptysis (Am. hemoptysis). Mr U informed the medical staff that he had been diagnosed HIV positive 3 years earlier but had declined antiretroviral therapy.

On examination he appeared pale, and thin and he indicated that he had lost a considerable amount of weight over the past 2 months. He was pyrexial (Temp. 39.1°C), tachycardic (121 beats/min), and tachypnoeic (Am. tachypneic) (28 breaths/min).

Examination of his mouth revealed white patches with surrounding inflammation indicative of a severe candidiasis; swabs were taken and sent for analysis. He was short of breath with poor lung expansion and a chest X-ray showed diffuse bilateral shading. His serum biochemistry and liver function were normal.

Mr U was admitted to the ward with a clinical diagnosis of PCP or other atypical pneumonia and started on the antibacterial co-trimoxazole in two daily doses and the antibiotic erythromycin given as an infusion over 1 hour. He was also given an intravenous steroid methylprednisolone to reduce inflammation in his alveoli and improve gaseous exchange.

The next day a bronchoscopy was performed, and the washings sent to the microbiology laboratory for culture and sensitivity testing. The results confirmed the diagnosis of *Pneumocystis carinii* infection and haematology reported a CD4 count of less than 50 cells mm^{-3}, indicating Mr U had developed AIDS. His mouth infection was confirmed as *Candida albicans* and he was prescribed the antifungal itraconazole.

Following administration of his high dose of co-trimoxazole Mr U developed severe nausea and was given the anti-emetic metoclopramide parenterally before his infusions.

Two weeks later he was clinically much improved, and a pharmaceutical plan was devised prior to his discharge. He was advised that he required antiretroviral therapy and counselled on the possibility of side-effects. He was given a discharge medication of sufficient oral co-trimoxazole to complete his initial course of treatment and instructed on a prophylactic dose regimen.

WORD HELP

AIDS acquired immune deficiency syndrome

atypical not conforming to the usual type/in microbiology applied to strains of unusual type

bilateral pertaining to both sides

bronchoscopy technique of viewing/examining the bronchial tree

Candida albicans a yeast-like fungus belonging to the genus *Candida* that infects the digestive and reproductive systems

CD4 cluster designation/cluster of differentiation. Refers to clusters of chemicals (cell surface markers) found on the surface of leucocytes (Am. leukocytes). CD4 molecules found on lymphocytes called T-cells (helper T (T$_H$) cells or T4 cells) act as the receptor molecules for HIV. The depletion of CD4 lymphocytes by HIV leads to the development of AIDS

culture and sensitivity testing growing microorganisms in the laboratory and testing them for sensitivity to antibiotics

dyspnoea difficult/laboured breathing (Am. dyspnea)

haemoptysis (Am. hemoptysis) spitting/coughing up of blood

infusion slow introduction of a therapeutic agent into a vein

non-productive not producing (sputum)

HIV positive presence of antibodies to the human immunodeficiency virus in the blood, it indicates the virus has infected the body

parenterally the word means pertaining to beyond the intestine but in practice it means administered by injection into the skin or muscle

PCP *Pneumocystis carinii* pneumonia

Pneumocystis carinii a protozoa-like organism that causes pneumonia, an opportunistic infection commonly seen in AIDS patients

prophylactic pertaining to preventative treatment

pyrexial having a fever/elevation of body temperature above normal

regimen a regulated scheme (e.g. of taking drugs/medication)

tachycardic pertaining to a fast heart beat

tachypnoeic pertaining to fast breathing (Am. tachypneic)

washing a solution that has contacted a surface and is to be used for analysis

Now write the meaning of the following words from the case study without using your dictionary lists:

(a) antiretroviral

(b) candidiasis

(c) antibacterial

(d) antibiotic

(e) microbiology

(f) antifungal

(g) anti-emetic

(h) pharmaceutical plan

(Answers to the case history exercise are given in the Answers to Word Exercises beginning on page 301)

There is a more extensive list for reference on page 335.

Abbreviations

Some common abbreviations related to microbiology and infectious disease are listed below. Note some are not standard and their meaning may vary from one health care setting to another. There is a more extensive list for reference on page 335.

ABX	antibiotics
AFB	acid-fast bacilli
BCG	bacille (bacillus) Calmette–Guérin (causes tuberculosis)
C+S	culture and sensitivity test
EBV	Epstein–Barr virus
HBV	Hepatitis B virus
HSV	*Herpes simplex* virus
Hib	*Haemophilus influenzae* type b
HIV	human immunodeficiency virus
MRSA	methicillin resistant *Staphylococcus aureus*
NGU	non-gonococcal urethritis
PCN	penicillin

Quick Reference

Combining forms relating to the pharmacology and microbiology:

cocc/o	coccus (a berry-shaped bacterium)
bacill/o	bacillus (a rod-like bacterium)
bacteri/o	bacterium/bacteria
fung/i	fungus
helmint/h/o	worm
myc/o	fungus
pharmac/o	drug
spirill/o	a spiral-shaped bacterium of genus *Spirillum*
staphylococc/o	staphylococcus/a bunch of cocci
streptococc/o	streptococcus/a chain of cocci
toxic/o	poison
vibri/o	a comma-shaped bacterium of genus *Vibrio*
vir/o	virus/virion

NOW TRY THE WORD CHECK

WORD CHECK

This self-check exercise lists all the word components used in this unit. First write down the meaning of as many word components as you can. Then check your answers using the Exercise Guide and Quick Reference box or the Glossary of Word Components (pp. 347–371).

Prefixes

a-

an-

anti-

auto-

dia-

neo-

oxy-

retro-

Roots/Combining forms

acid/o

aesthet/o

anxi/o

alges/i/o

bacill/o	
bacteri/o	
bio-	
bronch/i/o	
cocc/o	
cycl/o	
cyt/o	
dynam/o	
epilept/o	
esthet/o (Am.)	
estr/o (Am.)	
fibrin/o	
fung/i	
gonad/o	
haem/o	
helmint/h/o	
hem/o (Am.)	
hypn/o	
immun/o	
kerat/o	
kinet/o	
lact/i/o	
muc/o	
oestr/o	
pharmac/o	
plas/m/o	
prurit/o	
psych/o	
(r)rhythm/o	
septic/o	
spasm/o/d	
spirill/o	
staphylococc/o	
streptococc/o	

thyroid/o	
tox/ic/o	
troph/o	
tuss/i	
ur/o	
vir/o	

Suffixes

-aemia	
-al	
-ase	
-cid(e)	
-emia (Am.)	
-form	
-gen	
-gnosy	
-ia	
-ic	
-ite	
-ive	
-logist	
-logy	
-lytic	
-oid	
-ose	
-osis	
-plegia	
-rrhea (Am.)	
-rrhoea	
-uria	
-y	

NOW TRY THE SELF-ASSESSMENT

SELF-ASSESSMENT

Test 21A

Prefixes and suffixes

Match each prefix or suffix in Column A with a meaning in Column C by inserting the appropriate number in Column B.

Column A	Column B	Column C
(a) an-		1. quick
(b) anti-		2. knowledge/process of judgment
(c) -ase		3. chemical derived from ammonia
(d) -cide		4. abnormal condition/disease
(e) -gen		5. condition of rhythm
(f) -gnosy		6. process/condition
(g) -ose		7. study of
(h) -ic		8. drug that breaks down . . . / pertaining to breakdown
(i) -in		9. without
(j) -ine		10. end-product
(k) -ite		11. excessive discharge/flow
(l) -ive		12. enzyme
(m) -logy		13. against
(n) -logist		14. non-specific suffix indicating a chemical
(o) -lytic		15. type of drug/pertaining to (i)
(p) -osis		16. type of drug/pertaining to (ii)
(q) oxy-		17. agent that kills
(r) -rrhoea (Am. rrhea)		18. specialist who studies
(s) -rrhythmia		19. precursor/agent that produces
(t) -y		20. sugar

Score [ ] / 20

Test 21B

Combining forms of word roots

Match each combining form of a word root from Column A with a meaning from Column C by inserting the appropriate number in Column B.

Column A	Column B	Column C
(a) acid/o		1. poison
(b) aesthet/o (Am. esthet/o)		2. worms
(c) alges/i/o		3. itching
(d) anxi/o		4. fungus (i)
(e) bacteri/o		5. fungus (ii)
(f) bio-		6. bacteria
(g) dynam/o		7. drug
(h) fung/i		8. life
(i) helmint/h/o		9. sensation
(j) hypn/o		10. mind
(k) kinet/o		11. nourish/stimulate
(l) muc/o		12. cough
(m) myc/o		13. anxiety
(n) pharmac/o		14. force/power of movement
(o) prurit/o		15. virus/virion
(p) psych/o		16. pain
(q) toxic/o		17. acid

Column A	Column B	Column C
(r) troph/o		18. motion/ movement
(s) tuss/i		19. sleep
(t) vir/o		20. mucus

Score

20

Test 21C

Write the meaning of:

(a) toxicology

(b) mycotoxicosis

(c) pharmacist

(d) chemotherapeutic agent

(e) microbiologist

Score

5

Test 21D

Build words that mean:

(a) specialist who studies bacteria

(b) drug that acts against living things

(c) the study of protozoa

(d) agent that stops the growth of bacteria

(e) pertaining to killing viruses

Score

5

Test 21E

Match each drug action from Column A with a drug classification from Column C by inserting the appropriate number in Column B.

Column A	Column B	Column C
(a) acts against worms		1. immuno-suppressant
(b) acts to reduce pain		2. cytotoxic
(c) reduces sensation		3. miotic
(d) acts to reduce coughing		4. antipsychotic
(e) neutralises stomach acid		5. anxiolytic
(f) acts to break up mucus		6. antipruritic
(g) acts to promote the excretion of urine		7. anthelmintic
(h) acts to dilate bronchi		8. antihistamine
(i) used to treat schizophrenia		9. antitussive
(j) used to induce labour		10. antibiotic
(k) acts to lower blood sugar of non-insulin dependent diabetics		11. gonadotrophin
(l) acts to kill cancer cells		12. analgesic
(m) reduces the immune response		13. hypnotic
(n) used to treat glaucoma		14. antihypertensive
(o) dilates the pupil for examination		15. contraceptive

Column A	Column B	Column C
(p) promotes evacuation of the bowels		16. anticoagulant
(q) prevents the effects of histamine		17. bronchodilator
(r) used to induce sleep		18. diuretic
(s) used to reduce high blood pressure		19. anaesthetic (Am. anesthetic)
(t) used to reduce anxiety		20. antacid
(u) used to prevent itching		21. mucolytic
(v) used to prevent conception/ pregnancy		22. mydriatic
(w) stimulates/ nourishes the reproductive organs		23. antidiabetic
(x) prevents blood clotting		24. laxative
(y) destroys bacteria and fungi		25. oxytocic

Score ⬜

25

Test 21F

Match each description from Column A with the name of an organism from Column C by inserting the appropriate number in Column B.

Column A	Column B	Column C
(a) a round, berry-like bacterium		1. staphylococci
(b) a rod-like bacterium		2. spirillum
(c) a comma-shaped bacterium		3. rhinovirus
(d) a spiral-shaped bacterium		4. bacillus
(e) a cancer forming virus that contains RNA		5. streptococci
(f) a plant (fungus) that infects the skin		6. diplococci
(g) round berry-like bacteria that occur in chains		7. a bacteriophage
(h) round berry-like bacteria that occur in bunches		8. coccus
(i) a virus that infects the nose		9. vibrio
(j) berry-like bacteria that group in pairs		10. dermatophyte

Column A	Column B	Column C
(k) a single-celled animal that causes malaria		11. a protozoan *Plasmodium*
(l) a virus that infects bacteria		12. oncornavirus

Check answers to Self-Assessment Tests on page 325.

Test your recall of the meanings of word components in Units 16–21 by completing the appropriate self-assessment tests in Unit 22 on page 298.

Score

12

UNIT **22**
FINAL SELF-ASSESSMENT TESTS

In this section you can assess your recall of the meaning of medical word components. The tests that follow each contain a selection of words relating to the topics studied in Units 1–21. Answers can be found on page 332.

FINAL SELF-ASSESSMENT TESTS FOR UNITS 1–5

Final test 1 prefixes

Match each prefix in Column A with a meaning in Column C by inserting the appropriate number in Column B.

Column A	Column B	Column C
(a) a-		1. around
(b) bi-		2. inside/within
(c) brady-		3. beside/near
(d) dextro-		4. below normal/ reduced
(e) dys-		5. slow
(f) endo-		6. right
(g) epi-		7. large (i)
(h) hyper-		8. large (ii)
(i) hypo-		9. all
(j) inter-		10. fast
(k) macro-		11. small
(l) mega-		12. upon/above in position
(m) micro-		13. many
(n) normo-		14. varied/irregular
(o) pan-		15. between
(p) para-		16. normal
(q) peri-		17. painful/difficult
(r) poikilo-		18. without
(s) poly-		19. above normal/ excessive
(t) tachy-		20. two

Score [ ]

[20]

Final test 2 combining forms of medical word roots

Match each combining form in Column A with a meaning in Column C by inserting the appropriate number in Column B.

Column A	Column B	Column C
(a) angi/o		1. abdomen/ abdominal wall
(b) ather/o		2. nose
(c) cardi/o		3. stomach
(d) cholecyst/o		4. platelet
(e) cost/o		5. tissue
(f) cyt/o		6. anus/rectum
(g) erythr/o		7. liver
(h) gastr/o		8. atheroma (fatty plaque)
(i) haem/o (Am. hem/o)		9. organ
(j) hepat/o		10. diaphragm
(k) hist/o		11. vessel
(l) lapar/o		12. vein
(m) laryng/o		13. cell
(n) leuc/o (Am. leuk/o)		14. lung
(o) myel/o		15. disease
(p) organ/o		16. pulse
(q) path/o		17. gallbladder
(r) phleb/o		18. rib
(s) phren/o		19. larynx
(t) pneumon/o		20. heart
(u) proct/o		21. myelocyte/ marrow
(v) reticul/o		22. red blood cell

Column A	Column B	Column C
(w) sphygm/o		23. blood
(x) rhin/o		24. white blood cell
(y) thrombocyt/o		25. immature erythrocyte

Score

25

Column A	Column B	Column C
(p) -stomy		16. pertaining to being poisonous
(q) -tomy		17. condition of
(r) -toxic		18. pertaining to stimulating/ inducing
(s) -tropic		19. technique of making a recording/X-ray
(t) -uria		20. inflammation of

Score

20

Final test 3 suffixes

Match each suffix in Column A with a meaning in Column C by inserting the appropriate number in Column B.

Column A	Column B	Column C
(a) -algia		1. condition of the urine
(b) -clysis		2. opening into/an opening
(c) -genesis		3. enlargement
(d) -gram		4. breakdown
(e) -graphy		5. disease of
(f) -ia		6. study of
(g) -ic		7. specialist
(h) -ist		8. condition of pain
(i) -itis		9. a recording/ X-ray
(j) -logy		10. pertaining to
(k) -lysis		11. technique of viewing/ examining
(l) -megaly		12. infusion/ injection into
(m) -pathy		13. incision into
(n) -scope		14. formation of
(o) -scopy		15. instrument to view/examine

Final test 4 suffixes

Match each suffix in Column A with a meaning in Column C by inserting the appropriate number in Column B.

Column A	Column B	Column C
(a) -aemia (Am. -emia)		1. formation of
(b) -ary		2. a cutting instrument
(c) -centesis		3. condition of paralysis
(d) -chromia		4. condition of narrowing
(e) -cytosis		5. tumour (Am. tumor)/ swelling
(f) -desis		6. surgical repair/ reconstruction
(g) -dynia		7. pertaining to
(h) -ectasis		8. excessive discharge/ excessive flow
(i) -meter		9. surgical fixation (i)
(j) -metry		10. surgical fixation (ii)

Column A	Column B	Column C
(k) -oma		11. involuntary contraction
(l) -osis		12. stopping/ cessation of movement
(m) -penia		13. puncture to remove fluid
(n) -pexy		14. condition of pain
(o) -plasty		15. dilation/stretching
(p) -plegia		16. structure/ anatomical part
(q) -poiesis		17. condition of/ disease of
(r) -ptysis		18. technique of measuring
(s) -rrhage		19. a measuring instrument
(t) -rrhoea (Am. -rrhea)		20. condition of cells (too many)
(u) -spasm		21. condition of blood
(v) -stasis		22. bursting forth of blood
(w) -stenosis		23. condition of deficiency
(x) -tome		24. spitting up
(y) -um		25. condition of haemoglobin (Am. hemoglobin)/ colour

Score

25

FINAL SELF-ASSESSMENT TESTS FOR UNITS 6–10

Final test 5 prefixes

Match each prefix in Column A with a meaning in Column C by inserting the appropriate number in Column B.

Column A	Column B	Column C
(a) agora-		1. deficiency/few
(b) ambly-		2. grey (grey matter of the CNS)
(c) auto-		3. through
(d) bin-		4. open place
(e) di-		5. out/away from
(f) dia-		6. same/equal
(g) diplo-		7. four (i)
(h) en-		8. four (ii)
(i) ex-		9. under
(j) hemi-		10. beside/near
(k) intra-		11. dry
(l) iso-		12. after/behind
(m) meso-		13. old man/old age
(n) mono-		14. in/within (i)
(o) oligo-		15. in/within (ii)
(p) para-		16. one (i)
(q) polio-		17. one (ii)
(r) post-		18. self
(s) pre-		19. middle
(t) presby-		20. before/in front of
(u) quadri-		21. dull/dim
(v) sub-		22. half
(w) tetra-		23. two/double (i)
(x) uni-		24. two/double (ii)
(y) xero-		25. two/double (iii)

Score 25

Final test 6 combining forms of medical word roots

Match each word combining form in Column A with a meaning in Column C by inserting the appropriate number in Column B.

Column A	Column B	Column C
(a) adenoid-		1. kidney (i)
(b) aesthesi/o (Am. esthesi/o)		2. kidney (ii)
(c) alges/i		3. dura mater
(d) azot/o		4. thymus gland
(e) cyst/o		5. pain
(f) dur/o		6. bladder (i)
(g) encephal/o		7. bladder (ii)
(h) immun/o		8. lymph vessel
(i) lith/o		9. nerve
(j) lymphaden/o		10. sensation
(k) lymphangi/o		11. serum
(l) nephr/o		12. ureter
(m) neur/o		13. urinary tract/urine
(n) phag/o		14. spleen
(o) psych/o		15. stone
(p) pyel/o		16. brain
(q) py/o		17. mind
(r) ren/o		18. adenoids
(s) ser/o		19. renal pelvis
(t) splen/o		20. urethra
(u) thym/o		21. lymph node
(v) ureter/o		22. pus
(w) urethr/o		23. eating/consuming
(x) ur/o		24. immunity
(y) vesic/o		25. urea/nitrogen

Score 25

Final test 7 combining forms of medical word roots

Match each combining form in Column A with a meaning in Column C by inserting the appropriate number in Column B.

Column A	Column B	Column C
(a) audi/o		1. Eustachian tube/ auditory tube
(b) aur/i		2. angle of anterior chamber of the eye
(c) auricul/o		3. pupil
(d) blephar/o		4. sclera
(e) chromat/o		5. auricle/ear flap
(f) cochle/o		6. lens
(g) cor/e/o		7. malleus (an ear ossicle)
(h) cycl/o		8. ear drum/ear membrane
(i) dacry/o		9. stapes (an ear ossicle)
(j) goni/o		10. uvea
(k) incud/o		11. iris
(l) irid/o		12. ear (i)
(m) lacrim/o		13. ear (ii)
(n) malle/o		14. eye (i)
(o) myring/o		15. eye (ii)
(p) ocul/o		16. middle ear/ tympanum
(q) ophthalm/o		17. hearing
(r) opt/o		18. cochlea
(s) ot/o		19. incus (an ear ossicle)
(t) phac/o		20. ciliary body
(u) scler/o		21. sight
(v) salping/o		22. tear (i)
(w) stapedi/o		23. tear (ii)
(x) tympan/o		24. colour/ haemoglobin (Am. hemoglobin)
(y) uve/o		25. eyelid

Score [ ] / 25

Final test 8 suffixes

Match each suffix in Column A with a meaning in Column C by inserting the appropriate number in Column B.

Column A	Column B	Column C
(a) -al		1. abnormal condition/ disease of
(b) -cele		2. stitching/suturing
(c) -eal		3. act of crushing
(d) -ectomy		4. tumour (Am. tumor)/boil
(e) -ferous		5. condition of softening
(f) -genic		6. condition of urine (excretion of)
(g) -iasis		7. presence of stones/ abnormal condition of stones
(h) -ity		8. swelling/protrusion
(i) -lapaxy		9. pertaining to carrying
(j) -lithiasis		10. instrument that fragments e.g. using shock-waves
(k) -malacia		11. instrument that crushes
(l) -phyma		12. condition of bursting forth of blood/bleeding
(m) -ptosis		13. pertaining to (i)

Column A	Column B	Column C
(n) -rrhagia		14. pertaining to (ii)
(o) -rrhaphy		15. pertaining to (iii)
(p) -tic		16. removal of
(q) -tripsy		17. falling/displacement
(r) -triptor		18. pertaining to forming
(s) -trite		19. to wash out/ evacuate
(t) -uresis		20. state/condition of

Score

20

Final test 9 suffixes

Match each suffix in Column A with a meaning in Column C by inserting the appropriate number in Column B.

Column A	Column B	Column C
(a) -agogic		1. thing/a structure
(b) -ar		2. to carve
(c) -chalasis		3. pertaining to circular motion
(d) -conus		4. heat
(e) -graph		5. instrument that records

Column A	Column B	Column C
(f) -emphraxis		6. pertaining to (i)
(g) -erysis		7. pertaining to (ii)
(h) -gyric		8. cone-like protrusion
(i) -iatry		9. prick/puncture
(j) -kinesis		10. splitting/parting
(k) -metrist		11. drag/draw/suck out
(l) -mileusis		12. wasting away
(m) -nyxis		13. nourishment/ development
(n) -ous		14. blocking/stopping up
(o) -phthisis		15. medical treatment
(p) -plasia		16. slackening/loosening
(q) -schisis		17. pertaining to inducing/stimulating
(r) -thermy		18. specialist who measures
(s) -trophy		19. condition of movement
(t) -us		20. condition of growth (of cells)

Score

20

FINAL SELF-ASSESSMENT TESTS FOR UNITS 11–15

Final test 10 prefixes

Match each prefix in Column A with a meaning in Column C by inserting the appropriate number in Column B.

Column A	Column B	Column C
(a) a-		1. large
(b) an-		2. under/below
(c) crypto-		3. above normal/excessive
(d) dys-		4. inside/within
(e) endo-		5. below normal/reduced
(f) epi-		6. beside/near
(g) hyper-		7. yellow
(h) hypo-		8. little/small amount
(i) macro-		9. hidden
(j) oligo-		10. difficult/painful
(k) ortho-		11. many
(l) pachy-		12. straight/correct
(m) para-		13. after
(n) peri-		14. dry
(o) poly-		15. across/through
(p) post-		16. without/not (i)
(q) sub-		17. without/not (ii)
(r) trans-		18. around
(s) xantho-		19. upon/above in position
(t) xero-		20. thick

Score 20

Final test 11 combining forms of medical word roots

Match each combining form in Column A with a meaning in Column C by inserting the appropriate number in Column B.

Column A	Column B	Column C
(a) arthr/o		1. sweat
(b) balan/o		2. movement
(c) cheil/o		3. jaw
(d) chondr/o		4. epidermis
(e) dermat/o		5. bone
(f) gingiv/o		6. foreskin/prepuce
(g) gnath/o		7. cartilage
(h) hidr/o		8. muscle
(i) kerat/o		9. lip
(j) kinesi/o		10. joint
(k) kyph/o		11. glans penis
(l) lei/o		12. vas deferens
(m) my/o		13. vertebra
(n) onych/o		14. smooth (muscle)
(o) orchi/o		15. striated muscle
(p) oste/o		16. penis
(q) phall/o		17. testis/testicle
(r) posth/o		18. skin
(s) rhabd/o		19. crooked/hunched
(t) rhin/o		20. tendon
(u) spondyl/o		21. scaly
(v) squam/o		22. hair
(w) tendin/o		23. nail
(x) trich/o		24. gum
(y) vas/o		25. nose

Score 25

Final test 12 suffixes

Match each suffix in Column A with a meaning in Column C by inserting the appropriate number in Column B.

Column A	Column B	Column C
(a) -agogue		1. condition of softening
(b) -auxis		2. condition of muscle tone
(c) -blast		3. increase
(d) -cide		4. condition of eating
(e) -clasis		5. slipping
(f) -clast		6. a plant-like growth/a plant e.g. a fungus
(g) -dynia		7. slight paralysis
(h) -globin		8. condition of having voice
(i) -ism		9. immature germ cell/cell that forms
(j) -kymia		10. condition of pain
(k) -malacia		11. formation
(l) -oid		12. breakdown/ surgical breakdown
(m) -olisthesis		13. agent that kills/ killing
(n) -paresis		14. agent that induces/ stimulates
(o) -phagia		15. protein
(p) -phonia		16. condition of involuntary muscle twitching
(q) -phyte		17. resembling
(r) -poiesis		18. a cell that breaks something

Column A	Column B	Column C
(s) -rrhexis		19. rupturing
(t) -tonia		20. process of/state or condition of

Score

20

FINAL SELF-ASSESSMENT TESTS FOR UNITS 16–21 (EXCLUDING UNIT 20)

Final test 13 prefixes

Match each prefix in Column A with a meaning in Column C by inserting the appropriate number in Column B.

Column A	Column B	Column C
(a) acro-		1. before (i)
(b) an-		2. before (ii)
(c) ana-		3. before (iii)
(d) ante-		4. against
(e) anti-		5. without/not
(f) auto-		6. through/across
(g) dia-		7. first
(h) eu-		8. many
(i) hypo-		9. extremity/point
(j) meta-		10. beyond
(k) multi-		11. none
(l) neo-		12. self
(m) nulli-		13. second
(n) oxy-		14. below normal/reduced
(o) pre-		15. new
(p) primi-		16. good
(q) pro-		17. quick
(r) retro-		18. backward (i)
(s) secundi-		19. backward (ii)
(t) ultra-		20. changed in form or position

Score

20

Final test 14 combining forms of medical word roots

Match each combining form in Column A with a meaning in Column C by inserting the appropriate number in Column B.

Column A	Column B	Column C
(a) aden/o		1. vagina
(b) andr/o		2. breast (i)
(c) cine/o		3. breast (ii)
(d) colp/o		4. birth
(e) echo-		5. slice/section
(f) endometr/i		6. pregnancy
(g) -gravida		7. labour (Am. labor)
(h) helmint/h/o		8. fungus
(i) hyster/o		9. gland
(j) kal/i		10. midwifery/obstetrics
(k) lact/o		11. Fallopian tube/uterine tube
(l) mamm/o		12. to bear/bring forth (as in pregnancy)
(m) mast/o		13. drug
(n) myc/o		14. potassium (K^+)
(o) nat/o		15. uterus
(p) obstetr-		16. ovary
(q) oophor/o		17. milk
(r) -para		18. worm
(s) pharmac/o		19. echo/ultrasound echo
(t) radi/o		20. movement/motion picture
(u) salping/o		21. thyroid gland

Column A	Column B	Column C
(v) toc/o		22. endometrium
(w) tom/o		23. virus/virion
(x) thyr/o		24. X-ray/radiation
(y) vir/o		25. male

Score [25]

Final test 15 suffixes

Match each suffix in Column A with a meaning in Column C by inserting the appropriate number in Column B.

Column A	Column B	Column C
(a) -arche		1. agent that suppresses or removes
(b) -ase		2. pertaining to stopping/agent that stops or controls
(c) -cidal		3. condition of small size
(d) -er		4. beginning
(e) -form		5. treatment
(f) -fuge		6. condition of holding back/reducing
(g) -gnosy		7. stopping

Column A	Column B	Column C
(h) -ischia		8. pertaining to a tube or a uterine tube
(i) -ite		9. enzyme
(j) -ive		10. having the form/structure of
(k) -micria		11. carbohydrate/sugar/starch
(l) -ose		12. condition of the urine (excretion of)
(m) -pathia		13. process of/state or condition of
(n) -pause		14. dripping
(o) -static		15. type of drug
(p) -staxis		16. end-product
(q) -therapy		17. condition of disease
(r) -tubal		18. process of judging/having knowledge of
(s) -uresis		19. one who
(t) -y		20. pertaining to killing

Score [20]

FINAL SELF-ASSESSMENT TEST FOR UNIT 20

Final test 16 locative prefixes

Match each locative prefix in Column A with a meaning in Column C by inserting the appropriate number in Column B.

Column A	Column B	Column C
(a) ab-		1. around
(b) ad-		2. between
(c) circum-		3. against
(d) contra-		4. inside
(e) de-		5. middle
(f) dextro-		6. through/across (i)
(g) dorso-		7. through/across (ii)
(h) epi-		8. away from e.g. the midline
(i) extra-		9. back/dorsal
(j) in-		10. right

Column A	Column B	Column C
(k) infra-		11. left
(l) inter-		12. outside
(m) laevo- (Am. levo-)		13. side
(n) later-		14. down
(o) medi-		15. backwards
(p) per-		16. upon
(q) retro-		17. to/towards e.g. the midline
(r) supra-		18. below
(s) trans-		19. front/ventral
(t) ventr-		20. above

Score ☐

20

ANSWERS TO WORD EXERCISES

Introduction

Word Exercise 1

(a) Gastropathy
(b) Gastroscopy
(c) Hepatitis
(d) Hepatomegaly
(e) Hepatoma

Word Exercise 2

(a) Duodenojejunostomy
(b) Tracheobronchitis
(c) Gastroenterostomy
(d) Laryngopharyngectomy
(e) Osteoarthropathy

Word Exercise 3

(a) Endodontic
(b) Prosthodontist
(c) Pararectal
(d) Monocular
(e) Perisplenitis

Unit 1 Levels of organization

Word Exercise 1

(a) Cyt – word root meaning cell, o – combining vowel, pathy – suffix meaning disease
(b) Disease of cells
(c) Study of disease
(d) Study of disease of cells
(e) Breakdown/disintegration of cells
(f) Pertaining to poisonous to cells
(g) Specialist who studies cells

Word Exercise 2

(a) Erythr – word root meaning red, o – combining vowel, cyte – word root meaning cell (here used as a suffix)
(b) Red cell

Word Exercise 3

(a) Melanocyte
(b) Fibrocyte
(c) Lympho/lymphocyte (lymph cell)
Spermato/spermatocyte (sperm cell)
Oo/oocyte (egg cell)
Granulo/granulocyte (granular cell)
Chondro/chondrocyte (cartilage cell)

Word Exercise 4

(a) Bone forming cell/immature bone cell
(b) Fibre forming cell/immature fibre cell
(c) Immature blood cell/cell that forms blood cells

Word Exercise 5

(a) The chemistry of tissues (refers to the study of)
(b) Study of diseased tissues
(c) Person who specializes in study of tissues
(d) Breakdown/disintegration of tissues

Word Exercise 6

(a) Small
(b) Instrument to view small objects
(c) Technique of viewing very small objects with a microscope
(d) Specialist who views small things (a specialist in microscopy)
(e) Study of small life/microorganisms

Word Exercise 7

(a) The formation of organs
(b) Pertaining to formation of organs
(c) Pertaining to nourishing/stimulating organs

Case History 1

(a) The study of tissues/a department that studies tissues
(b) Specialist who studies disease/diseased organs
(c) Pertaining to the study of cells
(d) Technique of viewing small things (here cells)
(e) White (blood) cell
(f) Lymph cell
(g) Study of small forms of life i.e. bacteria, fungi and protozoa etc.
(h) Pertaining to causing disease

Unit 2 The digestive system

Word Exercise 1

(a) Instrument to view the oesophagus (Am. esophagus)
(b) Removal of oesophagus (Am. esophagus)
(c) Incision into the oesophagus (Am. esophagus)
(d) Inflammation of the oesophagus (Am. esophagus)

Word Exercise 2

(a) Instrument to view the stomach
(b) Removal of part or all of the stomach
(c) Incision into the stomach
(d) Inflammation of the stomach, especially the lining
(e) Gastropathy
(f) Gastrology
(g) Epigastric
(h) Gastrologist
(i) Gastroscopy

Word Exercise 3

(a) Inflammation of the intestines
(b) Disease of the intestines
(c) Incision into the intestine
(d) Opening into the intestine (often to connect to stomach, ileum, jejunum or abdominal wall)
(e) Intestinal stone (compacted material in intestine)
(f) Enterology
(g) Enterologist
(h) Study of intestines and stomach (plus associated structures, e.g. liver and pancreas)
(i) Disease of intestines and stomach
(j) Inflammation of the intestines and stomach (often due to infection)
(k) Technique of viewing the intestines and stomach

Word Exercise 4

(a) Removal of stomach and pylorus
(b) Technique of viewing pylorus (with an endoscope)

Word Exercise 5

(a) Formation of an opening (anastomosis) between the intestine and duodenum
(b) Formation of an opening (anastomosis) between one part of the jejunum and another part of the jejunum
(c) Pertaining to the jejunum and duodenum
(d) Ileostomy
(e) Ileitis

Word Exercise 6

(a) Large colon
(b) Inflammation of the appendix
(c) Removal of the colon
(d) Opening into the colon (usually a connection between the colon and the abdominal wall; it acts as an artificial anus)

(e) Caecostomy (Am. cecostomy)
(f) Appendicectomy (Am. appendectomy)
(g) Gastrocolostomy

Word Exercise 7

(a) Technique of viewing the sigmoid colon
(b) Pertaining to beside the rectum
(c) Inflammation around the anus/rectum
(d) Administration of fluid into the anus/rectum (enema)
(e) Condition of pain in the anus/rectum
(f) Proctoscope
(g) Proctocaecostomy (Am. proctocecostomy)
(h) Caecosigmoidostomy (Am. cecosigmoidostomy)

Word Exercise 8

(a) Inflammation of the peritoneum
(b) Infusion/injection into the peritoneum

Word Exercise 9

(a) Breaking down of the pancreas
(b) Enlargement of the liver
(c) Liver tumour (Am. tumor)
(d) Pertaining to poisonous to the liver
(e) Formation of an opening between the stomach and hepatic duct
(f) Pertaining to the duodenum and pancreatic duct

Word Exercise 10

(a) Condition of absence of bile
(b) Bile stone
(c) Abnormal condition of stones in the bile duct (or gallbladder)
(d) Condition of bile in the blood
(e) Condition of bile in the urine
(f) Incision into the gallbladder
(g) Removal of the gallbladder
(h) Abnormal condition of stones in the gallbladder
(i) X-ray film demonstrating bile ducts (vessels)
(j) Technique or process of making a cholangiogram
(k) Abnormal condition of stones in the common bile duct
(l) Incision into the common bile duct to remove stones

Word Exercise 11

(a) Visual examination of the abdomen (i.e. abdominal cavity) with a laparoscope
(b) Incision through the abdominal wall

Word Exercise 12

(a) Enteroscope (4)
(b) Endoscope (6)
(c) Enteroscopy (7)
(d) Endoscopy (9)
(e) Endoscopist (8)
(f) Colonoscopy (3)

(g) Proctoscope (1)
(h) Sigmoidoscopy (10)
(i) Panendoscopy (5)
(j) Photoendoscopy (2)

Case History 2

(a) Abnormal condition of stones in the bile (in the gallbladder or bile duct)
(b) Pertaining to the region upon/above the stomach (epigastrium)
(c) Pertaining/relating to bile
(d) Study of the intestines and stomach
(e) Pertaining to using a laparoscope (instrument to view the abdomen)
(f) Removal of the gallbladder
(g) Inflammation of the gallbladder
(h) Pertaining to the stomach and nose (here a tube passed through the nose into the stomach)

Unit 3 The respiratory system

Word Exercise 1

(a) Technique of viewing the nose
(b) Disease of the nose
(c) Condition of pain in the nose
(d) Inflammation of the nose
(e) Excessive flow/discharge from the nose
(f) Surgical repair of the nose

Word Exercise 2

(a) A tube that passes from nose to stomach (for suction or feeding)
(b) A tube that passes from nose to oesophagus (Am. esophagus) (for suction or feeding)

Word Exercise 3

(a) Condition of pain in the pharynx
(b) Excessive flow/discharge from the pharynx
(c) Pharyngoplasty
(d) Pharyngorhinitis

Word Exercise 4

(a) Study of the larynx
(b) Removal of the pharynx and larynx
(c) Laryngoscopy
(d) Laryngorhinology

Word Exercise 5

(a) Incision into the trachea
(b) Formation of an opening into the trachea (to establish a safe airway) or the opening itself

Word Exercise 6

(a) Bronchorrhoea (Am. bronchorrhea)
(b) Bronchogram

(c) Bronchography
(d) Bronchoscope
(e) A structure – the bronchus
(f) Condition of paralysis of the bronchi
(g) Stitching/suturing of the bronchi
(h) Dilatation of the bronchi
(i) Abnormal condition of fungi in the bronchi
(j) Originating in the bronchi/pertaining to formation of the bronchi
(k) Involuntary contraction of the bronchi (smooth muscle)
(l) Pertaining to the bronchi and trachea
(m) Inflammation of bronchi, trachea and larynx
(n) Formation of an opening between the oesophagus (Am. esophagus) and bronchus

Word Exercise 7

(a) Incision into the lung
(b) Suturing of the lung
(c) Disease/abnormal condition of the lungs
(d) Pneumonectomy
(e) Pneumonopathy
(f) Puncture of the lung (by surgery)
(g) Fixation of a lung by surgery (to thoracic wall)

Word Exercise 8

(a) Blood and air in the thorax (in the pleural cavity)
(b) Technique of making an X-ray after injection of air
(c) Without breathing (temporary, due to low levels of carbon dioxide in blood)
(d) Difficult/painful breathing
(e) Above normal breathing (higher rate and depth)
(f) Below normal breathing (low rate and depth)
(g) Fast breathing

Word Exercise 9

(a) Lobotomy
(b) Lobectomy

Word Exercise 10

(a) Pertaining to the lungs
(b) Pertaining to the lungs

Word Exercise 11

(a) Inflammation of the pleura
(b) Puncture of the pleura
(c) Pleurography
(d) Condition of pain in the pleura
(e) Adhesion/fixation of pleura

Word Exercise 12

(a) Pertaining to the stomach and diaphragm
(b) Pertaining to the liver and diaphragm
(c) Condition of paralysis of the diaphragm

Word Exercise 13

(a) Thoracopathy
(b) Thoracotomy
(c) Puncture of the thorax (by surgery)
(d) Instrument used to view the thorax
(e) Abnormal condition of narrowing of the thorax

Word Exercise 14

(a) Pertaining to between the ribs
(b) Pertaining to originating in the ribs/pertaining to forming ribs
(c) Inflammation of the cartilage of the ribs

Word Exercise 15

(a) Bronchoscope (3)
(b) Laryngoscopy (4)
(c) Rhinoscope (8)
(d) Pharyngoscope (6)
(e) Bronchoscopy (7)
(f) Rhinologist (1)
(g) Tracheostomy tube (5)
(h) Laryngoscope (2)

Word Exercise 16

(a) Thoracoscope (5)
(b) Stethoscope (7)
(c) Spirometer (6)
(d) Spirography (3)
(e) Nasal speculum (1)
(f) Nasogastric tube (8)
(g) Pleurography (2)
(h) Spirometry (4)

Case History 3

(a) Pertaining to the lungs
(b) Removal of a lobe (here of the lung)
(c) Difficult/painful breathing
(d) Abnormal condition of blue (appearance of skin and mucous membranes)
(e) Spasmodic (involuntary) contractions of the bronchi/bronchial tubes
(f) Condition of below normal supply of oxygen (to tissues)
(g) Condition of above normal carbon dioxide (in the blood)
(h) Condition of the lung (in which there is inflammation of the spongy tissue of the lung due to infection)

Unit 4 The cardiovascular system

Word Exercise 1

(a) Pertaining to the heart
(b) Condition of pain in the heart
(c) Instrument used to view the heart (obsolete)
(d) Instrument that records the heart (beat – force and form of)

(e) Tracing/recording made by a cardiograph
(f) Condition of fast heart rate
(g) Cardiomegaly
(h) Cardioplasty
(i) Cardiopathy
(j) Cardiology
(k) A structure – the heart muscle
(l) Disease of heart muscle
(m) Stitching/suturing of the heart
(n) Instrument that records electrical activity of the heart
(o) Inflammation inside the heart (its lining)
(p) Inflammation of all of the heart
(q) Condition of slow heart beat
(r) Condition of right heart (heart displaced to right)
(s) Technique of recording heart sounds
(t) Technique of recording (ultrasound) echoes of the heart
(u) A tracing of the electrical activity of the heart

Word Exercise 2

(a) Pericarditis
(b) Fixation of the pericardium to the heart
(c) Puncture of the pericardium (by surgery)
(d) Removal of the pericardium (part of)

Word Exercise 3

(a) Valvoplasty
(b) Valvectomy
(c) Instrument for cutting a heart valve
(d) Pertaining to a valve
(e) Incision into a valve

Word Exercise 4

(a) Sudden contraction of a blood vessel
(b) Pertaining to without blood vessels
(c) Vasculitis
(d) Vasculopathy

Word Exercise 5

(a) X-ray picture of blood vessels (usually arteries)
(b) X-ray picture of the heart and (major) vessels
(c) Technique of making an angiocardiogram
(d) Angiology
(e) Angioplasty
(f) Tumour (Am. tumor) formed from blood vessels (non-malignant)
(g) Dilatation of blood vessels
(h) Formation of blood vessels
(i) Abnormal condition of hardening of blood vessels

Word Exercise 6

(a) Aortopathy
(b) Aortography

Word Exercise 7

(a) Arteriorrhaphy
(b) Arteriosclerosis

(c) Removal of the lining of an artery
(d) Abnormal condition of decay of arteries
(e) Abnormal condition of narrowing of arteries

Word Exercise 8

(a) X-ray picture of a vena cava
(b) Technique of making an X-ray/tracing of the venae cavae

Word Exercise 9

(a) Dilatation of a vein (a varicosity or varicose vein)
(b) Injection or infusion into a vein (of nutrients or medicines)
(c) Pertaining to veins/of the nature of veins
(d) Venogram
(e) Venography

Word Exercise 10

(a) Dilatation of arteries and veins
(b) Injection/infusion into a vein
(c) Incision into vein
(d) Cessation of movement of blood in a vein
(e) Instrument used to measure pressure within a vein
(f) Concretion or stone within a vein

Word Exercise 11

(a) Formation of a clot
(b) Inflammation of a vein associated with a thrombus
(c) Removal of the lining of an artery and a thrombus
(d) Thrombosis
(e) Thrombectomy
(f) Formation of clots
(g) Disintegration/breakdown of clots

Word Exercise 12

(a) Formation of atheroma
(b) Blockage caused by atheroma and an embolus

Word Exercise 13

(a) Surgical repair of an aneurysm
(b) Suturing/stitching of an aneurysm

Word Exercise 14

(a) Instrument that measures the force of the pulse (pressure and volume)
(b) Instrument that measures pressure of the pulse (arterial blood pressure)
(c) Technique of measuring the pulse
(d) Instrument that records the pulse
(e) Tracing/picture/recording of the pulse
(f) Instrument that records the heart beat and pulse

Word Exercise 15

(a) Cardioscope (6)
(b) Cardiograph (4)

(c) Electrocardiograph (5)
(d) Cardiovalvotome (2)
(e) Angiocardiography (3)
(f) Sphygmomanometer (1)

Word Exercise 16

(a) Echocardiography (6)
(b) Sphygmocardiograph (5)
(c) Stethoscope (2)
(d) Phonocardiogram (1)
(e) Electrocardiogram (3)
(f) Phlebomanometer (4)

Case History 4

(a) Study of the heart
(b) Pertaining to veins/of the nature of veins
(c) Condition of fast heart beat
(d) Instrument that records the electrical activity of the heart
(e) Enlargement of the heart
(f) Pertaining to two ventricles (right and left)
(g) Pertaining to the heart
(h) Drug that induces dilatation of blood vessels

Unit 5 The blood

Word Exercise 1

(a) The study of blood
(b) Study of diseases of the blood
(c) Pertaining to the force and movement of the blood (study of)
(d) Formation of the blood
(e) Cessation of blood flow/stopping of bleeding by clotting
(f) Blood in the pericardial sac (a structure containing blood in the pericardium)
(g) Spitting up of blood
(h) Haematoma (Am. hematoma)
(i) Haemolysis (Am. hemolysis)
(j) Haematuria (Am. hematuria)
(k) Haemorrhage (Am. hemorrhage)
(l) Condition of too many blood cells (it refers to conditions in which there is an increase in the number of circulating red blood cells)
(m) Condition of without blood (it refers to condition of reduced number of red cells and/or quantity of haemoglobin (Am. hemoglobin))
(n) Condition of decay of blood (due to infection)
(o) Instrument that measures haemoglobin (Am. hemoglobin)
(p) Blood protein
(q) Condition of haemoglobin (Am. hemoglobin) in the urine
(r) Condition of abnormal decrease of haemoglobin (colour) (Am. hemoglobin)
(s) Condition of abnormal increase of haemoglobin (colour) (Am. hemoglobin)
(t) Pertaining to normal concentration of haemoglobin (colour) (Am. hemoglobin)

Word Exercise 2

(a) Condition of reduction in number of red blood cells
(b) Formation of red blood cells
(c) Immature germ cell that gives rise to red blood cells
(d) Formation of red blood cells
(e) Breakdown of red blood cells
(f) Condition of erythrocyte blood, i.e. too many red blood cells
(g) Abnormal condition of too many small cells (small erythrocytes)
(h) Abnormal condition of too many large cells (large erythrocytes)
(i) Abnormal condition of too many elliptical cells (elliptical erythrocytes)
(j) Abnormal condition of too many unequal cells (unequal sized erythrocytes)
(k) Abnormal condition of too many irregular/varied cells (variable shaped erythrocytes)
(l) Pertaining to normal cells (red blood cells of normal size)

Word Exercise 3

(a) Reticuloblast
(b) Reticulocytosis
(c) Reticulopenia

Word Exercise 4

(a) Leucopenia (Am. leukopenia)
(b) Leucopoiesis (Am. leukopoiesis)
(c) Formation of white blood cells
(d) Condition of white blood (synonymous with leukocythaemia, a malignant cancer of white blood cells)
(e) Abnormal condition of white cells (an increase in white blood cells, usually transient in response to infection)
(f) Tumour (Am. tumor) of leucocytes (Am. leukocytes)
(g) Immature germ cell that gives rise to leucocytes (Am. leukocytes)
(h) Abnormal condition of too many white germ cells (results in proliferation of leucocytes (Am. leukocytes))
(i) Pertaining to poisonous to white cells

Word Exercise 5

(a) Marrow cell (a cell that forms white blood cells called polymorphonuclear granulocytes)
(b) Condition of fibres in marrow
(c) Myeloblast
(d) Myeloma

Word Exercise 6

(a) Condition of reduction in the number of platelets
(b) Formation of platelets
(c) Breakdown of platelets

(d) Disease of platelets
(e) Instrument that measures the volume of thrombocytes in a sample, or the actual value of the measured volume of thrombocytes in a sample of blood
(f) Withdrawal of blood, removal of red cells and retransfusion of the remainder
(g) Withdrawal of blood, removal of thrombocytes and retransfusion of the remainder
(h) Withdrawal of blood, removal of leucocytes and retransfusion of the remainder

Word Exercise 7

(a) Plasmapheresis (4)
(b) Differential count (3)
(c) Haematocrit (2)
(d) Haemoglobinometer (5)
(e) Blood count (1)

Case History 5

(a) Spitting/coughing up of blood
(b) Condition of reduction of all cells (i.e. all types of cells in the blood)
(c) Pertaining to leukaemia/white blood (a cancer of the white blood cells)
(d) Pertaining to normal colour (here meaning normal haemoglobin)
(e) Pertaining to normal cells (here normocyte refers to an erythrocyte of a typical shape and size)
(f) Condition of a reduction in granulocytes (types of white blood cells)
(g) Condition of reduction in thrombocytes/platelets
(h) Condition of without blood (actually a reduction in erythrocytes and haemoglobin (Am. hemoglobin)

Unit 6 The lymphatic system and immunology

Word Exercise 1

(a) Abnormal condition of lymph cells (too many cells)
(b) Condition of bursting forth of lymph (from lymph vessels)
(c) Technique of making an X-ray/tracing of lymphatic vessels
(d) X-ray picture/tracing of a lymph vessel
(e) Dilatation of lymph vessels
(f) Tumour (Am. tumor) of a lymph node
(g) Removal of a lymph node
(h) Disease of a lymph node
(i) Inflammation of a lymph node

Word Exercise 2

(a) Enlargement of the spleen
(b) Enlargement of the liver and spleen
(c) Surgical fixation of the spleen
(d) Hernia/protrusion of the spleen
(e) Condition of softening of the spleen

(f)   Breakdown/disintegration of the spleen
(g)   X-ray picture of the spleen
(h)   X-ray picture of the portal vein and spleen

Word Exercise 3

(a)   Tonsillitis
(b)   Tonsillectomy
(c)   Pertaining to the pharynx and tonsils
(d)   Instrument used to cut the tonsils

Word Exercise 4

(a)   Thymocyte
(b)   Thymopathy
(c)   Thymocele
(d)   Abnormal condition of ulceration of the thymus
      gland
(e)   Pertaining to the lymphatics and the thymus gland

Word Exercise 5

(a)   Immunology
(b)   Immunopathology
(c)   Formation of immunity
(d)   Self immunity (the immune system acts against
      itself, producing an autoimmune disease)
(e)   A protein of the immune system (an antibody)

Word Exercise 6

(a)   Serology

Word Exercise 7

(a)   Condition of pus in the blood (infection in blood)
(b)   Pertaining to generating pus
(c)   Flow of pus (usually referring to pus flowing
      from the teeth sockets)
(d)   Formation of pus

Word Exercise 8

(a)   Tonsillotome (3)
(b)   Lymphangiography (4)
(c)   Lymphadenography (6)
(d)   Lymphogram (2)
(e)   Splenoportogram (1)
(f)   Lymphography (5)

Case History 6

(a)   Inflammation of the tonsils
(b)   Enlargement of the spleen
(c)   Disease of the lymph glands i.e. the lymph nodes
(d)   Pertaining to a lymph node
(e)   Study of disease of tissues (here refers to a
      section of the pathology laboratory)
(f)   Tumour (Am. tumor) of the lymph (tissue)
(g)   Lymph cell
(h)   Type of lymphocyte that secretes antibodies
      (named after the Bursa of Fabricus in birds)

Unit 7 The urinary system

Word Exercise 1

(a)   Pertaining to the stomach and kidney
(b)   X-ray/tracing of the kidney
(c)   Technique of making an X-ray/tracing of the kidney

Word Exercise 2

(a)   Falling kidney (downward displacement)
(b)   Abnormal condition of water in a kidney (a
      swelling)
(c)   A swelling/hernia of a kidney
(d)   Condition of pain in a kidney
(e)   Nephropexy
(f)   Nephroplasty
(g)   Nephrotomy
(h)   Nephrolithiasis
(i)   Nephrectomy
(j)   Inflammation of glomeruli (producing pus)
(k)   Disease of glomeruli
(l)   Abnormal condition of hardening of glomeruli

Word Exercise 3

(a)   Inflammation of a kidney and renal pelvis
(b)   Incision to remove a stone from the renal pelvis
(c)   Disease/abnormal condition of a kidney and
      renal pelvis
(d)   Pyeloplasty
(e)   Pyelogram

Word Exercise 4

(a)   Hernia/protrusion of the ureter
(b)   Removal of a ureterocele
(c)   Condition of excessive flow of blood from the
      ureter
(d)   Stitching/suturing of the ureter
(e)   Dilatation of a ureter
(f)   Visual examination of the kidney and ureters
(g)   Formation of an opening into the ureter
(h)   Ureteroenterostomy
(i)   Ureterocolostomy

Word Exercise 5

(a)   Inflammation of the bladder
(b)   Removal of stones from the bladder
(c)   Inflammation of the renal pelvis and bladder
(d)   Falling/displacement of the bladder
(e)   Instrument used to view the bladder
(f)   Formation of an opening between rectum/anus
      and bladder
(g)   Cystometer
(h)   Cystometry
(i)   Cystometrogram

Word Exercise 6

(a)   Vesicostomy
(b)   Vesicotomy

(c) Infusion/injection into the bladder
(d) Pertaining to the bladder
(e) Opening between the sigmoid colon and bladder (to drain urine)
(f) Pertaining to the ureter and bladder

Word Exercise 7

(a) Process of measuring the urethra
(b) Inflammation of the trigone and urethra
(c) Fixation (by surgery) of the urethra
(d) Urethralgia
(e) Urethrorrhagia
(f) Urethroscopy
(g) Tumour (Am. tumor)/boil in the urethra
(h) Instrument for cutting the urethra
(i) Abnormal condition of narrowing of the urethra
(j) Condition of pain in the urethra

Word Exercise 8

(a) Of the nature of/pertaining to carrying urine
(b) Urine splitting/separating for analysis
(c) Instrument used to measure urine

Word Exercise 9

(a) Technique of recording the urinary tract (X-ray)
(b) Person specializing in the study of the urinary tract
(c) Formation of urine
(d) Condition of little urine (diminished secretion of)
(e) Condition of albumin in the urine
(f) Condition of urea (too much) in the urine
(g) Condition of much urine
(h) Condition of painful difficult (flow) of urine
(i) Condition of blood in the urine
(j) Condition of pus in the urine
(k) Condition of too much calcium in the urine

Word Exercise 10

(a) Inflammation of kidney due to stones
(b) Condition of calculi or stones in the urine
(c) Formation of stones
(d) Instrument used to crush stones
(e) Washing of stones from bladder following crushing
(f) Instrument that uses shock waves to destroy stones
(g) The procedure of breaking stones using shock waves from a lithotriptor
(h) Excretion of stones in the urine

Word Exercise 11

(a) Diathermy (8)
(b) Cystoscope (10)
(c) Lithotriptor (7)
(d) Urinometer (9)
(e) Haemodialyser (2)
(f) Ureteroscopy (4)
(g) Urethrotome (3)
(h) Cystometer (5)

(i) Urethroscope (6)
(j) Lithotrite (1)

Case History 7

(a) Abnormal condition of stones in the urinary tract
(b) Pertaining to the urethra
(c) Condition of painful/difficult urine (urination)
(d) Condition of blood in the urine
(e) Disease of the urinary tract
(f) Technique of making a tracing/X-ray of the renal pelvis
(g) Technique of breaking up stones using a lithotriptor
(h) Condition of above normal calcium in the urine

Unit 8 The nervous system

Word Exercise 1

(a) Study of the nerves/nervous system
(b) Disease of the nervous system
(c) Condition of pain in nerves
(d) A nerve fibre tumour (Am. tumor) (arises from connective tissue around nerves)
(e) Inflammation of many nerves
(f) Pertaining to formation of nerves/originating in nerves
(g) Neurosclerosis
(h) Neuromalacia
(i) Neurologist
(j) Wasting/decay of nerves
(k) Pertaining to affinity for/stimulating nervous tissue
(l) Injury to nerves
(m) Nerve glue cell
(n) A tumour (Am. tumor) of gliocytes/gliacytes (nerve glue cells)

Word Exercise 2

(a) Disease of a plexus
(b) Pertaining to the formation of a plexus/originating in a plexus

Word Exercise 3

(a) Hernia/protrusion from the head
(b) Pertaining to without a head
(c) Pertaining to a tumour (Am. tumor) of blood within the head (actually a collection of blood in sub-periosteal tissue, the result of an injury)
(d) Thing (baby) with water in the head
(e) Microcephalic
(f) Cephalogram
(g) Cephalometry
(h) Thing (baby) with a large head
(i) Pertaining to a turning motion of the head

Word Exercise 4

(a) Tumour of the brain (Am. tumor)
(b) Abnormal condition of pus (infection) of the brain
(c) Pertaining to without a brain

(d) Instrument that records electrical activity of the brain
(e) Encephalography
(f) Electroencephalography
(g) Encephalopathy
(h) Encephalocele
(i) Tracing/picture of the brain made using reflected ultrasound (echoes)
(j) The middle brain
(k) Inflammation of the grey matter of the brain

Word Exercise 5

(a) Cerebrosclerosis
(b) Cerebromalacia
(c) Cerebrosis

Word Exercise 6

(a) Ventriculoscopy
(b) Ventriculotomy
(c) Technique of making an X-ray of the brain ventricles
(d) Opening between the cistern (subarachnoid space) and ventricles

Word Exercise 7

(a) Craniotomy
(b) Craniometry
(c) Intracranial

Word Exercise 8

(a) Ganglioma
(b) Pertaining to before a ganglion
(c) Pertaining to after a ganglion
(d) Removal of a ganglion

Word Exercise 9

(a) Meningitis
(b) Meningocele
(c) Meningorrhagia
(d) Hernia/protrusion of the brain through the meninges
(e) Inflammation of the brain and meninges
(f) Disease of the brain and meninges
(g) Tumour (Am. tumor) of the meninges
(h) Pertaining to above/upon the dura
(i) Swelling/tumour (Am. tumor) of blood beneath the dura

Word Exercise 10

(a) Inflammation of the ganglia and spinal roots
(b) Inflammation of nerves and spinal nerve roots
(c) Incision into a spinal root

Word Exercise 11

(a) Inflammation of the meninges and spinal cord
(b) Hernia/protrusion of the spinal cord through the meninges

(c) Inflammation of spinal nerve roots and spinal cord
(d) Inflammation of the brain and spinal cord
(e) Wasting of the spinal cord
(f) Inflammation of the grey matter of the spinal cord
(g) Myelosclerosis
(h) Myelomalacia
(i) Myelography
(j) Condition of abnormal/difficult development/ growth (of cells) of the spinal cord
(k) Without nourishment of the spinal cord (wasting away/poor growth)
(l) Abnormal condition of tubes (cavities) in the spinal cord

Word Exercise 12

(a) Instrument used to measure the spine (curvature)
(b) Puncture of the spine
(c) Splitting of the spine

Word Exercise 13

(a) Condition of paralysis of all four limbs
(b) Condition of paralysis of half the body, right or left side
(c) Condition of near/beside/beyond paralysis (lower limbs)
(d) Condition of two parts paralyzed (similar parts on either side of the body)
(e) Condition of paralysis of four limbs (synonymous with quadriplegia)

Word Exercise 14

(a) Condition of without sensation/state of being anaesthetized (Am. anesthetized)
(b) Pertaining to a drug that reduces sensation
(c) Study of anaesthesia (Am. anesthesia)
(d) Person who administers anaesthesia/specialist in anaesthesia (Am. anesthesia)
(e) Condition of without sensation of half the body (one side)
(f) Condition of decreased sensation
(g) Condition of increased sensation
(h) Post-anaesthesic/anaesthetic/anaesthesia (Am. post- anesthesic/anesthetic/anesthesia)
(i) Pre-anaesthesic/anaesthetic/anaesthesia (Am. pre-anesthesic/anesthetic/anesthesia)

Word Exercise 15

(a) Abnormal condition of stupor/deep sleep (drug induced)
(b) Treatment with narcotics

Word Exercise 16

(a) Condition of sensing pain
(b) Condition of without sensation of pain
(c) Condition of excessive/above normal sensation of pain
(d) Pertaining to a loss of pain/a drug that reduces pain

Word Exercise 17

(a) Study of the mind (behaviour)
(b) Pertaining to the mind
(c) Disease of the mind
(d) Abnormal condition/disease of the mind
(e) Drug that acts on/has an affinity for the mind
(f) Pertaining to body and mind (actually body symptoms of mental origin)
(g) Study/treatment of the mind/mental illness/treatment of the mind by a doctor

Word Exercise 18

(a) Condition of fear of heights (peaks, extremities)
(b) Condition of fear of open spaces
(c) Condition of fear of water
(d) Condition of fear of cancer
(e) Condition of fear of death/dead bodies

Word Exercise 19

(a) Pertaining to forming/causing epileptic fits
(b) Pertaining to following/after an epileptic fit
(c) Having the form of epilepsy

Word Exercise 20

(a) Encephalography (5)
(b) Positron emission tomography (4)
(c) Ventriculoscopy (6)
(d) Tendon hammer (1)
(e) Tomograph (2)
(f) Craniometry (3)

Word Exercise 21

(a) MRI (3)
(b) Lumbar puncture (6)
(c) Myelography (5)
(d) CAT (1)
(e) Electroencephalography (2)
(f) Ventriculography (4)

Case History 8

(a) Pertaining to the (blood) vessels of the cerebrum/brain
(b) Condition of half paralysis (it refers to one side of the body)
(c) Condition of beyond sensation (numbness) of half (one side) of the body/it refers to abnormal sensations
(d) Loss of sensation of half (one side) of the body
(e) Pertaining to the cerebrum/cerebral hemispheres
(f) Pertaining to within the cranium/skull
(g) Study of nerves or the nervous system, here it refers to a department that studies and treats disorders of the nervous system
(h) Pertaining to above normal/exaggerated reflexes

Unit 9 The eye

Word Exercise 1

(a) Ophthalmoscope
(b) Ophthalmologist
(c) Ophthalmoplegia
(d) Ophthalmitis
(e) Ophthalmomycosis
(f) Pertaining to pain in the eye
(g) Pertaining to circular movement of the eye
(h) Inflammation of the optic nerve
(i) Inflammation of all of the eye
(j) Instrument used to measure tension (pressure) within the eye
(k) Condition of inflammation of the eye with mucus discharge
(l) Condition of inflammation due to dryness of the eye
(m) In eye (displacement of the eyes into their sockets)
(n) Out eye (bulging eyes)

Word Exercise 2

(a) Pertaining to one eye
(b) Pertaining to one eye
(c) Pertaining to two eyes
(d) A nerve that stimulates eye movement/action
(e) Pertaining to the nose and eye
(f) Picture/tracing of the electrical activity of the eye
(g) Pertaining to a circular movement of the eye

Word Exercise 3

(a) Instrument that measures sight
(b) Technique of measuring sight
(c) Person who measures sight (specializes in optometry)
(d) Instrument for measuring the muscles of sight (the power of the ocular muscles)
(e) Condition of sensation of sight (ability to perceive visual stimuli)

Word Exercise 4

(a) Condition of double vision
(b) Condition of old man's vision
(c) Condition of dim vision
(d) Condition of half colour vision (faulty colour vision in half the field of view)
(e) Condition of painful/difficult/bad vision
(f) Condition of without half vision (blindness in one half of the visual field in one or both eyes)

Word Exercise 5

(a) Blepharoplegia
(b) Blepharospasm
(c) Blepharoptosis
(d) Blepharorrhaphy
(e) Flow of pus from the eyelid
(f) Inflammation of the eyelid glands (meibomian glands)

(g) Condition of sticking together of the eyelids
(h) Slack, loose eyelids (causes drooping)

Word Exercise 6

(a) Incision into the sclera
(b) Dilatation of the sclera
(c) Instrument to cut the sclera

Word Exercise 7

(a) Inflammation of the cornea and sclera
(b) Measurement of the cornea (actually the curvature of the cornea)
(c) Instrument to cut the cornea
(d) Surgical repair of the cornea (a corneal graft)
(e) Puncture of the cornea
(f) Abnormal condition of ulceration of the cornea
(g) Puncture of the cornea
(h) To carve the cornea
(i) A cone-like protrusion of the cornea

Word Exercise 8

(a) Iridoptosis
(b) Iridokeratitis
(c) Motion/movement of the iris (contraction and expansion)
(d) Separation of the iris
(e) Hernia/protrusion of the iris (through the cornea)
(f) Separation of the iris and sclera
(g) Incision into the iris and sclera
(h) Inflammation of the iris and cornea

Word Exercise 9

(a) Inflammation of the ciliary body and iris
(b) Condition of paralysis of the ciliary body
(c) Heating through the ciliary body (to destroy tissue)

Word Exercise 10

(a) Goniometer
(b) Gonioscope
(c) Goniotomy

Word Exercise 11

(a) Condition of paralysis of the pupil
(b) Measurement of pupils (diameter)

Word Exercise 12

(a) Condition of equal pupils
(b) Condition of unequal pupils
(c) Surgical fixation of the pupil into a new position
(d) Surgical repair of the pupil

Word Exercise 13

(a) Inflammation of the ciliary body and choroid
(b) Inflammation of the choroid and sclera

Word Exercise 14

(a) Tumour (Am. tumor) of germ cells of the retina
(b) Condition of softening of the retina
(c) Splitting (separation of the retina)
(d) Disease of the retina
(e) Technique of viewing the retina
(f) Electroretinogram
(g) Retinochoroiditis
(h) Choroidoretinitis

Word Exercise 15

(a) Swelling of the optic disc
(b) Retinopapillitis

Word Exercise 16

(a) Phacomalacia
(b) Phacoscope
(c) Phacosclerosis
(d) Aphakia
(e) Removal of the lens bladder (capsule)
(f) Sucking out of the lens

Word Exercise 17

(a) Instrument to measure scotomas
(b) Technique of measuring scotomas
(c) Instrument to record scotomas

Word Exercise 18

(a) Lacrimotomy
(b) Nasolacrimal

Word Exercise 19

(a) Tear bladder (the lacrimal sac)
(b) Technique of making an X-ray of the lacrimal sac
(c) Formation of an opening between the nose and lacrimal sac
(d) A tear stone
(e) Abnormal condition of narrowing of the lacrimal duct (or lacrimal apparatus)
(f) Pertaining to stimulation of tears
(g) Flow of mucus from the lacrimal sac
(h) Condition of pus in the lacrimal sac

Word Exercise 20

(a) Ophthalmoscope (4)
(b) Dacryocystogram (1)
(c) Keratome (5)
(d) Pupillometry (8)
(e) Optometry (7)
(f) Scotometry (2)
(g) Ophthalmotonometer (3)
(h) Optomyometer (6)

Word Exercise 21

(a) Sclerotome (5)
(b) Optometer (4)
(c) Keratometry (6)
(d) Pupillometer (8)
(e) Phacoscope (7)
(f) Retinoscopy (1)
(g) Tonography (2)
(h) Dacryocystography (3)

Case History 9

(a) Specialist who measures sight
(b) Condition of double vision
(c) Condition of pain in the eye
(d) Inflammation of the optic nerve
(e) Inflammation of the optic disc
(f) A dark area/region of reduced vision within a visual field
(g) Pertaining to the eye
(h) Condition of paralysis of the eye

Unit 10 The ear

Word Exercise 1

(a) Otology
(b) Otoscope
(c) Otosclerosis
(d) Otopyosis
(e) Technique of viewing the ear (with an otoscope)
(f) Study of the larynx, nose and ear
(g) Abnormal condition of fungi in the ear
(h) Excessive flow of pus from the ear
(i) Condition of small ears
(j) Condition of large ears

Word Exercise 2

(a) Auriscope
(b) Pertaining to two ears
(c) Pertaining to within the ear
(d) Pertaining to having two ear flaps (pinnae)

Word Exercise 3

(a) Myringotomy
(b) Myringotome
(c) Myringomycosis

Word Exercise 4

(a) Tympanoplasty
(b) Tympanocentesis
(c) Tympanostomy
(d) Inflammation of the middle ear and/or ear drum
(e) Incision into the middle ear and/or ear drum

Word Exercise 5

(a) Blocking up of the Eustachian tube/pharyngotympanic tube
(b) Pertaining to the pharynx and Eustachian tube/pharyngotympanic tube

Word Exercise 6

(a) Stapedectomy
(b) Cutting of the tendon of the stapes

Word Exercise 7

(a) Incision into the malleus

Word Exercise 8

(a) Pertaining to the malleus and incus
(b) Pertaining to the stapes and incus
(c) Pertaining to the incus and malleus

Word Exercise 9

(a) Cochleostomy
(b) Electrocochleography

Word Exercise 10

(a) Labyrinthitis
(b) Labyrinthectomy

Word Exercise 11

(a) Incision into the vestibule
(b) Pertaining to originating in the vestibule

Word Exercise 12

(a) Mastoidalgia
(b) Mastoidotomy
(c) Mastoidectomy
(d) Tympanomastoiditis

Word Exercise 13

(a) Audiology
(b) Instrument that measures hearing
(c) A tracing/recording made by an audiometer
(d) Technique of measuring hearing/using an audiometer

Word Exercise 14

(a) Audiometer (6)
(b) Audiometry (1)
(c) Aural speculum (7)
(d) Auriscope (2)
(e) Otoscopy (3)
(f) Aural syringe (4)
(g) Grommet (5)

Case History 10

(a) Condition of pain in the ear
(b) Technique of viewing/examining the ear
(c) Technician who measures hearing

(d) A tracing/recording of hearing (ability)
(e) Study of the ear and its disorders
(f) Technique of measuring the tympanic membrane (actually the measurement of the mobility and impedance of the membrane)
(g) Incision into the tympanic membrane/ear drum
(h) Opening into the tympanum/tympanic membrane

Unit 11 The skin

Word Exercise 1

(a) Abnormal condition of the skin
(b) Above/upon the skin, the outer layer of the skin
(c) A skin plant (fungus that infects skin)
(d) Thick skin
(e) Yellow skin
(f) Self surgical repair of skin (using one's own skin for a graft)
(g) Condition of dry skin
(h) Specialist who studies skin and diseases of the skin
(i) Dermatomycosis
(j) Dermatome
(k) Hypodermic/subdermal
(l) Intradermal

Word Exercise 2

(a) Abnormal condition of the epidermis caused by excessive exposure to the sun
(b) Abnormal condition of the epidermis (above normal thickening)
(c) Tumour (Am. tumor) of the epidermis
(d) Breakdown/disintegration of the epidermis

Word Exercise 3

(a) A nerve that produces a hair action (it erects the hair in cold conditions)

Word Exercise 4

(a) Abnormal condition of hair plants (fungal infection)
(b) Abnormal condition of hair
(c) Condition of sensitive hairs
(d) Condition of split hairs
(e) Broken/ruptured hairs

Word Exercise 5

(a) Excessive flow of sebum
(b) A sebaceous stone (actually hardened sebum)
(c) Pertaining to stimulating the sebaceous glands

Word Exercise 6

(a) Abnormal condition of sweating (excess)
(b) Condition of increased/above normal sweating
(c) Formation of sweat
(d) Abnormal condition of without sweating
(e) Inflammation of sweat glands

Word Exercise 7

(a) Abnormal condition of a hidden nail (ingrowing)
(b) Condition of increased growth of nails
(c) Difficult/poor growth of nails (malformation)
(d) Without nourishment/wasting away of nails
(e) Condition beside a nail (inflammation)
(f) Splitting/parting of nails
(g) Condition of nail eating (actually biting)
(h) Onycholysis
(i) Onychomycosis
(j) Onychitis
(k) Rupture/breaking of nails
(l) Condition of without nails
(m) Condition of thickened nails

Word Exercise 8

(a) Melanocyte
(b) Melanosis
(c) Tumour (Am. tumor) of melanin (melanocytes), highly malignant

Word Exercise 9

(a) Excision biopsy (4)
(b) Dermatome (5)
(c) Medical laser (2)
(d) PUVA (6)
(e) Epilation (1)
(f) Electrolysis (3)

Case History 11

(a) Study of the skin
(b) Specialist who studies the skin and its disorders
(c) Pertaining to above normal epidermis i.e. a thickening of the epidermis
(d) Pertaining to the skin/of the nature of skin
(e) Disintegration/breakdown of the nails
(f) Pertaining to the epidermis or keratin
(g) Tumour (Am. tumor) formed from an epithelium/epithelial cell
(h) Tumour (Am. tumor) of melanin/melanocytes

Unit 12 The nose and mouth

Word Exercise 1

(a) Study of the mouth
(b) Condition of excessive flow (of blood) from mouth
(c) Disease of the mouth
(d) Stomatodynia/stomatalgia
(e) Stomatomycosis

Word Exercise 2

(a) Pertaining to the mouth
(b) Pertaining to inside the mouth
(c) Pertaining to the pharynx and mouth
(d) Pertaining to the nose and mouth

Word Exercise 3

(a) Glossology
(b) Glossodynia
(c) Glossopharyngeal (e.g. glossopharyngeal nerve IX)
(d) Condition of paralysis of the tongue
(e) Condition of hairy tongue
(f) Protrusion/swelling of the tongue
(g) Condition of a large tongue
(h) Surgical repair of the tongue

Word Exercise 4

(a) Removal of a salivary gland
(b) Technique of making X-ray/tracing of salivary vessels/ducts
(c) Condition of much saliva (excess secretion)
(d) X-ray of the salivary glands and ducts
(e) Sialolith
(f) A drug that stimulates saliva (production)
(g) Condition of eating air and saliva (excessive swallowing)

Word Exercise 5

(a) Pertaining to formation of saliva/originating in saliva
(b) Excessive flow of saliva
(c) Stone in the saliva

Word Exercise 6

(a) Gnathalgia/gnathodynia
(b) Gnathoplasty
(c) Gnathology
(d) Stomatognathic
(e) Instrument that measures force of jaw (closing force)
(f) Split or cleft jaw
(g) Inflammation of the jaw

Word Exercise 7

(a) Surgical repair of the mouth and lips
(b) Split/cleft lip
(c) Suturing of lips
(d) Cheilitis

Word Exercise 8

(a) Pertaining to the larynx, tongue and lips
(b) Labioglossopharyngeal

Word Exercise 9

(a) Gingivitis
(b) Gingivectomy
(c) Pertaining to the gums and lips

Word Exercise 10

(a) Palatoplegia
(b) Palatognathic
(c) Palatoschisis
(d) Pertaining to after the palate

Word Exercise 11

(a) Uvulectomy
(b) Uvulotomy

Word Exercise 12

(a) Condition of without speech/loss of voice
(b) Condition of difficult speech (difficulty speaking)

Word Exercise 13

(a) Odontology
(b) Odontopathy
(c) Odontalgia
(d) Pertaining to around the teeth (the study of tissues that support the teeth)
(e) Study of the inside of teeth (pulp, dentine, etc.)
(f) Pertaining to straight teeth (the branch of dentistry dealing with the straightening of teeth and associated facial abnormalities)
(g) Person who specializes in orthodontics
(h) Pertaining to adding teeth (the branch of dentistry dealing with the construction of artificial teeth and other oral components)

Word Exercise 14

(a) Condition of having a nasal voice (speech through the nose)
(b) Technique of measuring pressure (air flow) in the nose
(c) Tumour (Am. tumor)/swelling/boil of the nose
(d) Technique of viewing the nose (internally)
(e) Study of the larynx, nose and ear
(f) Condition of excessive flow of blood (from nose)

Word Exercise 15

(a) Hollow/cavity in bone/an anatomical part
(b) Inflammation of the bronchi and sinuses
(c) Inflammation of a sinus
(d) An X-ray/tracing of a sinus

Word Exercise 16

(a) Antroscope
(b) Antrotympanitis
(c) Incision into the antrum
(d) Pertaining to the nose and antrum
(e) Swelling/protrusion of the antrum
(f) Pertaining to the cheek and antrum
(g) Formation of an opening into the antrum

Word Exercise 17

(a) Pertaining to the face
(b) Condition of paralysis of the face
(c) Surgical repair of the face

Word Exercise 18

(a) Antroscope (3)
(b) Sialangiography (5)
(c) Gnathodynamometer (1)
(d) Rhinomanometer (6)
(e) Prosthesis (4)
(f) Glossography (2)

Case History 12

(a) Inflammation of the nose
(b) Technique of viewing/examining the nose
(c) Inflammation of a sinus
(d) Study of the larynx, nose and ears (here referring to the department that studies disorders of these areas)
(e) Pertaining to towards the back of the nose
(f) Pertaining to the antrum (here referring to the maxillary sinus or antrum of Highmore)
(g) Pertaining to within the nose
(h) Formation of an opening into the antrum (here into the maxillary sinus or antrum of Highmore)

Unit 13 The muscular system

Word Exercise 1

(a) Pertaining to nerve and muscle
(b) Disease of heart muscle
(c) Poor nourishment (growth) of muscle
(d) Inflammation of a muscle
(e) Abnormal condition of fibres in muscle
(f) Myosclerosis
(g) Myoma
(h) Myoglobin
(i) Myospasm
(j) Condition of involuntary twitching of muscle
(k) Condition of muscle tone (abnormal increased tone)
(l) Slight paralysis of muscle
(m) Rupture of a muscle
(n) Condition of softening of a muscle
(o) Myography
(p) Electromyography
(q) Myogram

Word Exercise 2

(a) Tumour (Am. tumor) of striated muscle
(b) Breakdown of striated muscle

Word Exercise 3

(a) Pertaining to affinity for/stimulating muscle
(b) Pertaining to the diaphragm muscles
(c) Poor nourishment (growth) of muscle. An inherited disease

Word Exercise 4

(a) Condition of sensation of movement
(b) Instrument that measures muscular movement

(c) Pertaining to forming movements
(d) Condition of above normal movement
(e) Dyskinesia

Word Exercise 5

(a) Condition of pain in a tendon
(b) Instrument used to cut tendons
(c) Inflammation of tendons
(d) Study of tendons
(e) Tenomyoplasty
(f) Tenomyotomy
(g) Suturing of an aponeurosis
(h) Inflammation of an aponeurosis

Word Exercise 6

(a) Pertaining to a straight child, now a branch of surgery that deals with the restoration of function in the musculoskeletal system

Word Exercise 7

(a) Myography (5)
(b) Electromyography (4)
(c) Myogram (2)
(d) Myokinesiometer (6)
(e) Orthosis (1)
(f) Electromyogram (3)

Case History 13

(a) Difficult/poor nourishment (of a tissue)
(b) False, above normal nourishment (here the muscles look large and over nourished but the enlargement is due to disease processes within the muscle)
(c) Pertaining to dystrophy
(d) Technique of recording the electrical activity of muscle
(e) Pertaining to disease of muscle
(f) A recording/tracing of the electrical activity of muscle
(g) Without nourishment (wasting away)
(h) Pertaining to heart muscle

Unit 14 The skeletal system

Word Exercise 1

(a) A bone plant (a plant-like growth of bone)
(b) Abnormal condition of passages (pores) in bone
(c) Condition of softening of the bones
(d) Abnormal condition of stone-like bones
(e) Breaking down of bone
(f) A cell that breaks down bone
(g) Bad nourishment of bone (poor growth)
(h) Osteoblast
(i) Osteolytic
(j) Osteotome
(k) Osteologist

Word Exercise 2

(a) Instrument used to view within a joint
(b) Abnormal condition of pus in a joint
(c) Technique of making an X-ray of joints
(d) Inflammation of many joints
(e) Fixation of a joint by surgery
(f) Breaking of a joint (actually breaking adhesions within a joint to improve mobility)
(g) Arthroscopy
(h) Arthrocentesis
(i) Arthrogram
(j) Arthropathy
(k) Arthrolith
(l) Arthroplasty

Word Exercise 3

(a) Inflammation of a synovial joint
(b) Removal of the synovial membranes/synovia
(c) Tumour (Am. tumor)/swelling of a synovial membrane

Word Exercise 4

(a) A plant-like growth of cartilage
(b) Pertaining to/of the nature of bone and cartilage
(c) Abnormal condition of passages (pores) in cartilage
(d) Bad nourishment of cartilage (poor growth)
(e) Condition of softening of cartilage
(f) Pertaining to rib cartilage
(g) Pertaining to within cartilage
(h) Chondralgia
(i) Chondrogenesis
(j) Chondrolysis
(k) Abnormal condition of calcified cartilage (an abnormal increase in calcium in cartilage)

Word Exercise 5

(a) Condition of pain in the vertebrae
(b) Abnormal condition of pus in vertebrae
(c) Spondylolysis
(d) Spondylopathy
(e) Slipping/dislocation of vertebrae

Word Exercise 6

(a) Resembling a disc
(b) Pertaining to forming a disc/originating in a disc
(c) Discography
(d) Discectomy

Word Exercise 7

(a) Inflammation of bone marrow
(b) Abnormal condition of fibres in marrow

Word Exercise 8

(a) Osteotome (4)
(b) Arthrodesis (3)

(c) Replacement arthroplasty (5)
(d) Arthrocentesis (1)
(e) Arthrography (2)

Word Exercise 9

(a) Claviculoplasty
(b) Craniomalacia
(c) Intercostal
(d) Phalangectomy
(e) Pelvic
(f) Olecranarthritis
(g) Tibiofemoral
(h) Scapulodesis
(i) Metatarsalgia
(j) Acetabuloplasty

Word Exercise 10

(a) Pertaining to between the phalanges (finger or toe bones)
(b) Condition of pain in a metatarsus or metatarsal bone
(c) Pertaining to a metatarsus and tarsus or metatarsal and tarsal bones
(d) Pertaining to a metacarpus or metacarpal bone

Case History 14

(a) Specialist who studies rheumatism
(b) Condition of pain in the joints
(c) Inflammation of a bursa
(d) Inflammation of many joints
(e) Pertaining to the phalanges and metacarpals
(f) Pertaining to between the phalanges
(g) Pertaining to the phalanges and the metatarsal bones
(h) Disease of joints

Unit 15 The male reproductive system

Word Exercise 1

(a) Disease of the testes
(b) Hernia/protrusion/swelling of testes (through scrotum)
(c) Process/condition of hidden testes, i.e. undescended
(d) Surgical fixation of the testes, i.e. into their normal position
(e) Orchiotomy/orchidotomy
(f) Orchioplasty/orchidoplasty
(g) Orchidectomy/orchiectomy
(h) Orchialgia/orchidalgia
(i) Surgical fixation of hidden testes, i.e. into their normal position

Word Exercise 2

(a) Scrotectomy
(b) Scrotoplasty
(c) Scrotocele
(d) Pertaining to through/across the scrotum

Word Exercise 3

(a) Phallitis
(b) Phallic
(c) Phallectomy

Word Exercise 4

(a) Balanitis
(b) Condition of bursting forth (of blood) from the glans penis
(c) Inflammation of the prepuce and glans penis

Word Exercise 5

(a) Epididymitis
(b) Epididymectomy
(c) Inflammation of the testes and epididymis

Word Exercise 6

(a) Removal of the vas deferens (a section of it to prevent transfer of sperm)
(b) Formation of an opening between the epididymis and the vas deferens
(c) Technique of making an X-ray of the epididymis and vas deferens
(d) Cutting/excision of the vas deferens
(e) Stitching/suturing of the vas deferens
(f) Formation of an opening between the testes and the vas deferens
(g) Formation of an opening between the vas deferens and another part of the vas deferens
(h) Incision into the vas deferens

Word Exercise 7

(a) Vesiculography
(b) Vesiculotomy
(c) Removal of the seminal vesicles and vas deferens

Word Exercise 8

(a) Incision into the bladder and prostate gland
(b) Enlargement of the prostate gland
(c) Removal of the prostate gland
(d) Removal of the seminal vesicles and prostate gland

Word Exercise 9

(a) Pertaining to carrying semen
(b) Condition of semen in the urine
(c) Tumour (Am. tumor) of semen (actually the germ cells of the testis)

Word Exercise 10

(a) Condition of being without sperm
(b) Condition of few sperm (low sperm count)
(c) Killing of sperms (actually an agent used as a contraceptive for killing sperm)
(d) Spermatopathia

(e) Spermatogenesis
(f) Spermatolysis
(g) Spermatorrhoea (Am. spermatorrhea)

Word Exercise 11

(a) Sperm count (5)
(b) Transurethral resection (4)
(c) Vasectomy (6)
(d) Orchidometer (3)
(e) In vitro fertilization (1)
(f) Vasoligature (2)

Case History 15

(a) Process/condition of hidden testicles (i.e. undescended testicles)
(b) Fixation of testicles by surgery (an operation to fix undescended testicles in their correct position)
(c) Inflammation of the testes/testicles
(d) Pertaining to within a testicle
(e) Removal of a testicle
(f) Pertaining to sperm/semen
(g) Pertaining to through the scrotum
(h) Tumour (Am. tumor) of the semen (arising from undifferentiated germ cells in the testis)

Unit 16 The female reproductive system

Word Exercise 1

(a) Germ cell that produces eggs
(b) Egg cell (ovum)
(c) Formation of eggs

Word Exercise 2

(a) Oophorectomy
(b) Oophoropexy
(c) Oophorotomy
(d) Removal of a bladder (cyst) from the ovary (an ovarian cyst)
(e) Opening into an ovary/formation of an opening into an ovary

Word Exercise 3

(a) Ovariectomy
(b) Ovariotomy
(c) Rupture/breaking of an ovary
(d) Pertaining to the oviduct and ovary
(e) Puncture of an ovary

Word Exercise 4

(a) Removal of an ovary and oviduct
(b) Removal of an oviduct and ovary
(c) Fixation of a Fallopian tube (by surgery)
(d) Hernia/protrusion/swelling of an oviduct
(e) Inflammation of an ovary and oviduct
(f) Salpingography

(g) Salpingolithiasis
(h) Salpingoplasty

Word Exercise 5

(a) Uteralgia/uterodynia
(b) Uterosclerosis
(c) Pertaining to the (Fallopian) tubes and uterus
(d) Technique of making an X-ray of the oviduct and uterus
(e) Pertaining to the bladder and uterus
(f) Pertaining to the rectum and uterus
(g) Pertaining to the placenta and uterus

Word Exercise 6

(a) Hysteroscope
(b) Hysteroptosis
(c) Hysterogram
(d) Technique of making an X-ray of the oviduct and uterus
(e) Formation of an opening between the oviduct and uterus
(f) Removal of ovaries, oviducts and uterus
(g) Suturing of the neck of the uterus
(h) Incision into the neck of the uterus

Word Exercise 7

(a) Excessive dripping/bleeding from the uterus
(b) Condition of disease of the uterus with excessive loss of blood
(c) Inflammation of the peritoneum around the uterus
(d) Inflammation of the veins of the uterus
(e) Abnormal condition of cysts in the uterus
(f) Abnormal condition of a falling/prolapsed uterus
(g) Metrostenosis
(h) Metromalacia
(i) Inflammation within the lining of the uterus (endometrium)
(j) Tumour (Am. tumor) of the endometrium
(k) Abnormal condition of the endometrium

Word Exercise 8

(a) Excessive dripping of menses/prolonged menstruation
(b) The beginning of menstruation
(c) Stopping of menstruation (occurs in women aged 45–50 years approximately)
(d) Without menstrual flow (menstruation), e.g. as in pregnancy
(e) Difficult/painful/bad menstruation
(f) Reduced flow of menses/infrequent menstruation
(g) Pertaining to before menstruation

Word Exercise 9

(a) Cervicitis
(b) Cervicectomy

Word Exercise 10

(a) Visual examination of the vagina
(b) Microscope used to view the lining of the vagina in situ
(c) Picture (in this case a differential list) of vaginal cells
(d) Suturing of the perineum and vagina
(e) Removal of the uterus through the vagina
(f) Hernia/protrusion/swelling of the uterus into the vagina
(g) Inflammation of the vagina and cervix
(h) Colpoperineoplasty
(i) Colpopexy

Word Exercise 11

(a) Incision into the perineum and vagina
(b) Suturing of the perineum and vagina
(c) Pertaining to the bladder and vagina
(d) Vaginomycosis
(e) Vaginopathy

Word Exercise 12

(a) Inflammation of the vagina and vulva
(b) Surgical repair of the vagina and vulva

Word Exercise 13

(a) Instrument to view the rectouterine pouch
(b) Technique of viewing the rectouterine pouch
(c) Puncture of the rectouterine pouch

Word Exercise 14

(a) Study of women (particularly diseases of the female reproductive tract)
(b) Pertaining to woman-forming (feminizing)

Word Exercise 15

(a) A woman's first pregnancy
(b) A woman's second pregnancy
(c) A woman who is pregnant and has been pregnant more than twice before

Word Exercise 16

(a) A woman who has had one pregnancy that resulted in a viable child
(b) A woman who has had two pregnancies that resulted in viable offspring
(c) A woman who has had more than two pregnancies that resulted in viable offspring
(d) A woman who has never borne a viable child

Word Exercise 17

(a) Study of the fetus
(b) Instrument to view the fetus
(c) Pertaining to the placenta and fetus
(d) Fetotoxic
(e) Fetometry

Word Exercise 18

(a) Instrument to cut the amnion
(b) Pertaining to the amnion and fetus
(c) Amniotomy
(d) Amnioscope
(e) Technique of making an X-ray of the amnion
(f) An X-ray picture of the amnion
(g) Puncture of the amnion to remove amniotic fluid
(h) Pertaining to the amnion and chorion (fetal membranes)
(i) Inflammation of the amnion and chorion

Word Exercise 19

(a) Placentography
(b) Placentopathy

Word Exercise 20

(a) Condition of difficult/painful/bad birth
(b) Study of labour (Am. labor)/birth
(c) Condition of good (normal) birth

Word Exercise 21

(a) Pertaining to a new birth
(b) Pertaining to before birth
(c) Pertaining to around/near birth
(d) Pertaining to before birth
(e) Study of neonates (new births)

Word Exercise 22

(a) Technique of making a breast X-ray
(b) Surgical reconstruction/repair of the breast
(c) Pertaining to affinity for/affecting the breast

Word Exercise 23

(a) Mastography
(b) Mastoplasty
(c) Mastectomy
(d) Condition of women's breasts (abnormal condition seen in males)

Word Exercise 24

(a) Agent stimulating/promoting milk production
(b) Pertaining to carrying milk
(c) Instrument used to measure milk (its specific gravity)
(d) Hormone that stimulates (and sustains) milk secretion
(e) Hormone that acts before milk, i.e. on the breast to stimulate lactation
(f) Agent that stops milk (secretion)
(g) Pertaining to forming milk/originating in milk

Word Exercise 25

(a) Agent that stimulates milk production
(b) Excessive flow of milk
(c) Condition of holding back/stopping milk (secretion)
(d) Formation of milk

Word Exercise 26

(a) Vaginal speculum (9)
(b) Colposcope (5)
(c) Pap test (7)
(d) Culdoscopy (3)
(e) Fetoscope (10)
(f) Hysteroscope (2)
(g) Amniotome (4)
(h) Lactometer (6)
(i) Obstetrical forceps (8)
(j) Tocography (1)

Case History 16

(a) Woman pregnant for the first time
(b) Without menstruation/menstrual flow
(c) Technique of recording labour (Am. labor) (uterine contractions) and the heart rate (of the fetus) during delivery
(d) Pertaining to before birth
(e) Pertaining to around birth
(f) A doctor who specializes in problems associated with childbirth/midwifery
(g) Period following birth when reproductive organs return to their normal condition (approx. 6 weeks)
(h) Pertaining to the amnion

Unit 17 The endocrine system
Word Exercise 1

(a) Process of secreting below normal level of pituitary hormones
(b) Process of secreting above normal level of pituitary hormones
(c) Condition of small extremities, i.e. hands and feet (due to deficiency of growth hormone)
(d) Large extremities, i.e. hands and feet (due to excess production of growth hormone in adults)

Word Exercise 2

(a) Pertaining to the tongue and thyroid gland
(b) Inflammation of the thyroid gland
(c) Thyroid protein
(d) Incision into the thyroid cartilage
(e) Condition of poisoning by the thyroid (due to overstimulation of thyroid gland)
(f) Near/beside the thyroid (the parathyroid gland)
(g) Removal of the parathyroid gland
(h) Process of secreting above normal levels of parathyroid hormones
(i) Enlargement of the thyroid gland
(j) Hyperthyroidism
(k) Hypothyroidism
(l) Thyroptosis
(m) Thyrotropic
(n) Thyrogenic

Word Exercise 3

(a) Pertaining to affinity for/acting on the pancreas
(b) Formation of insulin (from the Islets of Langerhans)
(c) Tumour (Am. tumor) of the Islets of Langerhans
(d) Inflammation of the Islets of Langerhans
(e) Process of secreting above normal levels of insulin
(f) Condition of below normal levels of sugar in blood
(g) Condition of above normal levels of sugar in blood
(h) Condition of sugar in the urine
(i) Pertaining to a constant glucose level (a controlled level)

Word Exercise 4

(a) Adrenomegaly
(b) Adrenotoxic
(c) Adrenotropic
(d) Condition of above normal levels of sodium in the blood
(e) Condition of below normal levels of potassium in the blood
(f) Secretion of excess sodium in the urine
(g) Pertaining to nourishing the adrenal cortex
(h) Condition of above normal growth of cells of adrenal cortex

Word Exercise 5

(a) Pertaining to male and female (hermaphroditic or of doubtful sex)
(b) Tumour (Am. tumor) of the germ cells of the male, i.e. the testis

Word Exercise 6

(a) Adrenal function test (4)
(b) Glucose tolerance test (3)
(c) PBI test (2)
(d) Glucose oxidase paper strip test (5)
(e) Thyroid scan (1)

Case History 17

(a) Condition of too much urine
(b) Condition of sugar in the urine
(c) Condition of above normal concentration of sugar in the blood
(d) Condition of ketones in the blood
(e) Abnormal acidity caused by ketones
(f) Pertaining to the pancreas
(g) Condition of below normal levels of sugar in the blood
(h) Pertaining to sugar

Unit 18 Radiology and nuclear medicine

Word Exercise 1

(a) Specialist who studies radiology (medically qualified)
(b) An X-ray picture
(c) Technique of making an X-ray
(d) One who makes an X-ray (a technician, not medically qualified)
(e) A specialist who treats disease using radiation (medically qualified)

Word Exercise 2

(a) Technique of making an X-ray/roentgenogram
(b) A specialist who studies roentgenology/X-rays (medically qualified)
(c) An X-ray picture
(d) X-ray picture of the heart
(e) Fluoroscope
(f) Fluorography

Word Exercise 3

(a) A moving X-ray picture
(b) Technique of making a moving X-ray
(c) Technique of making a moving X-ray of the heart and vessels
(d) A moving X-ray picture of the oesophagus (Am. esophagus)

Word Exercise 4

(a) An X-ray picture of a slice/section through the body
(b) Technique of making an X-ray of a slice/section through the body

Word Exercise 5

(a) A picture of sparks, i.e. distribution of radioactivity within the body (synonymous with a scintiscan, an image/tracing produced by a scintiscanner)
(b) Technique of making a scintigram

Word Exercise 6

(a) Treatment by radiation
(b) A specialist who treats disease with radiation (medically qualified)

Word Exercise 7

(a) A picture/tracing produced using ultrasound
(b) Technique of making a picture/tracing using ultrasound
(c) An instrument that uses ultrasound to make a picture/tracing/recording

Word Exercise 8

(a) A picture/tracing of the brain made using ultrasound echoes
(b) Echogenic
(c) Echogram
(d) Echoencephalograph
(e) Echocardiogram
(f) Echography

Word Exercise 9

(a) A picture/tracing/recording of infrared heat within body
(b) Technique of making a thermogram of infrared heat from the scrotum (used to detect testicular cancer)

Word Exercise 10

(a) Radiography (4)
(b) Fluoroscopy (7)
(c) Thermography (8)
(d) Ultrasonograph (5)
(e) Computerized tomograph (6)
(f) Radiotherapy (9)
(g) Cineradiography (10)
(h) Gamma camera (1)
(i) Echocardiography (2)
(j) Contrast medium (3)

Case History 18

(a) A recording/picture produced using X-rays
(b) Technique of recording/producing an image of a slice/cross-section through the body
(c) Specialist who treats disease using radiation (medically qualified)
(d) Treatment using radiation/X-rays etc.
(e) An X-ray picture of a slice/section through the body
(f) Pertaining to the killing of a tumour (Am. tumor)
(g) A device that produces high energy beams of electrons/X-rays for radiotherapy
(h) Technique of making a recording using high frequency sound waves

Unit 19 Oncology

Word Exercise 1

(a) Abnormal condition of tumours (Am. tumor)
(b) Formation of tumours (Am. tumor)
(c) Pertaining to affinity for a tumour (Am. tumor)
(d) Oncogenic
(e) Oncolysis
(f) Oncologist

Word Exercise 2

(a) Pertaining to the formation of a carcinoma (a malignant tumour of an epithelium)
(b) Destruction/disintegration of a carcinoma
(c) Pertaining to stopping the growth of a carcinoma

Word Exercise 3

(a) A malignant tumour (Am. tumor) of cartilage
(b) A malignant tumour of smooth muscle
(c) A malignant tumour of striated muscle
(d) A malignant tumour of meninges
(e) A malignant tumour of blood vessels
(f) Abnormal condition of sarcomas

Case History 19

(a) A new growth (of cancer cells)
(b) Parts of a tumour (Am.tumor) that have spread from one site to another
(c) Tumour of the meninges
(d) Lump of matter (here meaning a tumour)
(e) Tumour of glial cells (neurogliacytes) in the brain
(f) A specialist who studies tumours/cancers
(g) A specialist who treats disease using radiation/ X-rays etc. (medically qualified)
(h) Treatment using chemicals (cytotoxic drugs that kill cancer cells)

Unit 20 Anatomical position

Word Exercise 1

(a) Superior
(b) Inferior
(c) Lateral
(d) Medial
(e) Anterior
(f) Dorsal
(g) Distal
(h) Proximal
(i) Superficial

Word Exercise 2

(a) Inferior
(b) Superior
(c) Medial
(d) Proximal
(e) Anterior
(f) Dorsal

Word Exercise 3

(a) Pertaining to the region below cartilage (of the rib cage)
(b) Pertaining to the region upon/above the stomach
(c) Pertaining to the region of the flank/hip

Word Exercise 4

(a) 6
(b) 1
(c) 7
(d) 2
(e) 5
(f) 8
(g) 3
(h) 4

Word Exercise 5

Leg regions
(a) femoral region
(b) patellar region
(c) crural region
(d) tarsal region

(e) digital/phalangeal region
(f) hallux region
(g) pedal region

Arm regions
(a) brachial region
(b) antebrachial region
(c) pollex region
(d) axillary region
(e) carpal region
(f) palmar/volar region
(g) digital/phalangeal region

Word Exercise 6

(a) 2
(b) 4
(c) 1
(d) 3

Word Exercise 7

(a) Paranasal
(b) Intervertebral
(c) Epigastric
(d) Post-ganglionic
(e) Dextrocardia
(f) Infra-orbital/sub-orbital

Word Exercise 8

(a) Pertaining to around the heart
(b) Pertaining to within a vein
(c) Pertaining to between the ribs
(d) A uterus turned backwards
(e) Pertaining to above the liver
(f) Pertaining to below the sternum
(g) Pertaining to before/in front of a ganglion
(h) Pertaining to outside the placenta
(i) Pertaining to under the epidermis

Case History 20

(a) Pertaining to near the point of attachment/origin
(b) Pertaining to near the surface of the body or surface of a structure
(c) Towards the front
(d) Pertaining to the median line along the centre of the body
(e) Flexing/bending back
(f) Pertaining to the side
(g) Pertaining to further away from the point of attachment/origin
(h) From the front to the back

Unit 21 Pharmacology and microbiology

Word Exercise 1

(a) The (scientific) study of drugs
(b) A specialist who studies drugs

(c) Abnormal condition of a psychosis due to drugs/abnormal condition of a drugged mind

Word Exercise 2

(a) 3
(b) 1
(c) 5
(d) 2
(e) 4

Word Exercise 3

(a) Drug that acts against bacteria
(b) Drug that acts against life (actually against bacteria and fungi)
(c) Drug that acts against fungi
(d) Drug that acts against viruses/virions
(e) Drug that acts against itching
(f) Drug that acts against acid (neutralizes acid)
(g) Drug that acts against worms, e.g. thread worms/tapeworms

Word Exercise 4

(a) The word means without pain, therefore a drug that reduces pain
(b) The word means without sensation, therefore a drug that reduces sensation

Word Exercise 5

(a) Drug that acts against (reduces symptoms of) diarrhoea (Am. diarrhea)
(b) Drug that acts against (prevents) spasm, it reduces the motility of the intestines

Word Exercise 6

(a) Drug that breaks down mucus (it reduces viscosity of mucus)
(b) Drug that acts against (prevents) coughing
(c) Drug that dilates the bronchi

Word Exercise 7

(a) Drug that breaks down fibrin of blood clots (used to remove clots/thrombi)
(b) Drug that prevents the breakdown of fibrin/clots (used to promote clotting in severe haemorrhage (Am. hemorrhage))
(c) The word means against without rhythm, therefore a drug that acts against arrhythmias (an arrhythmia is an abnormal heart beat, i.e. one without rhythm)
(d) Drug that stops blood flow thereby stimulating the clotting of blood

Word Exercise 8

(a) The word means pertaining to sleep, therefore a drug that induces sleep

(b) The word means breaking down anxiety, therefore a drug that reduces anxiety
(c) Drug that acts against (prevents) epilepsy
(d) Drug that acts against (prevents) psychosis, e.g. schizophrenia

Word Exercise 9

(a) Drug that paralyzes the ciliary body of the eye

Word Exercise 10

(a) Drug that acts against (prevents) itching
(b) Drug that breaks down epidermis/keratin (used to remove warts – overgrowths of epidermis caused by a viral infection)

Word Exercise 11

(a) Drug that produces quick labour (Am.labor)/birth (used to induce birth)
(b) Drug that nourishes/stimulates the gonads
(c) Drug that acts against oestrogen (Am. estrogen), used for infertility treatment in women

Word Exercise 12

(a) Drug that acts against the thyroid (especially the synthesis of thyroid hormones)

Word Exercise 13

(a) Drug that is poisonous to cells and kills them, used to destroy cancer cells
(b) Drug that acts against new growths (tumours/ cancer cells) and kills them

Word Exercise 14

(a) Drug that suppresses the immune system or immune response
(b) Drug used to suppress the cell-mediated immune response by killing cells (used to prevent rejection of transplanted organs)

Word Exercise 15

(a) 5
(b) 3
(c) 6
(d) 2
(e) 1
(f) 7
(g) 4

Word Exercise 16

(a) A specialist who studies bacteria
(b) Pertaining to streptococci

(c) Condition of bacteria in the urine
(d) Pertaining to killing bacteria
(e) Pertaining to stopping bacteria (growing)
(f) Pertaining to breakdown/disintegration of bacteria
(g) Condition of bacilli in the blood
(h) Pertaining to the formation of bacilli
(i) Agent that kills streptococci
(j) Condition of blood poisoning (septicaemia (Am. septicemia)) caused by streptococci
(k) Abnormal condition/disease caused by spirilla

Word Exercise 17

(a) Abnormal condition/disease of fungi (fungal infection)
(b) Pertaining to fungi
(c) A toxin/poison produced by fungi
(d) Abnormal condition/disease due to a fungal toxin/ fungal poison

Word Exercise 18

(a) Having the form of a fungus
(b) Pertaining to being toxic/poisonous to fungi
(c) Agent that kills fungi
(d) Pertaining to stopping fungi (growth)
(e) Resembling fungi
(f) State/condition of fungi

Word Exercise 19

(a) Agent that kills viruses
(b) Specialist who studies viruses
(c) Agent that acts against retroviruses (e.g. HIV)
(d) Condition of (excreting) viruses in urine
(e) Condition of viruses in the blood
(f) Condition of (excreting) viruses in milk

Case History 21

(a) Drug that acts against retroviruses (e.g. HIV)
(b) Abnormal condition resulting from Candida (a yeast-like fungal infection)
(c) Drug that acts against bacteria
(d) Drug that acts against life (antibiotics are derived or are derivatives of chemicals produced by living microorganisms and have the capacity to kill other organisms)
(e) The study of small organisms (bacteria, fungi, protozoa etc.)
(f) Drug that acts against fungi (e.g. Candida albicans)
(g) Drug that acts to prevent vomiting
(h) Pertaining to a treatment regimen involving drugs

ANSWERS TO SELF-ASSESSMENT TESTS

Levels of organization

Test 1A

(a) 7	(h) 4	(o) 16
(b) 14	(i) 17	(p) 20
(c) 18	(j) 12	(q) 11
(d) 19	(k) 5	(r) 15
(e) 8	(l) 10	(s) 6
(f) 3	(m) 1	(t) 13
(g) 9	(n) 2	

Test 1B

(a) Breakdown of cartilage
(b) Breakdown of white cells
(c) Pertaining to poisonous to tissues
(d) Disease of bone
(e) Immature lymph cell/cell that forms lymphocytes

Test 1C

(a) Microcyte
(b) Pathologist
(c) Cytopathologist
(d) Chondrology
(e) Cytopathic

The digestive system

Test 2A

(a) 15	(f) 4	(k) 3
(b) 14	(g) 13/12	(l) 7
(c) 10/11	(h) 5	(m) 8
(d) 2	(i) 12	(n) 6
(e) 9	(j) 1	(o) 11

Test 2B

(a) 14	(h) 17	(o) 11
(b) 20	(i) 15	(p) 13
(c) 2	(j) 7	(q) 10
(d) 5	(k) 12	(r) 4
(e) 19	(l) 3	(s) 18
(f) 9	(m) 16	(t) 8
(g) 6	(n) 1	

Test 2C

(a) 6	(h) 7	(o) 18
(b) 20	(i) 5	(p) 3
(c) 17	(j) 12	(q) 10
(d) 14	(k) 19	(r) 1
(e) 16	(l) 4	(s) 9
(f) 8	(m) 15	(t) 2
(g) 11	(n) 13	

Test 2D

(a) Inflammation of colon, intestine and stomach
(b) Technique of making an X-ray/recording of liver
(c) Pertaining to the rectum and ileum
(d) Instrument used to view the sigmoid colon and rectum
(e) Enlargement of the pancreas

Test 2E

(a) Duodenitis
(b) Gastralgia
(c) Hepatotomy
(d) Proctology
(e) Ileoproctostomy

The respiratory system

Test 3A

(a) 3	(e) 4	(i) 9
(b) 10	(f) 7/6	(j) 1
(c) 5	(g) 2	
(d) 6/7	(h) 8	

Test 3B

(a) 14	(h) 18	(o) 15
(b) 16	(i) 4	(p) 20
(c) 7	(j) 1	(q) 9
(d) 12	(k) 19	(r) 3
(e) 8	(l) 5	(s) 10
(f) 2	(m) 6	(t) 17
(g) 11	(n) 13	

Test 3C

(a) 3	(h) 13	(o) 17
(b) 19	(i) 12	(p) 9
(c) 5	(j) 10/11	(q) 11/10
(d) 18	(k) 14	(r) 20
(e) 7	(l) 2	(s) 4
(f) 15	(m) 6	(t) 8
(g) 1	(n) 16	

Test 3D

(a) Originating in bronchi/pertaining to formation of bronchi
(b) Abnormal condition of narrowing of trachea
(c) Specialist who studies lungs
(d) Instrument that records the diaphragm (its movement)
(e) Condition of paralysis of the larynx

Test 3E

(a) Bronchoplasty
(b) Bronchoscopy
(c) Tracheorrhaphy
(d) Rhinology
(e) Costophrenic

The cardiovascular system

Test 4A

(a) 6	(c) 4	(e) 2
(b) 1	(d) 5	(f) 3

Test 4B

(a) 7	(h) 20	(o) 17
(b) 6	(i) 1/2	(p) 14
(c) 4	(j) 19	(q) 12
(d) 15	(k) 18	(r) 13
(e) 3	(l) 11	(s) 5
(f) 10	(m) 9	(t) 16
(g) 8	(n) 2/1	

Test 4C

(a) 12	(h) 1	(o) 18
(b) 9/10	(i) 13	(p) 20
(c) 6	(j) 14	(q) 17
(d) 2	(k) 3	(r) 5
(e) 7	(l) 15/16	(s) 10/9
(f) 8	(m) 4	(t) 16/15
(g) 11	(n) 19	

Test 4D

(a) Inflammation of heart valves
(b) Suturing of the aorta
(c) Instrument used to view vessels
(d) Abnormal condition of narrowing of veins
(e) Inflammation of the lining of an artery due to a clot

Test 4E

(a) Thromboarteritis
(b) Cardiocentesis
(c) Arteriopathy
(d) Phlebectomy
(e) Angiocardiology

The blood

Test 5A

(a) 5	(c) 3	(e) 4
(b) 1/3	(d) 2	

Test 5B

(a) 10	(i) 3	(q) 5
(b) 17	(j) 12	(r) 11
(c) 9	(k) 7	(s) 16
(d) 6	(l) 2	(t) 15
(e) 13	(m) 21	(u) 24
(f) 19	(n) 4	(v) 14
(g) 20	(o) 18	(w) 8
(h) 22	(p) 23	(x) 1

Test 5C

(a) Condition of white blood cells/leucocytes (Am. leukocytes) in urine
(b) Abnormal condition of marrow cells (too many)
(c) Condition of erythrocytes in urine
(d) Condition of blood with thrombocytes (too many platelets)
(e) Breakdown of phagocytes

Test 5D

(a) Haemopathy (Am. hemopathy)
(b) Erythrocytopenia
(c) Haematologist (Am. hematologist)
(d) Haemotoxic/haematotoxic (Am. hemotoxic/hematotoxic)
(e) Neutropenia

The lymphatic system and immunology

Test 6A

(a) 5	(c) 2	(e) 4
(b) 3	(d) 1	

Test 6B

(a) 14	(h) 10	(o) 15
(b) 5	(i) 3	(p) 11
(c) 8	(j) 13	(q) 9
(d) 4	(k) 18	(r) 20
(e) 2	(l) 17	(s) 7
(f) 1	(m) 19	(t) 12
(g) 16	(n) 6	

Test 6C

(a) Excessive flow of lymph
(b) Pertaining to the spleen
(c) Dilatation of a lymph node
(d) Breakdown of the thymus gland
(e) A specialist who studies sera

Test 6D

(a) Lymphoma
(b) Lymphography
(c) Splenectomy
(d) Splenorrhagia
(e) Lymphangioma

The urinary system

Test 7A

(a) 4	(d) 3	(g) 5
(b) 2	(e) 7	(h) 8
(c) 1	(f) 6	

Test 7B

(a) 9	(h) 17	(o) 10
(b) 7	(i) 18	(p) 6
(c) 15	(j) 2	(q) 20
(d) 16	(k) 5	(r) 1
(e) 14	(l) 13	(s) 3
(f) 11	(m) 8	(t) 4
(g) 12	(n) 19	

Test 7C

(a) 17	(h) 18	(o) 16
(b) 8/9	(i) 12	(p) 7
(c) 11	(j) 5	(q) 13
(d) 15	(k) 3/2	(r) 14
(e) 1	(l) 4	(s) 10
(f) 19	(m) 20	(t) 9 or 8
(g) 2/3	(n) 6	

Test 7D

(a) Incision to remove stones from the renal pelvis and kidney
(b) Abnormal condition of narrowing of the ureter
(c) Technique of recording/making an X-ray of the urethra and bladder
(d) Hernia/protrusion of the bladder
(e) Dilatation of the pelvis

Test 7E

(a) Ureterectasis
(b) Sigmoidoureterostomy
(c) Cystography
(d) Urogram
(e) Nephrosclerosis

The nervous system

Test 8A

(a) 3	(e) 6	(h) 8
(b) 1	(f) 4	(i) 7
(c) 9	(g) 2	(j) 5
(d) 10		

Test 8B

(a) 7/8	(h) 13	(o) 20
(b) 19	(i) 4/3	(p) 12
(c) 15	(j) 14	(q) 1
(d) 8/7	(k) 6	(r) 11
(e) 3/4	(l) 2	(s) 9/10
(f) 18	(m) 17	(t) 10/9
(g) 16	(n) 5	

Test 8C

(a) 20	(h) 7	(o) 3
(b) 10	(i) 18	(p) 2
(c) 13	(j) 6	(q) 1
(d) 8	(k) 17	(r) 14
(e) 11	(l) 16	(s) 5
(f) 19	(m) 4	(t) 9
(g) 12	(n) 15	

Test 8D

(a) 14	(h) 2	(o) 4
(b) 7	(i) 17	(p) 6
(c) 19	(j) 11	(q) 15
(d) 13	(k) 8	(r) 20
(e) 3	(l) 1	(s) 9
(f) 18	(m) 16	(t) 5
(g) 12	(n) 10	

Test 8E

(a) Inflammation of the spinal cord and nerves
(b) Incision into the spine
(c) Condition of softening of the meninges
(d) Disease of spinal cord and brain
(e) Instrument used to view ventricles (of the brain)

Test 8F

(a) Meningopathy
(b) Cephalometer
(c) Radiculomyelitis
(d) Encephalorrhagia
(e) Neurocytology

The eye

Test 9A

(a) 3	(e) 1	(h) 9
(b) 4	(f) 7	(i) 6
(c) 2	(g) 8	(j) 10
(d) 5		

Test 9B

(a)	12	(h)	20	(o)	8
(b)	10	(i)	15	(p)	7
(c)	18	(j)	6	(q)	17
(d)	19	(k)	16	(r)	2
(e)	1	(l)	4/5	(s)	9
(f)	14	(m)	3	(t)	5/4
(g)	13	(n)	11		

Test 9C

(a)	17	(h)	10	(o)	3
(b)	14	(i)	4	(p)	11
(c)	9	(j)	2	(q)	5
(d)	18	(k)	20/19	(r)	8
(e)	1	(l)	16/15	(s)	13
(f)	12	(m)	15/16	(t)	7
(g)	19/20	(n)	6		

Test 9D

(a) Surgical repair/reconstruction of the eye
(b) Surgical fixation of the retina
(c) Excessive flow of pus from tear ducts
(d) Inflammation of the iris and sclera
(e) Nerve that stimulates movement/action of the eye

Test 9E

(a) Ophthalmoscopy
(b) Blepharitis
(c) Keratopathy
(d) Retinoscope
(e) Iridoplegia

The ear

Test 10A

(a)	8	(e)	3	(h)	1
(b)	5	(f)	4	(i)	6
(c)	7/5	(g)	10	(j)	2
(d)	9				

Test 10B

(a)	8/9/10	(h)	3	(o)	11
(b)	9/8/10	(i)	15	(p)	13
(c)	14	(j)	17	(q)	2
(d)	16	(k)	6	(r)	5
(e)	10/9/8	(l)	18	(s)	4
(f)	19	(m)	7	(t)	1
(g)	12	(n)	20		

Test 10C

(a)	12	(h)	17	(o)	3
(b)	5/6	(i)	11	(p)	4
(c)	7	(j)	13	(q)	1
(d)	15	(k)	18	(r)	14
(e)	20	(l)	6/5	(s)	8
(f)	2	(m)	16	(t)	9
(g)	10	(n)	19		

Test 10D

(a) Study of the larynx and ear
(b) Condition of hardening within the middle ear (around the ear ossicles)
(c) Pertaining to the vestibular apparatus and stapes
(d) Pertaining to the malleus and tympanic membrane
(e) Pertaining to the cochlea and vestibular apparatus

Test 10E

(a) Mastoidocentesis
(b) Myringectomy
(c) Otoplasty
(d) Otalgia
(e) Tympanogenic

The skin

Test 11A

(a)	5	(c)	1	(e)	2
(b)	4	(d)	6	(f)	3

Test 11B

(a)	18	(h)	4	(o)	20
(b)	19	(i)	3	(p)	1
(c)	17	(j)	14	(q)	7
(d)	8	(k)	6	(r)	12
(e)	13	(l)	5	(s)	15
(f)	2	(m)	10	(t)	9
(g)	16	(n)	11		

Test 11C

(a)	11	(e)	12	(i)	8
(b)	7	(f)	2	(j)	4/5
(c)	9	(g)	3	(k)	10
(d)	1	(h)	6	(l)	5/4

Test 11D

(a) Abnormal condition of skin plants (a fungal infection)
(b) Epidermal cell
(c) Condition of without hair sensation
(d) Tumour (Am. tumor) of a sweat gland
(e) Abnormal condition of fungi in the epidermis

Test 11E

(a) Dermatitis
(b) Onychosis
(c) Melanonychia
(d) Dermatology
(e) Pachyonychia

The nose and mouth

Test 12A

(a) 4	(d) 5	(g) 3
(b) 8	(e) 2	(h) 1
(c) 6	(f) 7	

Test 12B

(a) 19	(h) 8	(o) 6
(b) 14	(i) 7	(p) 11
(c) 13	(j) 9	(q) 20
(d) 15	(k) 18	(r) 10
(e) 16	(l) 5	(s) 3
(f) 4	(m) 1	(t) 2
(g) 17	(n) 12	

Test 12C

(a) 9	(h) 12	(o) 8
(b) 13	(i) 16/15	(p) 20/19
(c) 15/16	(j) 5	(q) 3
(d) 17	(k) 4	(r) 11
(e) 18	(l) 2	(s) 10
(f) 1	(m) 14	(t) 6
(g) 7	(n) 19/20	

Test 12D

(a) Instrument used to measure the power/force of the tongue
(b) Measurement of saliva
(c) Inflammation of the tongue and mouth
(d) Splitting of the palate and jaw
(e) Pertaining to formation of or originating in teeth

Test 12E

(a) Sialadenotomy
(b) Palatorrhaphy
(c) Rhinomycosis
(d) Labial
(e) Palatoplasty

The muscular system

Test 13A

(a) 18	(h) 17/16	(o) 7
(b) 15	(i) 3	(p) 10
(c) 8	(j) 19	(q) 20
(d) 13	(k) 1	(r) 11
(e) 9	(l) 5	(s) 12
(f) 2	(m) 4	(t) 14
(g) 16/17	(n) 6	

Test 13B

(a) Instrument that measures the electrical activity of muscle
(b) Study of movement
(c) Incision into a tendon and muscle
(d) Without nourishment of muscle (muscle wasting)
(e) Pertaining to an aponeurosis and muscle

Test 13C

(a) Myomalacia
(b) Myogenic
(c) Myopathy
(d) Tenorrhaphy
(e) Tenotomy

The skeletal system

Test 14A

(a) 4	(c) 2	(e) 6
(b) 3	(d) 1	(f) 5

Test 14B

(a) 14/15	(h) 13	(o) 3
(b) 4	(i) 15/14	(p) 2
(c) 18	(j) 20	(q) 6
(d) 12	(k) 11	(r) 16
(e) 7	(l) 8	(s) 5
(f) 19	(m) 9	(t) 10
(g) 17	(n) 1	

Test 14C

(a) 5	(h) 15	(o) 19
(b) 7	(i) 16	(p) 18
(c) 9	(j) 11	(q) 4
(d) 12	(k) 10	(r) 13
(e) 17	(l) 2	(s) 6
(f) 20	(m) 1	(t) 3
(g) 14	(n) 8	

Test 14D

(a) Inflammation of the cartilage of a joint
(b) Stone in a bursa
(c) Binding together of vertebrae
(d) A cell that breaks down cartilage
(e) Pertaining to having a humped/hunched back

Test 14E

(a) Arthralgia
(b) Osteosynovitis
(c) Spondylomalacia
(d) Osteoarthropathy
(e) Synovial

The male reproductive system

Test 15A

(a) 3	(d) 6	(g) 4
(b) 7	(e) 2	(h) 8
(c) 5	(f) 1	

Test 15B

(a) 16	(h) 13	(o) 14
(b) 18	(i) 20	(p) 19
(c) 3	(j) 12/11	(q) 2
(d) 9	(k) 1	(r) 5
(e) 15	(l) 7	(s) 6
(f) 17	(m) 10	(t) 4
(g) 11/12	(n) 8	

Test 15C

(a) 4	(f) 15	(k) 13
(b) 14	(g) 2	(l) 7
(c) 8	(h) 3	(m) 9
(d) 1	(i) 6	(n) 10
(e) 12	(j) 5	(o) 11

Test 15D

(a) Removal of the epididymes and testes
(b) Flow from the penis (abnormal)
(c) Removal of the vas deferens and epididymes
(d) Tying off of the vas deferens
(e) Condition of sperm in the urine

Test 15E

(a) Orchidorrhaphy/orchiorrhaphy
(b) Prostatalgia
(c) Epididymovasostomy
(d) Scrotitis
(e) Prostatorrhoea (Am. prostatorrhea)

The female reproductive system

Test 16A

(a) 3	(d) 6	(g) 8
(b) 4	(e) 2	(h) 7
(c) 1	(f) 5	

Test 16B

(a) 5	(h) 17	(o) 18
(b) 10/11	(i) 7	(p) 8
(c) 12	(j) 15	(q) 16
(d) 19	(k) 3	(r) 1
(e) 20	(l) 13	(s) 14
(f) 2	(m) 6	(t) 9
(g) 4	(n) 11/10	

Test 16C

(a) 22	(j) 4	(r) 9
(b) 17/18	(k) 13/12/14	(s) 7
(c) 16	(l) 5	(t) 23
(d) 8	(m) 10	(u) 15
(e) 1	(n) 19	(v) 14/12/13
(f) 12/13/14	(o) 20/21	(w) 18/17
(g) 24	(p) 21/20	(x) 25
(h) 2/3	(q) 11	(y) 6
(i) 3/2		

Test 16D

(a) An instrument that measures labour (Am. labor), it measures uterine contractions
(b) Removal of the uterus and ovaries
(c) Surgical fixation of the breasts
(d) Rupture of the uterus
(e) Disease of the uterus

Test 16E

(a) Culdoplasty
(b) Salpingostomy
(c) Amniorrhexis
(d) Colpoptosis
(e) Colpocytology

The endocrine system

Test 17A

(a) 4	(d) 2	(g) 1
(b) 3	(e) 5	(h) 8
(c) 7	(f) 6	

Test 17B

(a) 16	(h) 10	(o) 9
(b) 11	(i) 15	(p) 4
(c) 20	(j) 2	(q) 5
(d) 1	(k) 7	(r) 12
(e) 19	(l) 3	(s) 14
(f) 8	(m) 17	(t) 13
(g) 18	(n) 6	

Test 17C

(a) Removal of the parathyroid and thyroid gland
(b) A pituitary cell
(c) Enlargement of the adrenal
(d) Pertaining to acting on/affinity for sugar
(e) Condition of above normal level of ketones in the blood

Test 17D

(a) Hyperinsulinism
(b) Hyponatraemia (Am. hyponatremia)
(c) Thyrotrophic
(d) Adrenotropic
(e) Hypoparathyroidism

Radiology and nuclear medicine

Test 18A

(a) 11	(h) 19	(o) 10
(b) 13	(i) 9	(p) 7
(c) 15	(j) 3	(q) 4
(d) 20	(k) 1	(r) 8
(e) 17	(l) 2	(s) 6
(f) 14	(m) 18	(t) 5
(g) 12	(n) 16	

Test 18B

(a) Treatment with X-rays
(b) A specialist who studies sound (ultrasound images)
(c) Treatment with X-rays and heat
(d) Instrument that produces a moving X-ray picture
(e) Technique of making a recording/picture of a slice through the body using ultrasound

Test 18C

(a) Ultrasonotherapy
(b) Fluoroscopic
(c) Scintiangiography
(d) Thermograph
(e) Echoencephalography

Oncology

Test 19A

(a) 9	(h) 16	(o) 11
(b) 20	(i) 17	(p) 6
(c) 10	(j) 18	(q) 5
(d) 14	(k) 4	(r) 15
(e) 12	(l) 2	(s) 7
(f) 3	(m) 19	(t) 8
(g) 1	(n) 13	

Test 19B

(a) Malignant tumour (Am. tumor) of fibrous tissue
(b) Malignant glandular tumour of stomach
(c) Malignant tumour of liver cells
(d) Malignant, disordered tumour of the thyroid (refers to appearance of backward growth, i.e. becoming disordered)
(e) Malignant tumour originating in the bronchus

Test 19C

(a) Lymphosarcoma
(b) Chondroma
(c) Osteosarcoma
(d) Neoplasia
(e) Oncotherapy

Anatomical position

Test 20A

(a) 13	(h) 8/9	(o) 10
(b) 18	(i) 12	(p) 9/8
(c) 17	(j) 3	(q) 11
(d) 20	(k) 19	(r) 4
(e) 1	(l) 5/6	(s) 15
(f) 14	(m) 7	(t) 6/5
(g) 2	(n) 16	

Test 20B

(a) 9	(h) 15	(o) 8/7
(b) 12	(i) 19	(p) 13
(c) 7/8	(j) 5	(q) 10
(d) 14	(k) 18	(r) 3
(e) 1/2	(l) 6	(s) 17
(f) 20	(m) 11	(t) 4
(g) 16	(n) 2/1	

Test 20C

(a) Pertaining to between the phalanges (fingers and toes)
(b) A turning to the right
(c) Pertaining to behind/back of the cheek
(d) Pertaining to above the ribs
(e) Pertaining to within the nose

Test 20D

(a) Lateral
(b) Laevoversion (Am. levoversion)
(c) Post ganglionic
(d) Infrahepatic
(e) Transdermal

Pharmacology and microbiology

Test 21A

(a) 9	(h) 15/16	(o) 8
(b) 13	(i) 14	(p) 4
(c) 12	(j) 3	(q) 1
(d) 17	(k) 10	(r) 11
(e) 19	(l) 15/16	(s) 5
(f) 2	(m) 7	(t) 6
(g) 20	(n) 18	

Test 21B

(a) 17	(h) 4/5	(o) 3
(b) 9	(i) 2	(p) 10
(c) 16	(j) 19	(q) 1
(d) 13	(k) 18	(r) 11
(e) 6	(l) 20	(s) 12
(f) 8	(m) 5/4	(t) 15
(g) 14	(n) 7	

Test 21C

(a) Study of poisons
(b) Abnormal condition/disease caused by poisoning with fungi/fungal toxins
(c) A drug specialist (a person who dispenses drugs)
(d) Chemical/drug used for treatment of disease (used in treatment of cancer – chemotherapy)
(e) A specialist who studies microorganisms

Test 21D

(a) Bacteriologist
(b) Antibiotic
(c) Protozoology
(d) Bacteriostatic
(e) Virucidal

Test 21E

(a) 7	(h) 17	(o) 22	(v) 15
(b) 12	(i) 4	(p) 24	(w) 11
(c) 19	(j) 25	(q) 8	(x) 16
(d) 9	(k) 23	(r) 13	(y) 10
(e) 20	(l) 2	(s) 14	
(f) 21	(m) 1	(t) 5	
(g) 18	(n) 3	(u) 6	

Test 21F

(a) 8	(h) 1
(b) 4	(i) 3
(c) 9	(j) 6
(d) 2	(k) 11
(e) 12	(l) 7
(f) 10	
(g) 5	

Final self-assessment tests

Final test 1

(a) 18	(f) 2	(k) 7/8	(p) 3
(b) 20	(g) 12	(l) 8/7	(q) 1
(c) 5	(h) 19	(m) 11	(r) 14
(d) 6	(i) 4	(n) 16	(s) 13
(e) 17	(j) 15	(o) 9	(t) 10

Final test 2

(a) 11	(f) 13	(k) 5	(p) 9	(u) 6
(b) 8	(g) 22	(l) 1	(q) 15	(v) 25
(c) 20	(h) 3	(m) 19	(r) 12	(w) 16
(d) 17	(i) 23	(n) 24	(s) 10	(x) 2
(e) 18	(j) 7	(o) 21	(t) 14	(y) 4

Final test 3

(a) 8	(f) 17	(k) 4	(p) 2
(b) 12	(g) 10	(l) 3	(q) 13
(c) 14	(h) 7	(m) 5	(r) 16
(d) 9	(i) 20	(n) 15	(s) 18
(e) 19	(j) 6	(o) 11	(t) 1

Final test 4

(a) 21	(f) 9/10	(k) 5	(p) 3	(u) 11
(b) 7	(g) 14	(l) 17	(q) 1	(v) 12
(c) 13	(h) 15	(m) 23	(r) 24	(w) 4
(d) 25	(i) 19	(n) 10/9	(s) 22	(x) 2
(e) 20	(j) 18	(o) 6	(t) 8	(y) 16

Final test 5

(a) 4	(h) 14/15	(n) 16/17	(t) 13
(b) 21	(i) 5	(o) 1	(u) 7/8
(c) 18	(j) 22	(p) 10	(v) 9
(d) 23/24/25	(k) 15/14	(q) 2	(w) 8/7
(e) 24/25/23	(l) 6	(r) 12	(x) 17/16
(f) 3	(m) 19	(s) 20	(y) 11
(g) 25/23/24			

Final test 6

(a) 18	(f) 3	(k) 8	(p) 19	(u) 4
(b) 10	(g) 16	(l) 1/2	(q) 22	(v) 12
(c) 5	(h) 24	(m) 9	(r) 2/1	(w) 20
(d) 25	(i) 15	(n) 23	(s) 11	(x) 13
(e) 6/7	(j) 21	(o) 17	(t) 14	(y) 7/6

Final test 7

(a) 17	(f) 18	(k) 19	(p) 14/15	(u) 4
(b) 12/13	(g) 3	(l) 11	(q) 15/14	(v) 1
(c) 5	(h) 20	(m) 23/22	(r) 21	(w) 9
(d) 25	(i) 22/23	(n) 7	(s) 13/12	(x) 16
(e) 24	(j) 2	(o) 8	(t) 6	(y) 10

Final test 8

(a) 13/14/15	(f) 18	(k) 5	(p) 15/13/14
(b) 8	(g) 1	(l) 4	(q) 3
(c) 14/15/13	(h) 20	(m) 17	(r) 10
(d) 16	(i) 19	(n) 12	(s) 11
(e) 9	(j) 7	(o) 2	(t) 6

Final test 9

(a) 17	(f) 14	(k) 18	(p) 20
(b) 6/7	(g) 11	(l) 2	(q) 10
(c) 16	(h) 3	(m) 9	(r) 4
(d) 8	(i) 15	(n) 7/6	(s) 13
(e) 5	(j) 19	(o) 12	(t) 1

Final test 10

(a) 16/17	(f) 19	(k) 12	(p) 13
(b) 17/16	(g) 3	(l) 20	(q) 2
(c) 9	(h) 5	(m) 6	(r) 15
(d) 10	(i) 1	(n) 18	(s) 7
(e) 4	(j) 8	(o) 11	(t) 14

Final test 11

(a) 10	(f) 24	(k) 19	(p) 5	(u) 13
(b) 11	(g) 3	(l) 14	(q) 16	(v) 21
(c) 9	(h) 1	(m) 8	(r) 6	(w) 20
(d) 7	(i) 4	(n) 23	(s) 15	(x) 22
(e) 18	(j) 2	(o) 17	(t) 25	(y) 12

Final test 12

(a)	14	(f)	18	(k)	1	(p)	8
(b)	3	(g)	10	(l)	17	(q)	6
(c)	9	(h)	15	(m)	5	(r)	11
(d)	13	(i)	20	(n)	7	(s)	19
(e)	12	(j)	16	(o)	4	(t)	2

Final test 13

(a)	9	(f)	12	(k)	8	(p)	7
(b)	5	(g)	6	(l)	15	(q)	3/1/2
(c)	18/19	(h)	16	(m)	11	(r)	19/18
(d)	1/2/3	(i)	14	(n)	17	(s)	13
(e)	4	(j)	20	(o)	2/3/1	(t)	10

Final test 14

(a)	9	(f)	22	(k)	17	(p)	10	(u)	11
(b)	25	(g)	6	(l)	2/3	(q)	16	(v)	7
(c)	20	(h)	18	(m)	3/2	(r)	12	(w)	5
(d)	1	(i)	15	(n)	8	(s)	13	(x)	21
(e)	19	(j)	14	(o)	4	(t)	24	(y)	23

Final test 15

(a)	4	(f)	1	(k)	3	(p)	14
(b)	9	(g)	18	(l)	11	(q)	5
(c)	20	(h)	6	(m)	17	(r)	8
(d)	19	(i)	16	(n)	7	(s)	12
(e)	10	(j)	15	(o)	2	(t)	13

Final test 16

(a)	8	(f)	10	(k)	18	(p)	6/7
(b)	17	(g)	9	(l)	2	(q)	15
(c)	1	(h)	16	(m)	11	(r)	20
(d)	3	(i)	12	(n)	13	(s)	7/6
(e)	14	(j)	4	(o)	5	(t)	19

ABBREVIATIONS

The abbreviations listed here have been extracted from recent health care publications and the medical records of patients. Students should be aware that whilst certain abbreviations are standard, others are not and their meaning may vary from one health care setting to another. Abbreviations with several meanings should be carefully interpreted to avoid confusion.

A	anaemia (Am. anemia)
AAA	abdominal aortic aneurysm/acute anxiety attack
AAAAA	aphasia, agnosia, agraphia, alexia and apraxia
AAFB	acid alcohol fast bacilli
AB1	one abortion
Ab, ab	abortion/antibody
ABC	airway, breathing, circulation
Abdo	abdomen
ABE	acute bacterial endocarditis
ABG	arterial blood gases
abor	abortion
ABR	auditory brainstem evoked responses
ABX	antibiotics
AC	air conduction
ac	ante cibum (before meals/food)
ACBS	aortocoronary bypass surgery
Accom	accommodation of eye
ACE	angiotensin converting enzyme
ACh	acetyl choline
ACS	acute confused state
ACTH	adrenocorticotrophic hormone
ACU	acute care unit
AD or ad	Alzheimer's disease/auris dextra (right ear)
ADA	adenosine deaminase
ADC	AIDS dementia complex
ADD	attention deficit disorder
add	adduction
ADH	antidiuretic hormone
ADHD	attention deficit hyperactivity disorder
ADL	aids to daily living
ad lib	as desired
ADR	adverse drug reaction
ADT	admission, discharge and transfer
ADU	acute duodenal ulcer
A&E	accident and emergency
AED	anti-epileptic drug
AEM	ambulatory electrocardiogram monitoring
AF	amniotic fluid/atrial fibrillation
AFB	acid-fast bacilli
AFP	alphafeto protein
A/G	albumin/globulin ratio
Ag	antigen
AGA	appropriate for gestational age
AGL	acute granulocytic leukaemia (Am. leukemia)
AGN	acute glomerulonephritis
AI	aortic incompetence/aortic insufficiency/artificial insemination
AID	artificial insemination by donor
AIDS	acquired immunodeficiency syndrome
AIED	autoimmune inner ear disease
AIH	artificial insemination by husband
A/K	above knee (amputation)
alb	albumin (protein)
ALD	alcoholic liver disease
ALG	anti-lymphocyte immunoglobulin
ALL	acute lymphocytic leukaemia (Am. leukemia)
ALS	amyotrophic lateral sclerosis (Lou Gehrig disease)
ALs	activities of living
ALT	alanine aminotransferase/alanine transaminase
amb	ambulant/ambulatory (walking)
AMI	acute myocardial infarction
AML	acute myeloid leukaemia (Am. leukemia)
ANC	absolute neutrophil count
ANF	antinuclear factor
ANS	autonomic nervous system
ANT or ant	anterior
antib	antibiotic
A&O	alert and orientated
AOB	alcohol on breath
AP	antepartum/anteroposterior/appendicectomy/auscultation and percussion
APB	atrial premature beat
APH	antepartum haemorrhage (Am. hemorrhage)
APPY	appendicectomy
APSAC	acylated plasminogen streptokinase activator complex (anistreplase)
APTT	activated partial thromboplastin time
aq	aqueous/water
A–R	apical–radial (pulse)
ARC	aids related complex
ARD	acute respiratory disease
ARDS	adult respiratory distress syndrome
ARF	acute renal failure

ARMD	age-related macular degeneration	BOR	bowels open regularly
AS	alimentary system/aortic stenosis/auris sinistra (left ear)	BP	blood pressure/British Pharmacopoeia/bypass
A–S	Adams–Stokes attack	BPD	bronchopulmonary dysplasia
5-ASA	5-aminosalicylic acid (aspirin)	BPH	benign prostatic hyperplasia
ASC	altered state of consciousness	BPM	beats per minute
ASCVD	arteriosclerotic cardiovascular disease	BPPV	benign paroxysmal positional vertigo
ASD	atrial septal defect	BRO	bronchoscopy
ASHD	arteriosclerotic heart disease	BS	blood sugar/bowel sounds/breath sounds
ASO	antistreptolysin O	BSA	body surface area
ASOM	acute suppurative otitis media	BSE	bovine spongiform encephalopathy/breast self-examination
AST	aspartate transaminase		
Astigm	astigmatism of eye		
ASX	asymptomatic		
ATG	anti-thymocyte immunoglobulin	BSS	blood sugar series
ATN	acute tubular necrosis	BT	bedtime/bone tumour (Am. tumor)/brain tumour/breast tumour/bleeding time
ATP	adenosine triphosphate		
ATS	antitetanus serum		
AU	auris uterque (both ears)		
Au	gold	BTS	blood transfusion service
aud	audiology	BUN	blood urea nitrogen
aur dextr	to the right ear	BW	body weight
AV	arteriovenous/atrioventricular bundle/ atrioventricular node/aortic valve	BX, Bx or bx.	biopsy
AVM	arteriovenous malformation	C	Celsius
AVP	vasopressin	c	with
AVR	aortic valve replacement	C 1–7	cervical vertebra
A&W	alive and well	CA, Ca or ca.	cancer/carcinoma/cardiac arrest/ coronary artery
AXR	abdominal X-ray		
AZT	azidothymidine	Ca	calcium
		CABG	coronary artery bypass grafting
Ba	barium	CACX	cancer of the cervix
BaE	barium enema	CAD	coronary artery disease
BAER	brainstem auditory evoked responses	CAG	closed angle glaucoma
BAL	blood alcohol level	CAH	chronic active hepatitis/congenital adrenal hyperplasia
baso	basophil		
BBA	born before arrival	CAL	computer assisted learning
BBB	blood brain barrier/bundle branch block	CAO	chronic airway obstruction
		CAPD	continuous ambulatory peritoneal dialysis
BBBB	bilateral bundle branch block		
BBT	basal body temperature	CAT	computed axial tomography
BBx	breast biopsy	Cath	catheter/catheterization
BC	birth control/bone conduction	CAVH	continuous arteriovenous haemofiltration (Am. hemofiltration)
BCC	basal cell carcinoma		
BCG	bacille Calmette–Guérin	CAVHD	continuous arteriovenous haemodialysis (Am. hemodialysis)
BD or b.d.	bis diurnal (twice a day)		
BDA	British Diabetic Association	CBC	complete blood count
BE	bacterial endocarditis/barium enema	CBE	clinical breast examination
		CBF	cerebral blood flow
BI	bone injury	CCCC	closed-chest cardiac compression
BID	brought in dead	CCF	chronic cardiac failure/congestive cardiac failure
bid	bis in die (twice daily)		
B/KA	below knee (amputation)	CCIE	counter current immuno electrophoresis
BM	bowel movement		
BMI	body mass index	CCU	coronary care unit
BMR	basal metabolic rate	CD	Crohn's disease/cluster designation
BM (T)	bone marrow (trephine)	CDH	congenital dislocation of the hip joint
BMT	bone marrow transplant	CEA	carcino embryonic antigen
BNF	British National Formulary	CF	cancer free/cardiac failure/cystic fibrosis
BNO	bowels not open		
		CFT	complement fixation test

CFTR	cystic fibrosis transmembrane regulator	CSF	cerebrospinal fluid
CGL	chronic granulocytic leukaemia	CSH	chronic subdural haematoma (Am. hematoma)
CGN	chronic glomerulonephritis		
cGy	centigray (one hundredth of a gray)	CSM	cerebrospinal meningitis
CH	cholesterol	CSOM	chronic suppurative otitis media
chemo	chemotherapy	CSR	Cheyne–Stokes respiration/correct sedimentation rate
CHD	coronary heart disease		
CHF	congestive heart failure	CSU	catheter specimen of urine
CHI	creatinine height index	CT	cerebral tumour (Am. tumor)/clotting time/computed tomography/continue treatment/coronary thrombosis
chol	cholesterol		
CHOP	cyclophosphamide, hydroxydaunorubicin, oncovin and prednisolone		
		CTS	carpal tunnel syndrome
CHR, chr	chronic	CUG	cystourethrogram
CI	cardiac index/cerebral infarction	CV	cardiovascular/cerebrovascular
CIBD	chronic inflammatory bowel disease/disorder	CVA	cerebrovascular accident (stroke)/costovertebral angle
CIN	cervical intraepithelial neoplasia	CVD	cardiovascular disease
CIS	carcinoma in situ	CVP	central venous pressure
CJD	Creutzfeldt–Jakob disease	CVS	cardiovascular system/chorionic villus sampling
CK	creatine kinase		
CL	clubbing	CVVH	continuous venovenous haemofiltration (Am. hemofiltration)
CLD	chronic liver disease/chronic lung disease		
		CVVHD	continuous venovenous haemodialysis (Am. hemodialysis)
CLL	chronic lymphocytic leukaemia (Am. leukemia)		
		Cx	cervical/cervix
CMF	cyclophosphamide, methotrexate, 5-fluorouracil	CXR	chest X-ray
		Cy	cyanosis
		cyclic AMP	cyclic adenosine monophosphate
CMG	cystometrogram	Cysto	cystoscopy
CML	chronic myeloid leukaemia (Am. leukemia)		
		D	diagnosis
CMV	cytomegalovirus	db	decibel
CN	cranial nerve	DBP	diastolic blood pressure
CNS	central nervous system	D&C	dilatation and curettage
CO	carbon monoxide/cardiac output/complains of	DC or d/c	decrease/direct current/discharge/discontinue
COAD	chronic obstructive airways disease	DCCT	diabetes control and complications trial
COD	cause of death		
COLD	chronic obstructive lung disease	DCIS	ductal carcinoma in situ
COPD	chronic obstructive pulmonary disease	DD	differential diagnosis/discharge diagnosis
COP	colloid osmotic pressure	DDA	Dangerous Drugs Act
C&P	cystoscopy and pyelogram	DDAVP	desmopressin (synthetic vasopressin)
CP	cor pulmonale/cerebral palsy/chest pain	ddC/DDC	dideooxycytidine/zalcitabine
		ddI/DDI	didanosine/dideoxyinosine
CPA	cardiopulmonary arrest/costophrenic angle	DDx	differential diagnosis
		D&E	dilatation and evacuation
CPAP	continuous positive airways pressure	Decub	decubitus (lying down)
CPK	creatinine phosphokinase	Derm, derm	dermatology
CPN	community psychiatric nurse	DES	diethylstilbestrol
CPPV	continuous positive pressure ventilation	DH	delayed hypersensitivity/drug history
		DIC	disseminated intravascular coagulation
CPR	cardiopulmonary resuscitation		
CrCl	creatine clearance	DIDMOAD	diabetes insipidus, diabetes mellitus, optic atrophy and deafness
CRD	chronic renal disease		
CRF	chronic renal failure	diff	differential blood count (of cell types)
CRH	corticotrophin-releasing hormone	DIG	digitalis/digoxin
C + S	culture and sensitivity (test)	DIMS	disorders of initiating and maintaining sleep
C-sect, or c/sect	caesarean section (Am. cesarean)		
		DIOS	distal intestinal obstruction syndrome

DIP	distal interphalangeal	EMU	early morning urine
DJK	degenerative joint disease	EN	erythema nodosum
DKA	diabetics ketoacidosis	ENG	electronystagmogram
DLE	discoid lupus erythematosus/ disseminated lupus erythematosus	ENT	ear, nose and throat
		EOG	electrooculogram
DM	diabetes mellitus/diastolic murmur	EOM	extraocular movement
DMD	Duchenne muscular dystrophy	eos	eosinophil(s)
dmft	decayed missing and filled teeth (deciduous)	EP	ectopic pregnancy
		Epo	erythropoietin
DMFT	decayed missing and filled teeth (permanent)	EPSP	excitatory postsynaptic potential
		ERCP	endoscopic retrograde cholangiopancreatography
D/N	day/night (frequency of urine)		
DNA	deoxyribose nucleic acid/did not attend	ERG	electroretinogram
		ERT	estrogen replacement therapy (Am.)
DNR	do not resuscitate	ERV	expiratory reserve volume
DOA	dead on arrival	ESM	ejection systolic murmur
DOB	date of birth	ESN	educationally subnormal
DOD	date of death	ESP	end-systolic pressure
DOE	dyspnoea on exertion (Am. dyspnea)	ESR	erythrocyte sedimentation rate
DOES	disorders of excessive somnolence	ESRD	end-stage renal disease
DS	Down's syndrome	ESRF	end-stage renal failure
D/S	dextrose and saline	ESV	end-systolic volume
DSA	digital subtraction angiography	ESWL	extracorporeal shock wave lithotripsy
DT	delerium tremens	ET	embryo transfer/endotracheal/ endotracheal tube
DTP	diphtheria, tetanus and pertussis (vaccine)		
		ET CPAP	endotracheal continuous positive airways pressure
DTR	deep tendon reflex		
DU	duodenal ulcer	ETF	Eustachian tube function
DUB	dysfunctional uterine bleeding	ETT	endotracheal tube/exercise tolerance test
D&V	diarrhoea and vomiting		
DVT	deep venous thrombosis	EUA	examination under anaesthesia (Am. anesthesia)
Dx	diagnosis		
DXT	deep X-ray therapy	EX	examination
DXRT	deep X-ray radiotherapy	EXP	expansion
		Ez	eczema
EBM	expressed breast milk		
EBV	Epstein–Barr virus	F	Fahrenheit
ECF	extracellular fluid/extended care facility	FA	folic acid
		FAS	fetal alcohol syndrome
ECFV	extracellular fluid volume	FB	fasting blood sugar/finger breadth/foreign body
ECG	electrocardiogram		
ECHO	echocardiogram/echocardiography	FBC	full blood count
ECSL	extra corporeal shockwave lithotripsy	FBE	full blood examination
ECT	electroconvulsive therapy	FBS	fasting blood sugar
EDC	expected date of confinement	FDIU	fetal death in utero
EDD	expected date of delivery	Fe	iron
EDV	end-diastolic volume	FET	forced expiratory technique
EEG	electroencephalography/ electroencephalogram	FEV	forced expiratory volume
		FEV_1	forced expiratory volume in 1 second
EENT	eyes, ears, nose and throat	FFA	free fatty acids
EFM	electronic fetal monitoring	FFP	fresh frozen plasma
EGD	esophagogastroduodenoscopy (Am.)	FH	family history
ELBW	extremely low birth weight	FHR	fetal heart rate
ELISA	enzyme-linked immunosorbent assay	FLP	fasting lipid profile
Em	emmetropia (good vision)	FMH	family medical history
EMB	endometrial biopsy	FNAB	fine needle aspiration biopsy
EMD	electromechanical dissociation	FOB	faecal occult blood (Am. fecal)
EMG	electromyogram/electromyography	FOBT	faecal occult blood testing (Am. fecal)
EMI	elderly mentally infirm/etoposide- methotrexate-ifosfamide		
		FP	false positive

FRC	functional reserve capacity/functional residual capacity	H	hydrogen/hypodermic
FROM	full range of movement	HAV	hepatitis A virus
FSH	follicle stimulating hormone	HB	heart block
FSHRH	follicle stimulating hormone releasing hormone	Hb	haemoglobin (Am. hemoglobin)
		HBAg	hepatitis B antigen
FT	full term	HBGM	home blood glucose monitoring
FT_4	free thyroxine	HBO	hyperbaric oxygenation
FTI	free thyroxine index	HBP	high blood pressure
FTND	full term, normal delivery	HBsAg	hepatitis B surface antigen
F/u	follow up	HBV	hepatitis B virus
FUO	fever of unknown origin	HC	head circumference
FVC	forced vital capacity	HCG(hCG)	human chorionic gonadotrophin
FX, Fx or fx.	fracture	H/ct or /h.ct	haematocrit (Am. hematocrit)
		HCV	hepatitis C virus
		HCVD	hypertensive cardiovascular disease
g	gauge	HD	haemodialysis (Am. hemodialysis)/ Hodgkin's disease/Huntington's disease
G	gravid (pregnant) e.g. gravida I, a first pregnancy		
		HDLs	high density lipoproteins
GA	general anaesthesia (Am. anesthesia)/ general appearance	HDN	haemolytic disease of newborn (Am. hemolytic)
GABA	gamma-aminobutyric acid	HDV	hepatitis delta virus
GB	gall bladder/Guillain–Barré (syndrome)	HEENT	head, eyes, ears, nose and throat
		HF	heart failure
GC	gonococci	HGH or hGH	human growth hormone
GCSF	granulocyte colony stimulating factor	HGP	human genome project
GE	gastroenterology	HHNK	hyperglycaemic (Am. hyperglycemic) hyperosmolar nonketonic
GERD	gastro-esophageal reflux disease (Am.)		
GF	glomerular filtration/gluten-free	HHV	human herpes virus
GFR	glomerular filtration rate	Hib	*Haemophilus influenzae* type b
γGTP	gamma glutamyl transpeptidase	Hist.	histology (lab)
γGT	gamma glutamyl transferase	HIV	human immunodeficiency virus
GH	growth hormone	HIVD	herniated intervertebral disc
GHIH	growth hormone inhibiting hormone	H&L	heart and lungs
		HLA	human leucocyte antigen (Am. leukocyte)
GHRH	growth hormone releasing hormone		
GHRIH	growth hormone release-inhibiting hormone	HMG(hMG)	human menopausal gonadotrophin
		HOCM	hypertrophic obstructive cardiomyopathy
GI	gastrointestinal		
GIFT	gamete intrafallopian transfer	HO	house officer
ging	gingiva (gum)	H&P	history and physical
GIS	gastrointestinal system	HPC	history of present condition
GIT	gastrointestinal tract	HPEN	home parenteral and enteral nutrition
GKI	glucose/potassium/insulin		
GM	grand mal seizure	hpf	high power field
GN	glomerulonephritis	HPI	history of present illness
GNDC	Gram-negative diplococci	HPV	human papilloma virus
GnRH	gonadotrophin releasing hormone	HR	heart rate
GP	general practitioner	HRM	human resource management
GR1	pregnancy one	HRT	hormone replacement therapy
grav	gravid (pregnant)	HSA	human serum albumin
GS	general surgery/genital system	HSG	hysterosalpingography
G&S/XM	group and save/cross match	HSV	*Herpes simplex* virus
GTN	glyceryl trinitrate	5-HT	5-hydroxytryptamine
gtt	guttae (drops)	HT	hypertension
GTT	glucose tolerance test	HTLV	human T-cell leukaemia/lymphoma virus (Am. leukemia)
GU	gastric ulcer/genitourinary/gonococcal urethritis		
		HTN	hypertension
GUS	genitourinary system	HTVD	hypertensive vascular disease
GVHD	graft versus host disease	HUS	haemolytic uraemic syndrome (Am. hemolytic uremic syndrome)
Gyn	gynaecology (Am. gynecology)		

HVD	hypertensive vascular disease		IT	intrathecal
Hx	history		ITCP	idiopathic thrombocytopenia purpura
			ITP	idiopathic thrombocytopenic purpura
IABP	intra-aortic balloon pump		ITT	insulin tolerance test
IBC	iron binding capacity		ITU	intensive therapy unit
IBD	inflammatory bowel disease		IU	international units
IBS	irritable bowel syndrome		IUC	idiopathic ulcerative colitis
IC	intercostal/intracerebral/intracranial		IUCD	intrauterine contraceptive device
ICA	islet cell antibody		IUD	intrauterine death/intrauterine device
ICF	intracellular fluid		IUFB	intrauterine foreign body
ICH	intracerebral haemorrhage (Am. hemorrhage)		IUGR	intrauterine growth retardation
			IUP	intra-uterine pregnancy
ICM	intracostal margin		IV or i.v.	intravenous
ICP	intracranial pressure		IVC	inferior vena cava/intravenous cholecystogram
ICS	intercostal space		IVD	intervertebral disc
ICSH	interstitial cell stimulating hormone		IVF	in vitro fertilization/in vivo fertilization
ICU	intensive care unit			
ID or id	identity/intradermal/infectious disease		IVH	intraventricular haemorrhage (Am. hemorrhage)
I&D	incision and drainage		IVHP	intravenous high potency
IDDM	insulin dependent diabetes mellitus (Type 1)		IVI	intravenous infusion
			IVP	intravenous pyelogram/intravenous pyelography
IDL	intermediate-density lipoprotein		IVSD	interventricular septal defect
IFN	interferon		IVT	intravenous transfusion
Ig	immunoglobulin (e.g. IgA, IgG)		IVU	intravenous urography
IGT	impaired glucose tolerance			
IHD	ischaemic heart disease (Am. ischemic)		J	jaundice
IHR	intrinsic heart rate		JVD	jugular venous distension
i.m.	intramuscular		JVP	jugular vein pressure/jugular venous pressure
IM	infectious mononucleosis/intramuscular			
IMHP	intramuscular high potency		K	potassium /kalium (K$^+$)
IMI	inferior myocardial infarction		KA	ketoacidosis
IMP	impression		KCCT	kaolin-cephalin clotting time
IMV	intermittent mandatory ventilation		KCO	transfer factor for carbon monoxide
IN	internist (Am.)		Kg	kilogram (1000 grams)
inf	inferior		KJ	knee jerk
inf.MI	inferior myocardial infarction		KLS	kidney, liver, spleen
INR	international normalized ratio		KO	keep open
int	between/internal		KS	Karposi's sarcoma
I&O	intake and output		KUB	kidney, ureters and bladder
IOFB	intraocular foreign body		KVO	keep vein open
IOL	intraocular lens			
IOP	intraocular pressure		L	lymphadenopathy
in utero	within uterus		(L)	left/lower
i.p.	intraperitoneal		L 1–5	lumbar vertebrae
IPA	immunosuppressive acid protein		L&A	light and accommodation
IPD	idiopathic Parkinson's disease		LA	left arm/left atrium/local anaesthetic (Am. anesthetic)
IPF	idiopathic pulmonary fibrosis			
IPPA	inspection, palpation, percussion, auscultation		La	labial (lips)
			LAD	left axis deviation
IPPB	intermittent positive pressure breathing		LaG	labia and gingiva (lips and gums)
			LAS	lymphadenopathy syndrome
IPPV	intermittent positive pressure ventilation		LAT or lat.	lateral
			LAVH	laparoscopic assisted vaginal hysterectomy
IQ	intelligence quotient			
IRDS	idiopathic respiratory distress syndrome		LBBB	left bundle branch block
IRV	inspiratory reserve volume			
ISQ	idem status quo (i.e. unchanged)		LBM	lean body mass

LBW	low birth weight	M	male/married/murmur
LCCS	low cervical caesarean section (Am. cesarean)	MA	mental age
		MAb	monoclonal antibody
LD	lethal dose/loading dose	MABP	mean arterial blood pressure
LDH	lactic dehydrogenase	MAC	mid-arm circumference/*Mycobacterium avium* complex
LDL	low density lipoprotein		
L-dopa	levodopa (a drug used to treat Parkinson's disease)	MAMC	mid-arm muscle circumference
		mane	in the morning
LE	lupus erythematosus	MAOI	mono-amine oxidase inhibitor
LFT	liver function test	MAP	mean arterial pressure/muscle action potential
LGA	large for gestational age		
LH	luteinizing hormone	MAV	migraine associated vertigo
LHRH	luteinizing hormone releasing hormone	MBD	minimal brain dysfunction
		MCH	mean corpuscular (red cell) haemoglobin (Am. hemoglobin)
LIF	left iliac fossa		
LIH	left inguinal hernia	MCHC	mean corpuscular haemoglobin concentration (Am. hemoglobin)
LKKS	liver, kidney, kidney, spleen		
LL	left leg/left lower/lower lobe	MCL	mid clavicular line
LLETZ	large loop excision of the transformation zone	MCP	metacarpophalangeal
		MCV	mean corpuscular (cell) volume
LLL	left lower lid (eye)/left lower lobe (lung)	MD	maintenance dose/mitral disease/ muscular dystrophy
LLQ	left lower quadrant	MDI	metered dose inhaler
LMN	lower motor neuron	MDM	mid diastolic murmur
LMP	last menstrual period	MDRTB	multidrug resistant tuberculosis
LN	lymph node	ME	myalgic encephalopathy
LNMP	last normal menstrual period	med	medial
LOC	level of consciousness/loss of consciousness	MEN	multiple endocrine neoplasia
		meQ	milliequivalent
LOM	limitation of movement	mEq/L	milliequivalent per litre
LP	lumbar puncture	Metas	metastasis
LPA	left pulmonary artery	MF	mycoses fungoides/myocardial fibrosis
LPN	licensed practical nurse (Am.)		
LRI	lower respiratory infection	MFT	muscle function test
LS	left side/liver and spleen/ lumbosacral/lymphosarcoma	MG	myasthenia gravis
		MGN	membranous glomerulonephritis
LSB	long stay bed (geriatric)	MH	medical history/menstrual history
LSCS	lower section caesarean section (Am. cesarean)	MHC	major histocompatability complex
		MHz	megahertz (megacycles per second)
LSD	lysergic acid diethylamide	MI	mitral incompetence/mitral insufficiency/myocardial infarction
LSK	liver, spleen, kidneys		
LSM	late systolic murmur	MIBG	meta-iodobenzyl guanidine
LTB	laryngotracheal bronchitis	MIC	minimum inhibitory concentration
LTC	long term care	MID	multi-infarct dementia
LTOT	long term oxygen therapy	ML	middle lobe/midline
L&U	lower and upper	mL	millilitre
LUL	left upper lobe	MLT	medical laboratory technician/ technologist
LUQ	left upper quadrant		
LV	left ventricle	mm³	cubic millimetre
LVDP	left ventricular diastolic pressure	mmHg	millimetres of mercury
LVE	left ventricular enlargement	MMM	mitozantrone, methotrexate, mitomycin C
LVEDP	left ventricular end-diastolic pressure		
		mmol	millimole
LVEDV	left ventricular end-diastolic volume	MMR	measles, mumps and rubella (vaccine)
LVET	left ventricular ejection time		
LVF	left ventricular failure	MNJ	myoneural junction
LVH	left ventricular hypertrophy	MODY	maturity onset diabetes of the young
LVP	left ventricular pressure		
L&W	living and well	MOFS	multiple organ failure syndrome
Lymphos	lymphocytes	mono	monocyte(s)

MOPP	mustine, oncovin (vincristine), procarbazine, prednisolone	NREM	non-rapid eye movement (sleep)
MPJ	metacarpophalangeal joint	NRS	numerical rating scale
MPQ	McGill Pain Questionnaire	NS	nephrotic syndrome/nervous system/no specimen
MR	mitral regurgitation		
MRDM	malnutrition-related diabetes mellitus	NSAID	non-steroidal anti-inflammatory drug
MRI	magnetic resonance imaging	NSFTD	normal spontaneous full-term delivery
mRNA	messenger ribonucleic acid	NSR	normal sinus rhythm
MRSA	methicillin resistant *Staphylococcus aureus*	NST	non-shivering thermogenesis
		NSU	nonspecific urethritis
MS	mitral stenosis/multiple sclerosis/ muscle shortening/muscle strength/ musculoskeletal/musculo-skeletal system	NT	nasotracheal/nasotracheal tube
		N&T	nose and throat
		NTP	normal temperature and pressure
		N&V	nausea and vomiting
MSAFP	maternal serum alphafetoprotein	NVD	nausea, vomiting and diarrhoea
MSE	mental state examination		
MSH	melanocyte-stimulating hormone	O	oxygen/oedema (Am. edema)
MSL	midsternal line	O&A	observation and assessment
MSOF	multisystem organ failure	OA	on admission/osteoarthritis
MSSU	midstream specimen of urine	OAD	obstructive airway disease
MSU	midstream urine	OAG	open angle glaucoma
MTA	mid-thigh amputation	OB	occult blood
MTP	metatarsophalangeal	Ob-Gyn	obstetrics and gynaecology (Am. gynecology)
MV	mitral valve		
MVP	mitral valve prolapse	Obst-Gyn	obstetrics and gynaecology (Am. gynecology)
MVR	minute volume of respiration/mitral valve replacement		
		OC	oral cholecystogram/oral contraceptive
My, my	myopia		
		OCP	oral contraceptive pill
N	nitrogen/normal	OD	oculus dexter (right eye), oculo dextro (in the right eye)/overdose
Na	sodium/natrium (Na^+)		
NAD	nothing abnormal discovered/no acute distress/normal axis deviation	od	every day
		Odont	odontology
NAG	narrow angle glaucoma	ODQ	on direct questioning
NANB	non A, non B viruses	OE	on examination/otitis externa
NAP	neutrophil alkaline phosphatase	OGD	oesophago-gastro-duodenoscopy
NAS, nas	nasal/no added salt	OGTT	oral glucose tolerance test
NB	newborn	OH	occupational history
NBM	nil (nothing) by mouth	OHS	open heart surgery
NBS	normal bowel sounds/normal breath sounds	OM	olim mane (once daily in the morning)/otitis media
NCVs	nerve conduction velocities	OOB	out of bed
ND	normal delivery/normal development	OPA	outpatient appointment
NEC	necrotizing enterocolitis	OPD	outpatient department
NED	no evidence of disease	Ophth	ophthalmology
neg	negative	OPT	orthopantomogram
NFTD	normal full term delivery	OR	operating room
NG	nasogastric	ORT	operating room technician
NGU	non-gonococcal urethritis	Ortho	orthopaedics (Am. orthopedics)
NHL	non-Hodgkin lymphoma	Orthop	orthopnoea (Am. orthopnea)
NHS	national health service	OS	oculus sinister (left eye), oculo sinistro (in left eye)
NIDDM	non-insulin-dependent diabetes mellitus		
		Os	mouth
NK	natural killer (cells)	osteo	osteomyelitis
NMR	nuclear magnetic resonance	OT	occupational therapy/old tuberculin/oxytocin
NO	nitric oxide		
#NOF	fractured neck of femur	OTC	over the counter (remedies)
NP	nasopharynx	oto	otology
NPN	non-protein nitrogen	OU	oculus unitas (both eyes together)/ oculus uterque (for each eye)/oculus utro (in each eye)
NPO, npo	non per os/nothing by mouth		

P	phosphorus/posterior/pressure
PA	pernicious anaemia (Am. anemia)/posteroanterior/pulmonary artery
P&A	percussion and auscultation
PABA	para-aminobenzoic acid
PACG	primary angle closure glaucoma
PADP	pulmonary artery diastolic pressure
PAH	pulmonary artery hypertension/pregnancy induced hypertension
palp	palpable/palpation
PALS	paediatric (Am. pediatric) advanced life support
PAP	primary atypical pneumonia
Pap.	Papanicolaou smear test
Para	number of viable births e.g. Para 1 (unipara)
PAS	p-aminosalycilic acid
PAT	paroxysmal atrial tachycardia
PAWP	pulmonary artery wedge pressure
PBC	primary biliary cirrhosis
PBI	protein bound iodine
pc	post cibum (after meals/food)
PCA	patient controlled analgesia
PCAS	patient controlled analgesia system
PCN	penicillin
PCNL	percutaneous nephrolithotomy
PCO_2	partial pressure carbon dioxide
PCP	*Pneumocystis carinii* pneumonia
PCR	polymerase chain reaction
PCT	prothrombin clotting time
PCV	packed cell volume
PCWP	pulmonary capillary wedge pressure
PD	Parkinson's disease/peritoneal dialysis
PDA	patent ductus arteriosus
PE	physical examination/pleural effusion/pulmonary embolism
PEC	pneumoencephalogram
PED	paediatrics (Am. pediatrics)
PEEP	positive end expiratory pressure
PEF	peak expiratory flow
PEFR	peak expiratory flow rate
PEG	percutaneous endoscopic gastrostomy/pneumoencephalogram
PEJ	percutaneous endoscopic jejunostomy
PEM	protein-energy malnutrition
PERLAC	pupils equal, react to light, accommodation consensual
per os	by mouth
PERRLA	pupils equal, round, react to light, accommodation consensual
PET	positron emission tomography/pre-eclamptic toxaemia (Am. toxemia)
PF	peak flow
PFT	peak flow rate/ pulmonary function test
PG	prostaglandin
PGL	persistent generalized lymphadenopathy

PH	past history/patient history/prostatic hypertrophy/pulmonary hypertension
pH	hydrogen-ion concentration
PID	pelvic inflammatory disease/prolapsed intervertebral disc
PIH	prolactin inhibiting hormone/pregnancy induced hypertension
PIP	proximal interphalangeal
PIVD	protruded intervertebral disc
PKU	phenylketonuria
PM	post mortem
PMB	post menopausal bleeding
PMH	past medical history
PMI	past medical history/point of maximum impulse
PML	progressive multifocal leucoencephalopathy (Am. leukoencephalopathy)
PMN	polymorphonuclear leucocytes (Am. leukocyte)
PMS	premenstrual syndrome
PMT	premenstrual tension
PMV	prolapsed mitral valve
PN	percussion note/peripheral nerve/peripheral neuropathy
PND	paroxysmal nocturnal dyspnoea (Am. dyspnea)/post nasal drip
PNS	peripheral nervous system
PO or po	per os/by mouth/post operative
PO_2	partial pressure oxygen
POAG	primary open angle glaucoma
POLY	polymorphonuclear leucocytes (Am. leukocytes)
POP	plaster of Paris
pos	position
post	posterior
PPAM	pneumatic post-amputation mobility
PPD	packs per day/purified protein derivative (of tuberculin)
PPE	personal protective equipment
PPH	postpartum haemorrhage (Am. hemorrhage)
PPS	plasma protein solution
PPT	partial prothrombin time
PPV	positive-pressure ventilation
p.r. or PR	per rectum/plantar reflex/partial response
pre op	preoperative
PRH	prolactin releasing hormone
PRL	prolactin
PRN or p.r.n.	pro re nata (as required)
PROG	progesterone
PROM	premature rupture of membranes
PRV	polycythaemia rubra vera (Am. polycythemia)
procto	proctoscopy
pros	prostate
prox	proximal
PS	pulmonary stenosis/pyloric stenosis
PSA	prostate specific antigen

PSCT	pain and symptom control team
PSD	personal and social development
PSG	presystolic gallop
PSVT	paroxysmal supraventricular tachycardia
pt or PT	patient/physical therapy/prothrombin time/physical therapist (Am.)
PTA	prior to admission
PTC	percutaneous transhepatic cholangiogram/cholangiography
PTCA	percutaneous transluminal coronary angioplasty
PTD	permanent and total disability
PTH	parathormone/parathyroid hormone
PTR	prothrombin ratio
PTT	partial thromboplastin time
PTX	pneumothorax
PU	peptic ulcer/per urethra/pregnancy urine
PUO	pyrexia of unknown origin
PUVA	psoralen + ultraviolet light A
PV	per vagina
P&V	pyloroplasty and vagotomy
PVC	premature ventricular contraction
PVD	peripheral vascular disease
PVP	pulmonary venous pressure
PVT	paroxysmal ventricular tachycardia
PX	physical examination
Px	past history/prognosis
QDS or qds	quater diurnale summensum (four times a day)
qid	quater in die (four times a day)
qn	each night (quaque nox)
(R)	right/respiration
RA	rheumatoid arthritis/right auricle/right atrium
Ra	radium
RAD	radiation absorbed dose/right axis deviation
rad	radical
RAS	reticular activating system
RAST	radio-allergosorbent test
RBBB	right bundle branch block
RBC	red blood cell/red blood (cell) count
RBS	random blood sugar
RCC	red cell concentrate/red cell count
RDA	recommended dietary allowance
RDDA	recommended daily dietary allowance
rDNA	recombinant deoxyribose nucleic acid
RDS	respiratory distress syndrome
RE	rectal examination
REM	rapid eye movement (in sleep)
RES	reticulo endothelial system
RF	renal failure/rheumatoid factor/rheumatic fever
RFLA	rheumatoid factor-like activity
RFT	respiratory function tests
Rh	Rhesus factor (in blood)

RHD	rheumatic heart disease
RHL	right hepatic lobe
RIA	radioimmunoassay
RIF	right iliac fossa
RIND	reversible ischaemic (Am. ischemic) neurologic deficit
RK	radial keratotomy/right kidney
RL	right leg/right lung
RLC	residual lung capacity
RLD	related living donor
RLE	right lower extremity
RLL	right lower lobe
RLQ	right lower quadrant
RM	radical mastectomy
RML	right middle lobe (of the lung)
RN	registered nurse
RNA	ribose nucleic acid
R/O	rule out
ROM	range of movement (exercises)
ROS	review of symptoms
RP	radial pulse
RPE	retinal pigment epithelial (cells, layer)
RQ	respiratory quotient
RR	recovery room/respiratory rate
RR&E	round regular and equal
RRR	regular rate and rhythm
RS	respiratory system/Reye's syndrome
RSI	repetitive strain injury
RSV	respiratory syncytial virus
RT	radiologic technologist (Am.)/radiotherapy/right
RTA	renal tubular acidosis/road traffic accident
RUL	right upper lobe
RUQ	right upper quadrant
RV	residual volume/right ventricle
RVF	right ventricular failure
RVH	right ventricular hypertrophy
s	without
S1	first heart sound
S2	second heart sound
SA	sarcoma/sinoatrial (node)/sinus arrhythmia/Stokes-Adams (attacks)
SACD	subacute combined degeneration
SAD	seasonal affective disorder
SAH	subarachnoid haemorrhage (Am. hemorrhage)
SB	seen by
SBE	subacute bacterial endocarditis
SBO	small bowel obstruction
SBP	systolic blood pressure
s.c.	subclavian/subcutaneous
SCA	sickle-cell anaemia
SCC	squamous cell carcinoma
SCD	sequential pneumatic compression device/sudden cardiac death
SCID	severe combined immunodeficiency syndrome

SDH	subdural haematoma (Am. hematoma)	T&A	tonsils and adenoids or tonsillectomy/adenoidectomy
SDS	same day surgery	T.A.	toxin-antitoxin
SED	skin erythema dose	TAH	total abdominal hysterectomy
SEM	systolic ejection murmur	Tb or TB	tuberculosis (tubercle bacillus)
SG	skin graft/specific gravity	TBA	to be arranged
SGA	small for gestational age	TBG	thyroid binding globulin
SGOT	serum glutamic oxaloacetic transaminase, now serum aspartate transferase	TBI	total body irradiation
		TBW	total body water/total body weight
		T&C	type and crossmatch
SGPT	serum glutamic pyruvic transaminase	Tc	technetium
SF	synovial fluid	TCP	thrombocytopenia
SH	social history	TD	thymus dependent cells
SIADH	syndrome of inappropriate antidiuretic hormone	TDM	therapeutic drug monitoring
		TDS	ter diurnale summensum (three times a day)
SIDS	sudden infant death syndrome		
SIG	sigmoidoscope/sigmoidoscopy	TED	thromboembolic deterrent (stockings)
SIMV	synchronized intermittent mandatory ventilation		
		TENS	transcutaneous electrical nerve stimulation
s.l.	sublingual		
SLE	systemic lupus erythematosus	TFT	thyroid function test
SLS	social and life skills	TH	thyroid hormone (thyroxine)
SMD	senile macular degeneration	THR	total hip replacement
SNS	somatic nervous system	TI	thymus independent cells
SOA	swelling of ankles	TIA	transient ischaemic attack (Am. ischemic)
SOB	short of breath/stools for occult blood		
		TIBC	total iron-binding capacity
SOBOE	short of breath on exertion	t.i.d.	ter in die (three times daily)
SOS	swelling of sacrum	TIP	terminal interphalangeal
SP	systolic pressure	TIPS	transjugular intrahepatic portosystemic shunting
SPECT	single-photon emission computed tomography		
		TJ	triceps jerk
SPF	sun protection factor	TKVO	to keep vein open
SPP	suprapubic prostatectomy	TLC	tender loving care/total lung capacity
SR	sedimentation rate/sinus rhythm		
SS S/S	saline solution/signs and symptoms	TLD	thoracic lymph duct
ST	sinus tachycardia/skin test	TM	tympanic membrane
STD	sexually transmitted disease/skin test dose	TMJ	temporomandibular joint
		TMR	transmyocardial revascularization
Strep	streptococci	TNF	tumour necrosis factor (Am. tumor)
STS	serological tests for syphilis	TNM	tumour, node, metastases (Am. tumor)
STU	skin test unit		
Subcu	subcutaneous	TOP	termination of pregnancy
subling	sublingual/under the tongue	tPA	recombinant tissue-type plasminogen activator
sup	superior		
SV	stroke volume	TPHI	*Treponema pallidum* haemagglutination inhibition (Am. hemagglutination)
SVC	superior vena cava		
SVD	spontaneous vaginal delivery		
SVI	stroke volume index	TPI	*Treponema pallidum* immobilization
SVR	systemic venous resistance	TPN	total parenteral nutrition
SVT	supraventricular tachycardia	TPR	temperature, pulse, respiration
SWS	slow wave sleep	TRH	thyrotrophin-releasing hormone
Sx	symptoms	TRUS	transrectal ultrasound
syph.	syphilis	TSA	tumour specific antigen (Am. tumor)
		TSF	triceps skinfold thickness
T	temperature/tumour (Am. tumor)/time	TSH	thyroid stimulating hormone
		TSS	toxic shock syndrome
t	terminal	TT	tetanus toxoid/thrombin clotting time
T 1–12	thoracic vertebrae		
T_3, T_4	triiodothyronine, tetraiodothyronine (thyroid hormones)	TTA	transtracheal aspiration
		TTO	to take out (to home)

TUIP	transurethral incision of the prostate
TUR	transurethral resection (of prostate)
TURB	transurethral resection of bladder
TURP	transurethral resection of the prostate
TURT	transurethral resection of tumour (Am. tumor)
TV	tidal volume
TVH	total vaginal hysterectomy
Tx	therapy/transfusion/treatment
T&X	type and crossmatch
U	unit
UA	uric acid/urinalysis
UAC	umbilical artery catheter
UAO	upper airway obstruction
UC	ulcerative colitis/uterine contractions
UDO	undetermined origin
U&E	urea and electrolytes
UG	urogenital
UGH	uveitis1 glaucoma1 hyphaema syndrome (Am. hyphema)
UGI	upper gastrointestinal
UIBC	unsaturated iron-binding capacity
ung	ointment (unguentum)
U/O	urinary output
URI	upper respiratory (tract) infection
URT	upper respiratory tract
URTI	upper respiratory tract infection
US	ultrasonography/ultrasound/urinary system
USS	ultrasound scan
UTI	urinary tract infection
UVA	ultra violet light A
UVB	ultra violet light B
UVC	ultra violet light C
VA	visual acuity
VAC	vincristine, adriamycin, cyclophosphamide
VAS	visual analogue scale
VC	vital capacity/vulvovaginal candidiasis
VD	venereal disease
VDRL	venereal disease research laboratory (test)

VE	vaginal examination
VF	ventricular fibrillation/visual field
VHD	valvular heart disease
VLBW	very low birth weight
VLDL	very low density lipoprotein
VMA	vanillyl-mandelic acid
VP	venous pressure
VPC	ventricular premature contraction
VRS	verbal rating scale
VS	vital signs
VSD	ventricular septal defect
VT	ventricular tachycardia
VUR	vesicoureteric reflux
VWF	von Willebrand factor
VV	varicose veins/vulva and vagina
WBC	white blood (cell) count/white blood cell
WCC	white cell count
WNL	within normal limits
WPW	Wolff-Parkinson-White (syndrome)
WR	Wasserman reaction (test for syphilis)
X-match	cross-match
XR	X-ray
XRT	X-ray therapy
yrs	age in years
ZE	Zollinger-Ellison (syndrome)
ZN	Ziel-Nielsen Stain

Symbols

♂	male
♀	female
*	birth
α	alpha
β	beta
γ	gamma
Δ	delta/diagnosis
ΔΔ	differential diagnosis
#	fracture
†	dead

GLOSSARY

The glossary contains a list of prefixes, suffixes and combining forms used in common medical terms. The meaning of each word component is given with an example of its use in a medical term. Use the list to decipher the meaning of unfamiliar words. Note that a dash is added to indicate whether the component usually precedes or follows the other elements of a compound word; for example, ante- precedes the word root *nat* as in ante*nat*al whilst -ectomy follows the root *arter* as in end*arter*ectomy. Some word components are made from a root combined with a suffix; for example -**algia** contains the root **alg-** meaning pain and the suffix -**ia** meaning condition of. The vowels of combining forms are used or dropped by the application of the 'rules' described in the introduction of this book. Some roots are listed with more than one combining vowel, for example, **ren/i/o**; both vowels may be used in combination with the root as in **ren**ipelvic and **ren**ography.

Component	Meaning	Medical Term
a-	without, not (an is added before words beginning with a vowel)	**a**phasia
-a	noun ending/a name	**bursa**
ab-	away from	**ab**duct
abdomin/o	abdomen	**abdomino**pelvic
-able	capable of/having ability to	palp**able**
ac-	pertaining to/to/toward/near	**ac**cretion
acanth/o	spiny	**acanth**osis
acarin/o	mites of the order Acarina	**acarin**osis
acar/i/o	mites of the order Acarina	**acari**cide
acetabul/o	acetabulum	**acetabulo**plasty
acet/o	vinegar	*Aceto*bacter
aceton-	ketones/acetone	**aceton**aemia (Am. **aceton**emia)
achill/o	Achilles tendon	**achillo**tomy
acid/o	acid	**acido**phil
acin/i	sac-like dilatation	**acin**us
acne/o	acne/point/peak	**acne**genic
acou-	hear/hearing	**acou**metric
-acousia	condition of hearing	dys**acousia**
acoust/o	hear/hearing/sound	**acoust**ic
acro-	extremities, point	**acro**megaly
acromi/o	acromion (point of the shoulder)	**acromio**clavicular
act-	do, drive, act	**act**ion
actin/o	rays e.g. of sun/ultraviolet radiation	**actino**therapy
acu-	hear/hearing/severe/sudden	**acu**te
-acusia	condition/sense of hearing	dys**acusia**
ad-	to/toward/in the direction of the midline/near	**ad**duct
adamant/o	dental enamel	**adamant**ine
aden/o	gland	**aden**oid
adenoid-	adenoids	**adenoid**ectomy
adip/o	adipose tissue/fat	**adip**osity
adnex/o	bound to/conjoined	**adnex**a
adrenal/o	adrenal gland	**adrenal**ectomy
adren/o	adrenal gland	**adreno**genital
adrenocortic/o	adrenal cortex	**adrenocortic**al
-aem-	blood (Am. -em-)	an**aem**ia (Am. -an**em**ia)
-aemia	condition of blood (Am. -emia)	leuk**aemia**
aer/o	air/gas	**aero**phagia
aesthe/s/i/o	sensation/sensitivity (Am. esthe/s/i/o)	an**aesthesio**logy (Am. an**esthesio**logy)
aeti/o	cause (Am. eti/o)	**aeti**ology (Am. **eti**ology)

Component	Meaning	Medical Term
af-	to/towards/near	**af**ferent
ag-	to/towards/near	**ag**glutinate
agglutin/o	sticking/clumping together	**agglutin**ation
-ago	abnormal condition/disease	lumb**ago**
-agogic	pertaining to inducing/stimulating	dacry**agogic**
-agogue	inducing/promoting	lact**agogue**
agora-	market place open space	**agora**phobia
-agra	seizure/sudden pain	pod**agra**
-aise	comfort/ease	mal**aise**
-al^1	pertaining to	bronchi**al**
-al^2	used in pharmacology to mean a drug or drug action	antifung**al**
albin/o	white	**albin**ism
alb/i/o	white	**alb**us
album-	white	**album**in
albumin/o	albumin/albumen	**albumin**uria
aldosteron-	aldosterone	**aldosteron**ism
-algesia	condition of pain	an**algesia**
alges/i/o	sense of pain	**algesi**ometer
-algia	condition of pain	neur**algia**
alg/e/i/o	pain	**alg**aesthesia
aliment/o	to nourish	**aliment**ary
all/o	other/different from normal	**all**ogenic
alve/o	trough/channel/cavity	**alve**us
alveol/o	alveoli (of lungs)	**alveol**itis
ambi-	both/on both sides	**ambi**lateral
ambly/o	dull/dim	**ambly**opia
ameb/o (Am.)	ameba, a type of protozoan	**ameb**iasis
amel/o	dental enamel	**amel**oblast
-amine	nitrogen containing compound	catechol**amine**
amni/o	amnion/fetal membrane	**amnio**centesis
amnion/o	amnion/fetal membrane	**amnion**ic
amoeb/o	amoeba a type of protozoan (Am. ameb/o)	**amoeb**iasis (Am. **ameb**iasis)
amph/i	both/doubly/both sides	**amphi**gonadism
amyl/o	starch	**amyl**oid
an-	without/not	**an**encephalic
-an	pertaining to/characteristic of	ovari**an**
ana-	reversion/ going backward/apart/up/again	**ana**plastic
ancyl/o	crooked /stiffening/fusing/bent	**ancyl**ostomiasis
andr/o	male/masculine	**andr**ology
-ane	a saturated, open-chain hydrocarbon	meth**ane**
aneurysm/o	aneurysm	**aneurysmo**plasty
angi/o	vessel/blood vessel	**angio**plasty
an-iso-	unequal/dissimilar	**aniso**coria
ankyl/o	crooked /stiffening/fusing/bent	**ankyl**osis
an/o	anus	**ano**rectal
-ant	having the characteristic of/an agent that . . .	stimul**ant**
ante-	before in time or place/in front of/forward	**ante**natal
anter/o	front/in front of/anterior to	**antero**lateral
anthrac/o	coal dust	**anthrac**osis
anthrop/o	man/human	**anthrop**ometry
anti-	against	**anti**fungal
antr/o	antrum/maxillary sinus	**antro**tomy
anxi/o	anxiety	**anxio**lytic
aort/o	aorta	**aort**orrhaphy
ap-	to/towards/near/separated from	**ap**position
-aph-	touch	hyper**aph**ia
-apheresis	removal	leuk**apheresis**
aphth/o	ulcer	**aphth**ous

Component	Meaning	Medical Term
apic/o	apex	**apic**al
ap/o	away from/detached/derived from/separate	**apo**physis
aponeur/o	aponeurosis (flat tendon)	**aponeuror**rhaphy
append/ic/o	appendix	**appendic**ectomy
aqu/a/e/o	water	**aque**ous
-ar	pertaining to	lob**ar**
arachn/o	spider	**arachn**ophobia
arc/o	arch/bow-shaped	**arc**us
-arch/e-	beginning	men**arch**
arrhen/o	male/masculine	**arrheno**blastoma
arter/i/o	artery	**arterio**sclerosis
arteriol/o	arteriole	**arteriol**onecrosis
arthr/o	joint	**arthr**odesis
articul/o	joint	**articul**ate
-ary	pertaining to/connected with	pulmon**ary**
as-	to/towards/near	**as**sociation
-ase	an enzyme	amyl**ase**
-asia	state or condition	euthan**asia**
-asis	state or condition	elephant**iasis**
-asthenia	condition of weakness	my**asthenia**
asthen/o	weakness	**astheno**coria
astr/o	star-shaped/star	**astro**cyte
at-	to/towards/near	**at**traction
-ate	in a state/acted upon/possessing/chemical from a specific source/like	stimul**ate**
atel/o	imperfect/incomplete	**atelo**cardia
ather/o	atheroma, a fatty plaque lining a blood vessel	**athero**sclerosis
-ation	action/condition	ejacul**ation**
-atresia	condition of occlusion/closure/absence of opening	anal **atresia**
atret/o	closure of a normal opening/imperforation	**atreto**metria
atri/o	atrium	**atrio**ventricular
audi/o	hearing/sense of hearing	**audio**metry
audit/o	hearing/sense of hearing	**audit**ory
-aural	pertaining to the ear	mon**aural**
auricul/o	ear/pinna	**auriculo**plasty
aur/i/o	ear/hearing	**auri**scope
auto-	self	**auto**lysis
aux/i	increase	**auxi**lytic
-auxis	increase	onych**auxis**
aux/o	increase	**auxo**cardia
-ax	noun ending/a name	thor**ax**
axill/o	armpit	**axill**ary
ax/i/o	axis	**axi**petal
axon/o	axis/axon of neuron	**axon**al
azot/o	urea/nitrogen	**azot**aemia (Am. **azot**emia)
ba-	go/walk/stand	hypno**bat**ia
bacill/o	bacillus/a rod-shaped bacterium	**bacill**uria
bacter/i/o	baterium/bacteria	**bacterio**phage
balan/o	glans penis	**balan**itis
ballist/o	throw/movement	**ballisto**cardiograph
bar/o	pressure	**baro**trauma
bartholin/o	Bartholin's glands/greater vestibular glands of the vagina	**bartholin**itis
basi-	base/basic/alkaline	**basi**chromatin
baso-	base/basic/alkaline	**baso**phil
bathy-	deep	**bathy**pnoea (Am. **bathy**pnea)
bi-	two/twice/double/life	**bi**pedal

Component	Meaning	Medical Term
bili-	bile	**bili**ary
bilirubin/o	bilirubin	**bilirubin**uria
bin-	two each/double	**bin**ocular
bio-	life/living	**bio**logy
-blast	germ cell/immature cell/embryonic cell/developing stage	osteo**blast**
blast/o	germ cell/immature cell/embryonic cell/developing stage	retino**blast**oma
blenn/o	mucus	**blenn**oid
blephar/o	eyelid	**blephar**optosis
bol-	ball	**bol**us
brachi/o	arm	**brachi**al
brachy-	short	**brachy**gnathia
brady-	slow	**brady**cardia
brev/i	short	**brevi**flexor
bromidr/o	stench/smell of sweat	**bromidr**osis
bronch/i/o	bronchus/bronchial tube/windpipe	**broncho**scopy
bronchiol/o	bronchiole	**bronchiol**itis
bront/o	thunder	**bronto**phobia
bucca-	cheek	**bucca**l
bucc/o	cheek	**bucco**pharyngeal
bulb/o	bulb/medulla oblongata	**bulb**ar
burs/o	bursa (fluid filled sac)	**burs**itis
byssin/o	cotton dust	**byssin**osis
cac/o	bad/ill/abnormal	**cac**ocholia
caec/o	caecum (Am. cecum)	**caec**ocele (Am. cecocele)
calcane/o	calcaneus/heel bone	**calcaneo**plantar
calc/i/o	calcium/lime/heel	**calc**ipenia
calcin/o	calcium	**calcin**osis
calcul/o	calculus/stone/little stone	**calcul**us
calic-	calyx (Am. calix)/a cup-shaped organ or cavity	**calic**ectasis
calor/i	heat	**calor**imetry
calyc-	calyx (Am. calix)/a cup-shaped organ or cavity	**calyc**ulus
cancer/o	cancer (general term)	**cancero**phobia
canth/o	canthus (corner of the eye)	**cantho**plasty
capill/o	blood capillary/hair-like	**capill**ary
capit/o	head	**capit**ate
-capnia	condition of carbon dioxide	hyper**capnia**
caps-	container	**caps**itis
capsul/o	capsule	**capsul**ar
carb/o	carbon/bicarbonate	**carb**ohydrate
carcin/o	cancerous/malignant tumour of epithelial tissue	**carcin**oma
carcinomat-	carcinoma	**carcinomat**ous
-cardia	condition of the heart	tachy**cardia**
cardi/o	heart	**cardi**ologist
cari/o	rot/decay (of teeth)	**cari**ogenesis
carp/o	carpal/wrist bones	**carp**optosis
cary/o	nucleus	eu**cary**otic
cat/a	down/negative/wrong/back	**cat**abolic
caud/o	tail/towards the tail/lower part of body	**caud**al
caus-	burn/corrosive	**caus**tic
caut-	burn	**caut**ery
cav-	hollow	**cav**ity
cec/o (Am.)	cecum	**cec**ocele
-cele	swelling/protrusion/hernia	vesico**cele**
celi/o	hollow/abdomen	**celi**oscope
cell-	cell	**cell**ular
cellul-	cell	**cellul**ar
cel/o (Am.)	hollow/abdomen/celom	**cel**oschisis

Component	Meaning	Medical Term
cement/o	cementum of a tooth	**cemento**clasia
cen/o	new/empty/common	**cen**osis
-centesis	surgical puncture to remove fluid	amnio**centesis**
centi-	hundred/one hundredth	**centi**grade
centr/i/o	centre/central location	**centri**lobular
cephal/o	head	hydro**cephal**ic
cerat/o	horny/epidermis/cornea (syn: kerat/o)	**cerato**cricoid
cerebell/o	cerebellum	**cerebell**ar
cerebr/i/o	cerebrum/brain	**cerebr**oma
cer/o	wax	**cer**oma
cerumin/o	cerumen/ear wax	**cerumin**ous
cervic/o	cervix	**cervic**al
-chalasis	slackening/loosening	blepharo**chalasis**
chancr-	chancre, a destructive sore	**chancr**oid
cheil/o	lip	**cheil**oplasty
cheir/o	hand	**cheir**omegaly
chem/i/c/o	chemical	**chemo**receptor
-chezia	condition of defaecation, especially of foreign substances	uro**chezia**
chil/o	lip (cheil/o now used)	**chil**oplasty
chir/o	hand	**chir**opody
chlorhydr/o	hydrochloric acid	**chlorhydr**ia
chlor/o	green/chlorine	**chlor**oma
cholangi/o	bile vessel/bile duct	**cholangio**gram
cholecyst/o	gallbladder	**cholecysto**lithiasis
choledoch/o	common bile duct	**choledocho**lithiasis
chol/e/o	bile	**chol**uria
cholester/o	cholesterol	**cholester**osis
chondr/o	cartilage	**chondro**sarcoma
chord/o	string/cord	**chordo**tomy
chore/o	chorea/dance/jerky movement	**chore**a
chori/o	chorion/outer fetal membrane	**chorio**allantois
choroid/o	choroid layer of eye	**choroid**itis
chromat/o	colour	**chromat**opsia
-chromia	condition of haemoglobin/colour (Am. hemoglobin)	hypo**chromia**
chrom/o	colour	**chromo**cystoscopy
chron/o	time	**chron**ic
chrys/o	gold	**chryso**derma
chyl/e/o	chyle, a fluid formed by lacteals (lymphatics) in the intestine, a product of fat digestion	**chylo**thorax
chym/o	chyme, a creamy material produced by digestion of food	**chymo**poiesis
cib/o	meal	**cib**us
-cidal	pertaining to killing	bacterio**cidal**
-cide	agent that kills/killing	acari**cide**
cili/o	cilia/ciliary body of eye/eyelash	**cili**ectomy
cinemat/o	movement/motion (picture)	**cinemat**ography
cine/o	movement/motion	**cine**angiography
cinesi/o	movement/motion	**cinesi**ology
circum-	around	**circum**cision
cirrh/o	yellow	**cirrh**osis
cirs/o	varicose vein/varix	**cirs**ectomy
cis-	on the near side/this side	**cis** position
-cis-	cut/kill	ex**cis**ion
cistern/o	cistern/enclosed space (sub arachnoid space)	**cistern**ography
-clasia	condition of breaking	osteo**clasia**
-clasis	breaking	osteo**clasis**
-clast	a cell that breaks	osteo**clast**
claustr/o	barrier/enclosed	**claustr**ophobia
clavic/o	clavicle	**clavic**otomy
clavicul/o	clavicle	**clavicul**ar

Component	Meaning	Medical Term
-cle	small	vesicle
cleid/o	clavicle	cleidotomy
clin/o	bend/incline	clinodactyly
clitor/i/o	clitoris	clitorism
clon/o	clone of cells	monoclonal
-clonus	violent action	myoclonus
-clysis	infusion/injection/irrigation	venoclysis
co-	with/together	cofactor
coagul/o	clotting	anticoagulant
coccid/i	types of parasitic protozoa of the Order Coccidia	coccidiosis
cocc/i/o	a berry-shaped bacterium/a coccus	coccogenous
-coccus	a berry-shaped bacterium	streptococcus
coccyg/o	coccyx	coccygeal
cochle/o	cochlea	cochleovestibular
-coel(e)	hollow/abdomen	blastocoel(e)
coel/o	hollow/abdomen/ceolom (Am. celom)	coelom (Am. celom)
col-	with/together	collateral
coll/a	glue	collagen
collagen/o	collagen	collagenase
col/o	colon	colostomy
colon/o	colon	colonic
colp/o	vagina	colpohysterectomy
com-	with/together	commensal
con-	with/together	concentric
condyl/o	condyl	condylar
coni/o	dust	coniosis
conjunctiv/o	conjunctiva	conjunctivitis
contra-	against/opposed/opposite	contraception
-conus	cone-like protrusion	keratoconus
copr/o	faeces (Am. feces)	coprolith
cor-	with/together	corrosive
cord/o	a cord	cordotomy
cor/e/o	pupil	coreomorphosis
-coria	condition of the pupils	anisocoria
corne/o	cornea/horny (consisting of keratin)	corneoblepharon
coron/o-	crown-like projection/encircling/coronary vessels of the heart	coronary
corpor/o	body	corporal
-cortex-	outer part/bark	adrenal cortex
cortic/o	adrenal cortex/cortex/outer region	corticotrophic
cost/o	rib	intercostal
cox/o	hip/hip joint	coxofemoral
crani/o	cranium/skull	craniotomy
cren/o	crenated	crenocytosis
-crescent	crescent/sickle-shaped/shaped like a new moon	epithelial crescent
-crine	secrete	exocrine
crin/o	secrete	endocrinology
-crit	separate/device for measuring cells	haematocrit (Am. hematocrit)
crur/o	leg	crural
cry/o	relating to cold	cryostat
crypt/o	hidden	cryptorchism
cubit/o	elbow	cubitus
culd/o	Douglas pouch/rectouterine pouch/cul-de sac	culdoscope
-cule	small	animalcule
cult-	cultivate	culture
cune/i	wedge (shape)	cuneiform
cutane/o	skin	cutaneous
cut/i	skin	cuticle
cyan/o	blue	cyanosis

Component	Meaning	Medical Term
cycl/o	ciliary body/circle	**cyclo**tomy
cyes/i/o	pregnancy	**cyesio**logy
-cyesis	pregnancy	pseudo**cyesis**
cylindr/o	cylinder	**cylindr**oid
cyll/o	deformity	thoraco**cyll**osis
cyn/o	dog	**cyno**phobia
cyrt/o	curved/abnormal curvature	**cyrto**meter
cyst/i/o	bladder	**cyst**ostomy
-cyte	cell	melano**cyte**
cyt/o	cell	**cyto**logy
-cytosis	condition of cells, usually an abnormal increase	thrombo**cytosis**
dacry/o	tear/lacrimal apparatus	**dacryo**lith
dacryocyst/o	lacrimal sac	**dacryocysto**tomy
dactyl/o	digits/fingers or toes	**dactylo**megaly
de-	down/away from/loss of/reversing	**de**calcification
deca-	ten	**deca**gram
deci-	one tenth	**deci**litre
demi-	half	**demi**facet
dem/o	people	**demo**graphic
dendr/i/o	tree/tree-like (dendrite of neuron)	**dendr**itic
dentin/o	dentine of tooth (Am. dentin)	**dentino**genesis
dent/i/o	tooth	**dent**ist
derm/a/o	skin	**derm**abrasion
dermat/o	skin	**dermat**ology
descemet/o	Desçemet's membrane (of cornea)	**descemeto**cele
-desis	fixation/to bind together by surgery/sticking together	arthro**desis**
desm/o	band/ligament	**desmo**pathy
deuter/o	second	**deuter**anopia
dextro-	right	**dextro**cardia
di-	two/twice/double	**di**coria
dia-	through/apart/across/between	**dia**physis
-dialysis	separate	haemo**dialysis** (Am. hemo**dialysis**)
diaphor/o	sweating (excessive)	**diaphor**esis
diaphragmat/o	diaphragm	**diaphragmat**algia
diastol-	diastole	**diastol**ic
didym-	twins	epi**didym**is
digit/o	finger/toe	**digito**plantar
dipl/o-	double	**dipl**opia
dips/o	thirst	poly**dips**ia
dis-	apart/reversal/separation/duplication/free from	**dis**location
disc/o	intervertebral disc	**disco**graphy
disk/o (Am.)	intervertebral disk	**disk**ectomy
dist/o	far from point of origin	**dist**al
diverticul/o	diverticulum	**diverticul**itis
doch/o	duct/to receive	chole**doch**itis
dolich/o	long	**dolicho**cranial
dolor/i/o	pain (dol – unit of pain)	**doloro**genic
-dorsal	pertaining to the back (of the body)	ventro**dorsal**
dors/i/o	the back (of the body)/dorsal	**dorso**ventral
-drome	a course/conduction/flowing	syn**drome**
drom/o	a course/conduction/flowing	**dromo**tropic
-duct-	a tube to lead material toward or away from a structure	ovi**duct**
duoden/o	duodenum	**duodeno**stomy
dur/o	dura mater/hard	epi**dural**
dynam/o	force/power (of movement)	**dynam**ic
-dynia	condition of pain	pleuro**dynia**
dys-	difficult/disordered/painful/bad	**dys**phasia

Component	Meaning	Medical Term
e-	away from/out from/outside/without	emasculation
-e	noun ending/a name	trigone
-eal	pertaining to	oesophageal
ec-	away from/out from/outside/without	eccyesis
ech/o	echo/reflected sound	echolalia
ect-	out/outside/outer part	ectethmoid
ecto-	out/outside/outer part	ectoderm
ectopia-	condition of displacement	ectopia lentis
ectop/o	displaced away from normal position	ectopic
-ectasia	condition of dilation or stretching	pneumonectasia
-ectasis	dilatation, stretching	bronchiectasis
-ectomy	removal, excision	appendicectomy
ectro-	congenital absence/miscarriage	ectrodactylia
edema- (Am.)	condition of swelling due to fluid	edematous
ef-	out/away from	efferent
eikon/o	icon	eikonometer
elae/o	oil fat	elaeopathia
elast/o	elastic/elastic tissue/elastin	elastosis
electr/o	electrical	electrocardiograph
ellipto-	shaped like an ellipse	elliptocytosis
em-	in	empathy
-em- (Am.)	blood	anemia
-ema	condition	myxedema
embol/o	embolus/plug/blockage	embolism
embry/o	embryo	embryogenesis
-emesis	vomiting	haematemesis (Am. hematemesis)
emet/o	vomiting	emetic
-emia (Am.)	condition of blood	anemia
emmetr/o	in due measure/normally proportioned	emmetropia
-emphraxis	blocking/stopping up	salpingemphraxis
en-	within/in	ensheathed
encephal/o	brain	encephalitis
endo-	within/inside/inner	endoscope
endocardi/o	endocardium	endocarditis
endocrin/o	endocrine (gland)	endocrinologist
endometri/o	endometrium of uterus (the lining of the uterus)	endometriosis
endotheli/o	endothelium	endothelial
enter/o	intestine	enteritis
-ent	person/agent	diluent
ento-	within, inside	entocranial
eosin/o	red/dawn coloured/eosin, a red acid dye	eosinophil
ep-	above/upon/on	eparterial
epi-	above/upon/on/in addition	epidermis
epiderm/o	epidermis	epidermal
epididym/o	epididymis	epididymovasectomy
epiglott/o	epiglottis	epiglottitis
epilept/i/o	epilepsy	epileptiform
epipl/o	omentum	epiploplasty
episi/o	vulva/pudendum	episiotomy
epitheli/o	epithelium	epithelial
equin/o	horse	equine
-er	one who/a person/an agent	radiographer
erg/o/n/o	work	ergonometer
-erysis	drag/draw/suck out	phacoerysis
erythem/o	reddening of the skin/flushed/erythema	erythemogenic
erythr/o	red	erythrocyte
-esis	abnormal state/condition	uresis
es/o	within/inwards	esodeviation

Component	Meaning	Medical Term
esophag/o (Am.)	esophagus/gullet	**esophago**stomy
esthesi/o (Am.)	sensation	an**esthesio**logy
estr/o (Am.)	estrogen/female/estrus	**estro**genic
ethm/o	ethmoid bone	**ethm**oidonasal
ethmoid/o	ethmoid bone	**ethmoido**palatal
eti/o (Am.)	causation (of disease)	**etio**logy
eu-	good/normal/easily	**eu**tocia
eury-	wide/broad	**eury**cephalic
ex-	out/out of/away from	**ex**ophthalmos
exo-	out/away from/outside	**exo**gastic
-externa	external	otitis **externa**
extr/a/o	outside of/beyond/outward	**extra**hepatic
faci/o	face	**facio**maxillary
faec/o	faeces (Am. feces)	**faeco**lith (Am. **feco**lith)
falc/i	falx/sickle-shaped structure	**falci**form
fascicul/o	fascicle	**fascicul**ar
fasci/o	fascia/fibrous tissue e.g. covering muscles	**fascio**tomy
febr/o	fever	**febr**ile
fec/o (Am.)	feces/waste	**fec**al
femor/o	femur/thigh	**femor**al
-ferent	carrying/to carry/to bear	ef**ferent**
fer/o	to carry/to bear	urini**fer**ous
ferr/o	iron	**ferro**protein
fet/i/o (Am.)	fetus	**feto**metry
fibrill/o	muscular twitching	**fibrill**ation
fibrin/o	fibrinogen	**fibrino**lytic
fimbri/o	fringe	**fimbri**ate
fibr/o	fibre	**fibr**osis
fibul/o	fibula	**fibulo**calcaneal
-fida	split	spina. bi**fida**
fil/o	thread	**filo**pressure
fissur-	split/cleft	**fissur**al
fistul/o	tube/pipe	**fistul**a
flagell/o	flagellum/whip	**flagell**osis
flav/o	yellow	**flavo**protein
-flect	bend	re**flect**
-flex-	bend	**flex**ion
fluor/o	fluorescent/luminous/flow	**fluoro**scopy
foet/o	foetus (Am. fet/o)	**foet**al (Am. **fet**al)
follicul/o	small sac/follicle	**follicul**itis
fore-	before/in front of	**fore**brain
-form	having form/structure of	epilepti**form**
foss/o	depression	**foss**a
fove/o	pit/often used to mean the central fovea of the retina	**fove**a
fraen/o	fraenum or fraenulum/a restraining structure, e.g. fraenulum of the lip	**fraen**al (Am. **fren**al)
fren/o (Am.)	frenum or frenulum/a restraining structure, e.g. frenulum of the lip	**freno**plasty
front/o	front/forehead	**fronto**temporal
-fuge	agent that suppresses/gets rid of	lacti**fuge**
fund/o	bottom/base (of an organ)	**fund**us
fung/i	fungus	**fung**icide
furc/o	branching	bi**furc**ation
galact/o	milk	**galacto**poiesis
gamet/o	gametes/sperm or eggs	**gameto**genesis
gangli/o	ganglion/swelling/plexus	**gangli**form
ganglion-	ganglion/swelling/plexus	**ganglion**ectomy

Component	Meaning	Medical Term
gastr/o	stomach	**gastro**pathy
-gen	agent that produces/precursor	pepsino**gen**
-genesis	capable of causing/pertaining to formation	spermato**genesis**
-genic	pertaining to formation/originating in	oestro**genic**
genicul/o	knee	**genicul**ar
geni/o	chin	**geni**oglossal
genit/o	genitals/reproductive organs/produced by birth	**genit**al
gen/o	cause/produce/originate	**gen**ophobia
-genous	arising from/produced by/producing	andro**genous**
ger/i/o	old age/the aged	**ger**iatric
geront/o	old age/the aged	**geront**ology
gest/o	pregnancy	**gest**ation
gingiv/o	gum	**gingiv**itis
gli/a/o	glue-like/neuroglia, the supporting cells of the CNS	**gli**oma
glisson-	Glisson's capsule (around the liver)	**glisson**itis
-globin	protein	myo**globin**
-globulin	protein	immuno**globulin**
-globus	globe/like a small ball	kerato**globus**
glomerul/o	glomerulus of kidney	**glomerul**itis
gloss/o	tongue	**gloss**ectomy
glott-	glottis (the vocal apparatus and its opening)	**glott**al
gluc/o	glucose/sugar/sweet	**gluc**oneogenesis
glyc/o	glucose/sugar/sweet	**glyc**oprotein
glycogen/o	glycogen, a polysaccharide	**glycogen**osis
glycos-	sugar (an obsolete variant meaning glucose)	**glycos**uria
gnath/o	jaw	**gnath**oplasty
-gnomy	science or means of judging	patho**gnomy**
-gnos-	to know/known or knowledge of/judgment	**gnos**ia
-gnosia	condition of knowing/receiving/recognizing	hyper**gnosia**
-gnosis	to know/known or knowledge of/judgment	pro**gnosis**
gonad/o	gonads (the ovaries or testes)	**gonad**otrophin
gonecyst/o	seminal vesicle	**gonecysto**lith
gon/e/o	seed/semen/sperm/knee	**gono**coccus
goni/o	angle/corner	**goni**oscopy
gony/o	knee	**gony**oncus
-grade	to go	retro**grade**
-gram	X-ray/tracing/recording/one thousandth of a kilogram (g)	mammo**gram**
granul/o	granule/granular	**granul**oma
-graph	usually recording instrument/a recording/an X-ray picture /a mathematical curve representing data	electrocardio**graph**
-graphy	technique of recording/making X-ray	electrocardio**graphy**
-gravida	pregnancy/a pregnant woman	primi**gravida**
gravid/o	pregnancy	**gravido**cardiac
gynaec/o	gynaecology/female reproductive system/woman (Am. gynec/o)	**gynaec**ology (Am. **gynec**ology)
-gyne	woman/female	andro**gyne**
gynec/o (Am.)	gynecology/female reproductive system/woman	**gynec**ological
gyn/o	gynaecology (Am. gynecology)/female reproductive system/woman	**gyn**opathy
-gyric	pertaining to circular motion	oculo**gyric**
haemangi/o	blood vessel (Am. hemangi/o)	**haemangi**oma (Am. **hemangi**oma)
haem/a/o	blood (Am. hem/a/o)	**haemo**globin (Am. **hemo**globin)
haemat/o	blood (Am. hemat/o)	**haemat**ology (Am. **hemat**ology
haemoglobin/o	haemoglobin (Am. hemoglobin)	**haemoglobin**uria (Am. **hemoglobin**uria)

Component	Meaning	Medical Term
halit/o	breath	**halit**osis
hallucin/o	hallucination	**hallucin**ogenic
hallux	great toe	**hallux** rigidus
hal/o	salts	**hal**ogen
hapl/o	single/simple	**hapl**opia
hapt/o	touch	**hapt**ometer
hecto-	one hundred	**hecto**gram
helc/o	ulcer	**helc**osis
heli/o	sun	**heli**osis
helic/o	helix/spiral form	**helic**oid
helmint/h/o	worms	an**helminth**ic
hem/a/o (Am.)	blood	**hem**ocytoblast
hemat/o (Am.)	blood	**hemat**ology
hemi-	half/on one side	**hemi**plegia
hepatic/o	hepatic bile duct	**hepatico**stomy
hepat/o	liver	**hepat**ocyte
hept/a	seven	**hepta**chromic
herni/o	hernia	**herni**orrhaphy
heter/o	other/another/different	**heter**osexual
hex-	six/hold/being	**hex**ose
hidraden/o	sweat gland	**hidraden**itis
hidr/o	sweat/perspiration	**hidr**osis
histi/o	histiocyte, a type of macrophage	**histio**cytosis
hist/o	tissue	**hist**ology
hol/o	entire/whole	**hol**ocrine
homeo-	alike/unchanging/constant/resembling	**homeo**stasis
homo-	the same/resembling	**homo**zygous
humer/o	humerus	**humero**radial
hyal/o	glass-like	**hyal**oid
hydatid/i/o	hydatid cyst	**hydatid**osis
hydr/a/o	water	**hydr**onephrosis
hygr/o	moisture	**hygro**blepharic
hymen/o	hymen	**hymeno**tomy
hy/o	hyoid bone	**hyo**mandibular
hyp-	below/below normal/under	**hyp**hidrosis
hyper-	above/above normal/excessive/over	**hyper**chromia
hypn/o	sleep	**hypn**otic
hypo-	below normal/under	**hypo**thyroidism
hypophys-	hypophysis/pituitary gland	**hypophys**ectomy
hyster/o	uterus/womb	**hyster**ectomy
-ia	condition of/abnormal condition/disease	polyur**ia**
-iac	pertaining to	coel**iac** Am. cel**iac**
-ial	pertaining to	bronch**ial**
-ian	belonging to/characteristic of	physic**ian**
-iasis	abnormal condition/process or condition resulting from/disease	lith**iasis**
-iatrics	a medical specialty	paed**iatrics** (Am. ped**iatrics**)
iatr/o	medical treatment/doctor	**iatr**ogenic
-iatry	treatment by a doctor/specialty (of doctor)	psych**iatry**
-ible	capable of/able	flex**ible**
-ic[1]	pertaining to	gastr**ic**
-ic[2]	used in pharmacology to mean a drug or drug action	diuret**ic**
-ical	pertaining to/dealing with	cytolog**ical**
ichthy/o	fish-like/dry/scaly	**ichthy**osis
-ician	person associated with/specialist	techn**ician**
-icle	small	ves**icle**
-ics	art or science of	genet**ics**
-ictal	pertaining to seizure/attack	pre**ictal**

Component	Meaning	Medical Term
icter/o	jaundice	icterogenic
-ide	a binary chemical compound	glycoside
idi/o	self/one's own/peculiar to an organism/unknown	idiopathic
-igo	attack/abnormal condition	vertigo
il-	in/none	illegitimate
-ile	capable of/able	contractile
ile/o	ileum	ileocolitis
ili/o	ilium/flank	iliofemoral
im-	in/within/none/not	impotence
immun/o	immune/immunity	immunology
in-	in/none/not	incision
-in	used as suffix for various chemicals	glycerin
incud/o	incus (the anvil-shaped ear ossicle)/anvil	incudomalleal
-ine	pertaining to/a suffix used for chemicals derived or thought to be derived from ammonia	amine
infer/o	below/beneath/inferior to	inferolateral
infra-	below/inferior to	inframammary
inguin/o	groin	inguinal
insulin/o	insulin/islets of Langerhans	insulinogenesis
inter-	between	intercostal
-interna	internal	otitis interna
intestin/o	intestine	intestinal
intra-	within/inside	intranasal
intro-	into/within/inwards	introflexion
intus-	in/into	intussusception
iod/o	iodine	iodism
-ion	action/condition resulting from an action	ablation
ion/o	ion/to wander	ionic
-ior	pertaining to	posterior
ips/e/i/o	the same/self	ipsilateral
ir-	in/none/not	irreducible
irid/i/o	iris	iridoplegia
ir/o	iris	iritis
ischi/o	ischium	ischiococcygeal
isch/o	condition of holding back/reducing/suppressing	ischaemia (Am. ischemia)
-ism	process/state or condition/practice of/theory of	prostatism
-ismus	spasm/process/state or condition	strabismus
iso-	same/equal	isograft
-ist	specialist	optometrist
-ite	end product of a reaction	metabolite
-itic	relating to or having something specified	syphilitic
-itis	inflammation	tonsillitis
-ity	state/condition	severity
-ium	metallic element	calcium
-ive[1]	pertaining to/tendency	adhesive
-ive[2]	used in pharmacology to mean a drug or drug action	antitussive
-ize	use/subject to/to make/treat/combine with	neutralize
-ject	throw	projectile
jejun/o	jejunum	jejunostomy
juxta-	adjoining/near	juxtaposition
kal/i	potassium (K^+), from Latin kalium	kaliuresis
kary/o	nucleus	karyogram
kerat/o	epidermis/cornea/horny	keratoplasty
keratin/o	keratin (a protein present in skin, hair and nails)	keratinous
kern-	nucleus (of nerve cells)	kernicterus
ket/o/n	ketones/ketone bodies/carbonyl group	ketonuria

Component	Meaning	Medical Term
kin/e/o	motion/movement	kinesis
kinesi/o	motion/movement	kinesiology
-kinesis	a motion/movement	iridokinesis
kinet/o	motion/movement	kinetocardiography
kilo-	one thousand	kilocalorie
klept/o	thief/stealing	kleptomania
-kymia	condition of involuntary twitching of muscle/a wave of contraction in a muscle	myokymia
kyph/o	crooked/hump/forward curvature of the thoracic spine	kyphosis
labi/o	lip	labioplasty
labyrinth/o	labyrinth of ear	labyrinthitis
lachrym/o	tear/tear ducts/lacrimal apparatus	lachrymal
lacrim/o	tear/tear ducts/lacrimal apparatus	lacrimonasal
lact/i/o	milk	lactiferous
laevo-	left (Am. levo-)	laevocardia (Am. levocardia)
-lalia	condition of talking	dyslalia
lal/o	speech	laloplegia
lamell/a	thin leaf or plate	lamellar
lamin/o	lamina/thin plate/part of vertebral arch	laminectomy
lapar/o	abdomen/flank	laparotomy
-lapaxy	empty/wash out/evacuate	litholapaxy
-lapse	fall/slide/sag	prolapse
laryng/o	larynx	laryngectomy
later/o	side	laterotorsion
lei/o	smooth	leiodermia
leiomy/o	smooth muscle	leiomyoma
-lemma	sheath/covering	sarcolemma
lent/i	lens	lenticonus
-lepsy	seizure/fit	epilepsy
lept/o	thin/fine/slender	leptomeningitis
leuc/o	white	leucocyte (Am. leukocyte)
leukaem/o	leukaemia (Am. leukemia)	leukaemic
leukem/o (Am.)	leukemia/leukaemia	leukemogen
leuk/o	white	leukoblast
levo- (Am.)	left	levocardia
-lexia	condition of speech/words	dyslexia
lien/o	spleen	lienocele
-ligation	tying off of a vessel with a suture	vasoligation
lingu/a/o	tongue	linguogingival
lip/o	fat/fatty tissue	lipoma
-listhesis	slipping	spondylolisthesis
-lith	stone	ureterolith
-lithiasis	abnormal condition of stones	ureterolithiasis
lith/o	stone	lithotrite
lob/o	lobe	lobar
lochi/o	vaginal discharge (lochia)	lochiorrhagia
loc/o	place	locus
logad-	white of the eye	logadectomy
-logist	specialist who studies	cardiologist
log/o	words/speech/study/thought	logophasia
-logy	study of	laryngology
loph/o	ridge/tuft	lophodont
lord/o	bend forward/forward curvature of the lumbar spine	lordosis
lox/o	oblique/slanting	loxophthalmos
-lucent	to shine	radiolucent
lumb/o	loin/lower back	lumbocostal

Component	Meaning	Medical Term
lump-	lump/swelling	**lump**ectomy
lute/o	yellow/corpus luteum of ovary	**luteo**trophic
lymph/a/t/o	lymph	**lymph**oma
lymphaden/o	lymph node (lymph gland)	**lymphaden**itis
lymphangi/o	lymph vessel	**lymphangi**ography
lymphocyt/o	lymphocyte	**lymphocyt**osis
lymphomat-	lymphoma	**lymphomat**osis
lyo-	water soluble/solvent/dissolve	**lyo**phil
-lys/o	break down/disintegration/dissolving	**lys**in
-lysis	break down/disintegration/dissolving	auto**lysis**
-lytic	pertaining to break down/disintegration	haemo**lytic** (Am. hemo**lytic**)
macro-	large	**macro**phage
macul/o	spot/blotch	**maculo**papular
mal-	bad/diseased or impaired	**mal**nutrition
-malacia	condition of softening	myo**malacia**
malac/o	softening	**malac**ic
malign-	bad/harmful	**malign**ant
malleol/o	malleolus (the process on the side of the ankle)	**malleol**ar
malle/o	malleus (the hammer-shaped ear ossicle)/hammer	**malle**otomy
mamill/i/o	nipple	**mamill**iplasty
mamm/a/o	breast/mammary gland	**mamm**ography
mammill/i/o	nipple	**mammill**itis
mandibul/o	mandible (lower jaw bone)	**mandibul**oplasty
mani-	mental disorder/madness	**mani**ac
-mania	condition of mental disorder/psychosis (extreme excitment)	nympho**mania**
man/o	pressure	**mano**metry
manus-	hand	**manus** extensa
mast/o	breast/mammary gland	**mast**algia
mastoid/o	nipple-shaped/mastoid process/mastoid air cells	**mastoid**ectomy
maxill/o	maxilla (upper jaw bone)	**maxill**ofacial
meat/o	meatus/opening/external orifice e.g. of the urethra	**meat**otomy
medi/o	middle/midline	**medi**al
-media	middle	otitis **media**
medull/o	inner part/medulla	adrenal **medulla**
mega-	abnormally large	**mega**colon
megal/o	abnormally large	**megal**oglossia
-megaly	enlargement	acro**megaly**
melan/o	melanin/dark pigment	**melan**oma
melanomat-	melanoma	**melanomat**osis
melit/o	sugar/honey	**melit**uria
mel/o	limb/cheek	**mel**agra
melon/o	cheek	**melon**oplasty
mening/i/o	meninges, the protective membranes of the CNS	**mening**itis
menisc/o	meniscus/crescent-shaped	**menisc**ocyte
men/o	menses/menstruation/monthly flow	**men**orrhagia
ment/o	chin/mind	**ment**oplasty
mes/o	middle/intermediate	**meso**derm
meta-	change in form, position or order/after/next/between	**meta**plasia
metacarp/o	metacarpus/metacarpal or metacarpal bone	**metacarp**al
metatars/o	metatarsus/metatarsal or metatarsal bone	**metatars**algia
-meter	measuring instrument/a measure	audio**meter**
metr/a/i/o	uterus/womb	endo**metr**iosis
-metrist	person who measures	audio**metrist**
-metry	process of measuring	audio**metry**
micro-	small/one millionth	**micro**glia
mid-	middle	**mid**brain

Component	Meaning	Medical Term
-mileusis	to carve	keratomileusis
milli-	one thousandth	millilitre
-mimesis	simulation/imitation	pathomimesis
-mimetic	simulation of a specific effect	sympathomimetic
-mimia	condition of expressing through gestures	macromimia
mi/o	make smaller/less	miopia
-mission	to send	emission
mito-	thread-like/mitosis	mitotic
mono-	one/single	monosomy
monocyt/o	monocyte	monocytopenia
-morph	shape/form	ectomorph
morph/o	shape/form	morphogenesis
mort/o	death	mortal
-motor-	moving/action/set in motion	oculomotor
muc/o	mucus	mucous
multi-	many	multigravida
muscul/o	muscle	musculocutaneous
mut/a	change (genetic change)	mutagen
my-	(from myein) to close/squint	myopia
mycet/o	fungus	mycetoid
myc/o	fungus	bronchomycosis
myelin/o	myelin/myelin sheath	myelinated
myel/o	bone marrow/spinal cord/myelocyte	myeloma
myelomat/o	myeloma	myelomatosis
my/o	muscle	myoglobin
myocardi/o	myocardium (heart muscle)	myocardiopathy
myomat/o	myoma (muscle tumour)	myomatosis
myop-	short sighted	myopia
myos/o	muscle	myositis
myring/o	eardrum/tympanic membrane	myringotome
myx/o	mucus/mucoid tissue (embryonic connective tissue)	myxadenitis
myxomat-	myxoma	myxomatosis
nano-	one billionth/a quantity multiplied by (10^{-9})	nanometre (Am. nanometer)
narc/o	stupor/numbness	narcotic
nas/o	nose	nasopharyngitis
nasopharyng/o	nasopharynx	nasopharyngoscope
-natal	pertaining to birth	antenatal
nat/o	birth	neonatology
natr/i	sodium (Na^+), from Latin natrium	natriuresis
necr/o	death/death of tissue	necrosis
neo-	new/recent	neoplasia
nephr/o	kidney	nephritis
neur/o	nerve (rarely tendon)	neurology
neuron/o	neuron	neuronal
neutr/o	neutral	neutrophil
noc/i	harm	nociceptor
noct/i	night/darkness	nocturia
nod/o	knot/swelling	nodule
nom/o	distribute/law/custom	nomotopic
non-	without/no	non compos mentis
normo-	normal	normocytosis
nos/o	disease	nosology
not/o	back	notochord
nucle/o	nucleus	nucleoprotein
nulli-	none	nullipara
nyctal/o	night/darkness	nyctalopia

Component	Meaning	Medical Term
nyct/o	night/darkness	**nyct**algia
nymph/o	labia minora/nymphae	**nympho**mania
-nyxis	perforation/pricking/puncture	kerato**nyxis**
obstetr-	midwifery/obstetrics	**obstetr**ician
occipit/o	occiput, the posterior region of the skull	**occipito**cervical
occlus/o	shut/close up	**occlus**ion
oct/a/i/o-	eight	**oct**igravida
ocul/o	eye	bin**ocul**ar
odont/o	tooth/teeth	orth**odont**ics
-oedema	swelling due to fluid (Am. edema)	myx**oedema** (Am. myx**edema**)
oesophag/o	oesophagus/gullet (Am. esophago)	**oesophago**stomy (Am. **esophago**stomy)
oestr/o	oestrogen (a female sex-hormone)/oestrus (Am. estr/o)	**oestr**ogenic (Am. **estr**ogenic)
-oid	resembling	lip**oid**
-ola	small	arteri**ola**
-ole	small	arteri**ole**
olecran/o	elbow/olecranon (the bony projection of the ulna)	**olecran**arthropathy
ole/o	oil	**oleo**granuloma
olfact/o	sense of smell/smell	**olfact**ory
olig/o	deficiency/few/little	**olig**uria
-olisthesis	slipping	spondyl**olisthesis**
-oma	tumour/swelling	sarc**oma**
oment/o	omentum (peritoneal fold of stomach)	**omento**plasty
om/o	shoulder	**omo**clavicular
omphal/o	navel/umbilicus/umbilical cord	**omphalo**genesis
onc/o	tumour (Am. tumor)/mass	**onc**ology
-one	hormone	progester**one**
onych/o	nail	**onycho**dystrophy
oo-	egg	**oo**cyte
oophor/o	ovary	**oophor**ectomy
-opaque	obscure	radio-**opaque**
-op-	seeing/looking at	presby**op**ia
ophthalm/o	eye	**ophthalmo**scope
-ophthalmos	eye	ex**ophthalmos**
-opia	condition of vision/defective vision	ambly**opia**
opistho-	backward/behind	**opistho**gnathism
-opsia	condition of vision/defective vision	hemiachromat**opsia**
-opsy	to view/process of viewing	bi**opsy**
optic/o	vision/eye/optic nerve	**optic**al
opt/o	vision/eye	**opto**metry
orbit/o	orbit (the bony cavity of the eye)	**orbito**nasal
-or	a person or agent/a device	don**or**
orchid/o	testicle/testis	**orchid**opathy
orch/i/o	testicle/testis	**orchi**oplasty
-orexia	condition of appetite	an**orexia**
organ/o	organ	**organo**genesis
or/o	mouth	**or**al
orth/o-	correct/normal/straight	**orth**optics
-ory	pertaining to	sens**ory**
os-	bone/a mouth/an orifice	**os** uteri
osche/o	scrotum	**osche**oplasty
-ose	carbohydrate/sugar/starch/full of/pertaining to/having the form of	gluc**ose**
-osis	abnormal condition/disease of/abnormal increase	leucocyt**osis** (Am. leukocyt**osis**)
osm/o	odour/smell/osmosis	**osmo**dysphoria

Component	Meaning	Medical Term
osphresi/o	odour/smell/olfaction (the sense of smell)	osphresiology
osse/o	bone	osseous
oss/i	bone	ossicle
ossicul/o	ear ossicles/ear bones	ossiculectomy
ost/e/o	bone	osteoarthritis
ot/o	ear	otology
oul/o	scar/gum	oulectomy
-ous	pertaining to	uriniferous
ovari/o	ovary	ovariotomy
ov/i/o	egg/ovum	oviduct
-oxia	condition of oxygen	hypoxia
ox/i/o	oxygen	oximetry
oxy-	oxygen /sharp/quick	oxytocic
oxysm/o	sudden	paroxysmal
pachy-	thick	pachydermia
paed/o	child (Am. ped/o)	paediatric (Am. pediatric)
palae/o	old/primitive (Am. pale/o)	palaeocortex (Am. paleocortex)
palat/o	palate	palatoplasty
pale/o (Am.)	old/primitive	paleocortex
palm/o	palm	palmar
palpebr/a	eyelid	palpebritis
pan-	all	pancarditis
pancreatic/o	pancreatic duct	pancreaticoenterostomy
pancreat/o	pancreas	pancreatolysis
pannicul/o	fatty layer e.g. of abdomen	panniculitis
pant/o	all/entire	pantatrophy
papill/i/o	nipple-like/optic disc/optic papilla	papilloretinitis
para-	beside/near/beyond/accessory to/wrong	paranephric
-para	to bear/bring forth offspring/a woman who has borne viable young	primipara
parasympath/o	parasympathetic nervous system	parasympathomimetic
parathyr/o	parathyroid gland	parathyrotrophic
parathyroid/o	parathyroid gland	parathyroidectomy
-paresis	slight paralysis	juvenile paresis
-pareunia	sexual intercourse	dyspareunia
parotid/o	parotid gland	parotitis
-parous	pertaining to production of live young	nulliparous
-partum	birth/labour	post partum
parturi-	childbirth/labour/parturition	parturient
patell/o	patella/knee cap	patellofemoral
-pathia	condition of disease	psychopathia
pathic	pertaining to disease	idiopathic
path/o	disease	pathologist
-pathy	disease/emotion	gastropathy
-pause	stopping	menopause
pect-	chest/breast/thorax	pectus
pector/o	chest/breast/thorax	pectoral
pedicul/o	lice	pediculosis
ped/i/o (Am.)	foot/child (Am.)	pediatrics
pelli-	skin/hide	pellicle
pelv/i/o	pelvis	pelvimeter
pend/o	to hang	pendulous
-penia	condition of deficiency or lack of	erythropenia
pen/o	penis	penitis
peps-	digestion	dyspepsia
-pepsia	condition of digestion	bradypepsia

Component	Meaning	Medical Term
pepsin/o	pepsin (an enzyme)	**pepsin**ogen
pept/o	digestion/pepsin/peptone	**pept**ic
per-	through/completely/excessive	**per**cutaneous
perone/o	fibula	**perone**al
peri-	around	**peri**corneal
pericardi/o	pericardium	**pericardi**tis
perine/o	perineum	**perine**orrhaphy
periton/e/o	peritoneum	**periton**itis
petr/o	stone/rock	osteo**petr**osis
-pexis	surgical fixation/fix in place/storage	glyco**pexis**
-pexy	surgical fixation/fix in place/storage	arthro**pexy**
phac/o	lens	**phac**oscopy
phae/o	dusky/dark (Am. phe/o)	**phae**ochromocyte (Am. **pheo**chromocyte)
-phagia	condition of eating/swallowing	poly**phagia**
phag/o	eating/consuming/a phagocyte	**phag**ocytic
-phagy	eating or swallowing	copro**phagy**
phak/o	lens	**phak**itis
phalang/o	phalanx/finger/toe	**phalang**eal
phall/o	penis	**phall**ic
phaner/o	visible/manifesting	**phaner**ogenic
pharm/ac/o	drug/medicine	**pharmac**ology
pharyng/o	pharynx	**pharyng**itis
-phasia	condition of speaking/speech	dys**phasia**
phas/i/o	speech	a**phasi**ology
phe/o (Am.)	dusky/dark	**phe**ochromocyte
-phil	love/affinity for/a cell type with affinity for something	neutro**phil**
-philia	condition of love/affinity for something/an increase in (e.g. number of cells)	neutro**philia**
-phily	condition of love/affinity for	necro**phily**
phleb/o	vein	**phleb**ectomy
-phobia	condition of irrational fear/aversion	hydro**phobia**
-phonia	condition of having voice	a**phonia**
phon/o	speech/sound/voice	**phon**ocardiograph
-phony	sound/type of speech	tracheo**phony**
-phore	a carrier	chromato**phore**
-phoresis	movement in a specified way/bearing/carrying/driving ions	electro**phoresis**
-phoria	condition of mental state/feeling/bearing/deviation of the eyes (heterophoria)	eu**phoria**
phor/o	mental state/bearing/carrier (e.g. of disease)	**phor**ology
phosph/o	phosphate/phosphorus/phosphoric acid	**phosph**olipid
phot/o	light	**phot**osensitive
phrenic/o	diaphragm/mind/phrenic nerve	**phrenic**ectomy
phren/i/o	diaphragm/mind/phrenic nerve	**phren**ogastric
-phthisis	wasting away	neuro**phthisis**
-phylaxis	protection	pro**phylaxis**
-phyma	tumour/boil/swelling (Am. tumor)	rhino**phyma**
phys/i/o	nature/physical things/physiology	**physio**therapy
-physis	growth	hypo**physis**
-phyt/e/o	plant/fungus	dermato**phyte**
pico-	small/a quantity multiplied by 10^{-12}	**pico**gram
pil/o	hair	**pil**osebaceous
pineal/o	pineal body/pineal gland	**pineal**ocyte
pituitar-	pituitary gland	hypo**pituitar**ism
placent/o	placenta	**placent**ography
-plakia	condition of broad/flat (patch)	leuko**plakia**
-plania	condition of wandering e.g. a cell moving position	leucocyto**plania** (Am. leukocyto**plania**)
plan/o	flat	**plan**ocellular

Component	Meaning	Medical Term
plant/i	sole of foot	**plant**ar
-plasia	condition of growth due to formation of cells	hyper**plasia**
-plasm	formative substance/growth	cyto**plasm**
plasma-	plasma cell/plasma the fluid matrix of blood	**plasma**therapy
plasm/o	anything moulded, shaped or formed/formative substance/growth/plasma	**plasmo**cyte
-plastic	pertaining to formation of cells or moulding of tissues	neo**plastic**
-plasty	surgical repair/reconstruction	kerato**plasty**
platy-	flat	**platy**onychia
-plegia	condition of paralysis/stroke	para**plegia**
pleo-	more	**pleo**cytosis
plethysm/o	volume	**plethysmo**graph
pleur/o	pleural membranes/rib/side	**pleuro**dynia
-plexia	condition arising from a stroke or other occurrence	apo**plexia**
plex/o	network of nerves, blood or lymph vessels	**plex**us
-plexy	strike/paralyze	apo**plexy**
-ploid(y)	chromosome sets in a cell	di**ploid**
pluri-	several/more	**pluri**glandular
-pnea (Am.)	breathing	a**pnea**
pne/o	breath/breathing	**pneo**scope
pneum/a/o	gas/air/lung/breathing	**pneumo**thorax
pneumat/o	gas/air/lung/breathing	**pneumato**metry
pneumon/o	lung	**pneumon**ectomy
-pnoea	breathing (Am. pnea)	dys**pnoea** (Am. dys**pnea**)
pod/o	foot	**pod**iatry
pogon/o	beard	**pogon**iasis
-poiesis	formation	erythro**poiesis**
-poietin	substance that forms	erythro**poietin**
poikil/o	varied/irregular	**poikilo**cyte
polio-	grey matter (of CNS)	**polio**myelitis
pollex	thumb	**pollex** flexus
poly-	many/too much	**poly**uria
polyp/o	polyp/small growth	**polyp**ectomy
pont/o	pons (part of metencephalon of the brain)	**ponto**cerebellar
por/o	passage/pore	osteo**poro**sis
port/o	portal vein	**porto**graphy
post-	after/behind	**post**-ganglionic
poster/o	back of body/behind/posterior to	**postero**superior
posth/o	prepuce/foreskin	balano**posth**itis
-prandial	pertaining to a meal	post**prandial**
-praxia	condition of purposeful movement or conduct	a**praxia**
pre-	before/in front of	**pre**tracheal
preputi/o	prepuce/foreskin	**preputio**tomy
presby/o	old man/old age	**presby**opia
primi-	first	**primi**gravida
-privia	condition of loss or deprivation	calci**privia**
pro-	before/favouring/in front of	**pro**drome
proct/o	rectum/anus	**proct**algia
progest/o	progesterone	**progesto**gen
prosop/o	face	**prosopo**plegia
prostat/o	prostate gland	**prostat**ism
prosth-	adding (a replacement part)	**prosth**odontics
prote/o	protein	prote**ase**
proto-	first	**proto**diastole
protoz/o	protozoa	**protoz**oiasis
proxim/o	near	**proxim**al
prurit/o	itching	**pruri**tic
pseudo-	false	**pseudo**plegia

Component	Meaning	Medical Term
psych/o	mind	**psych**osis
psychr/o	cold	**psychr**algia
-ptosis	falling/displacement/prolapse	blepharo**ptosis**
-ptotic	pertaining to falling/displacement/prolapse/affected with a ptosis	nephro**ptotic**
ptyal/o	saliva	**ptyal**ography
-ptysis	spitting/coughing up	pyo**ptysis**
pub/o	pubis/pubic region	**pub**ovesical
pudend-	pudendum/vulva	**pudend**al
puerper/o	puerperium/time of childbirth	**puerper**al
pulm/o	lung	**pulmo**-aortic
pulmon/o	lung	**pulmon**ary
pupill/o	pupil	**pupillo**metry
purul/o	pus-filled	**purul**oid
pustul/o	infected pimple/pustule	**pustul**osis
pyel/o	the renal pelvis (the space in which urine collects in the kidney)	**pyelo**lithotomy
pykn/o	compact/thick/frequent	**pykn**osis
pyle/o	portal (vein)	**pyle**phlebitis
pylor/o	pylorus	**pylor**ic
py/o	pus	**pyo**genic
pyret/o	heat/fire/burning/fever	**pyret**ic
pyrex/o	heat/fire/burning/fever	**pyrex**ial
pyr/o	heat/fire/burning/fever	**pyro**gen
quadr/i/u-	four	**quadri**plegia
quinque-	five	**quinque**cuspid
quint-	five	**quint**an
rachi/o	backbone/spine/vertebral column	**rachio**pathy
radic/o	spinal nerve root	**radic**otomy
radicul/o	spinal nerve root	**radicul**itis
radi/o	radioactivity/radiation/X-ray/radius	**radio**therapy
re-	back/contrary/again	**re**position
rect/o	rectum	**recto**sigmoid
ren/i/o	kidney	**ren**ography
reticul/o	net-like/reticulum	**reticulo**cytosis
reticuloendotheli/o	reticuloendothelial system	**reticuloendotheli**um
retin/o	retina	**retino**blastoma
retro-	backwards/behind	**retro**verted
rhabd/o	rod/rod-shaped	**rhabd**oid
rhabdomy/o	striated muscle	**rhabdomy**oma
rhe/o	electric current/flow of fluid	**rhe**ology
rheumat/o	rheumatism	**rheumat**ism
rhin/o	nose	**rhino**plasty
rhiz/o	root/spinal nerve root	**rhizo**tomy
rhod/o	red	**rhod**opsin
rhytid/o	wrinkle	**rhytido**plasty
roentgen/o	X-ray/Roentgen ray	**roentgeno**graphy
rostr/i	superior/a rostrum/a beak	**rostr**al
-rrhage	bursting forth/excessive flow	haemo**rrhage** (Am. hemo**rrhage**)
-rrhagia	condition of bursting forth/excessive flow	oto**rrhagia**
-rrhaphy	stitching/suturing	teno**rrhaphy**
-rrhea (Am.)	excessive discharge/flow	rhino**rrhea**
-rrhexis	breaking/rupturing	ovario**rrhexis**
-rrhoea	excessive discharge/flow (Am. -rrhea)	rhino**rrhoea**
(r)rhythm/o	rhythm	ar**rhythm**ia
rubr-	red	**rubr**or
rug/o	wrinkle/fold/ridge	**rug**a

Component	Meaning	Medical Term
sacchar/o	sugar/sweet	**sacchar**olytic
saccul/o	saccule of the inner ear	**saccul**ar
sacr/o	sacrum	**sacro**coccygeal
salping/o	Eustachian (auditory) tube/Fallopian tube	**salping**ostomy
sanguin/o	blood/bloody	**sanguin**olent
sapr/o	decay/decayed matter	**sapr**odontia
sarc/o	flesh/connective tissue	**sarc**oid
-sarcoma	malignant (fleshy) tumour of connective tissue (Am. tumor)	Kaposi's **sarcoma**
sarcomat/o	sarcoma, a malignant tumour (Am. tumor) of connective tissue	**sarcomat**osis
scapul/o	scapula	**scapulo**clavicular
scat/o	faeces/faecal matter (Am. feces)	**scat**ology
-schisis	cleaving/splitting/parting	palato**schisis**
schist/o	cleaving/splitting/parting	**schisto**cephalus
schistosom/o	a parasitic worm of the Genus Schistosoma	**schistosom**iasis
schiz/o	split/cleft/divided	**schiz**otrichia
scint/i	scintillation/spark/flash of light	**scint**iscan
scirrh/o	hard	**scirrh**us
scler/o	hard/sclera (the white of the eye)	**scler**otome
-sclerosis	abnormal condition of hardening	arterio**sclerosis**
scoli/o	crooked/twisted/lateral curvature of the spine	**scoli**osis
-scope	instrument to view/examine	endo**scope**
-scopic	pertaining to examining/viewing	micro**scopic**
-scopist	specialist who examines or uses a viewing instrument	endo**scopist**
-scopy	visual examination/examination	endo**scopy**
scot/o	darkness/scotoma	**scot**opia
scotom/o	scotoma/ blind spot	**scotoma**graph
scrot/o	scrotum	**scroto**cele
seb/o	sebum/sebaceous gland	**sebo**lith
-sect(ion)	cut	re**section**
secundi-	second	**secundi**gravida
semi-	half/partly	**semi**comatose
semin/i	semen	**semin**oma
sen/i	old	**sen**ile
sens/o	sense	**senso**motor
sensor/i	sense/sensation	**sensor**ium
-sepsis	infection	a**sepsis**
septi-	seven	**septi**para
septic/o	sepsis/infection/putrefaction	**septic**aemia (Am. **septic**emia)
sept/o	septum e.g. nasal septum	**septo**tomy
sequestr-	sequestrum, a portion of dead bone	**sequestr**ectomy
ser/o	serum	**sero**positive
sex/i	six	**sexi**digital
sialaden/o	salivary glands	**sialaden**itis
sial/o	saliva/salivary gland or duct	**sial**ography
sider/o	iron	**sidero**penia
sigmoid/o	sigmoid colon	**sigmoido**scopy
silic/o	glass/silica	**silic**osis
sinistr/o	left/left side	**sinistro**cardia
sin/o	sinus	**sino**atrial
sinus-	sinus	**sinus** venosus
sinus/o	sinus	**sinus**itis
-sis	abnormal condition/action/state of	symbio**sis**
-sitia	condition of appetite for food	eu**sitia**
sit/o	food	**sito**phobia
-sol	solution	cyto**sol**
somatic/o	body	**somatico**splanchnic
somat/o	body	**somato**trophic

Component	Meaning	Medical Term
-some	body	lysosome
somn/i/o	sleep	somnial
son/o	sound/ultrasound	ultrasonography
-spadia(s)	condition of drawing out/cleft or rent of the male urethra	hypospadia
-spasm	involuntary contraction of muscle	blepharospasm
spasm/o	spasm/involuntary muscle contraction	spasmodic
spermat/o	sperm	spermatogenesis
sperm/i/o	sperm	spermicidal
sphen/o	sphenoid bone/wedge-shaped	sphenomandibular
spher/o	sphere-shaped/round	spherophakia
sphincter/o	sphincter/ring-like muscle	sphincteroplasty
sphygm/o	pulse	sphygmomanometer
-sphyx-	pulsation	asphyxia
spirill/i	spiral-shaped bacteria of the Genus Spirillum	*Spirillum minus*
spir/o	to breathe	spirometry
spirochaet/o	spirochaete (a spiral-shaped bacterium)	spirochaete (Am. spirochete)
spirochet/o (Am.)	spirochete (a spiral-shaped bacterium)	spirochete
splanchnic/o	splanchnic nerve	splanchnicectomy
splanchn/i/o	viscera/splanchnic nerve	splanchnic
splen/o	spleen	splenectomy
spondyl/o	vertebra	spondylitis
spongi/o	sponge	spongiform
spor/o	spore	sporomycosis
squam/o	scale/scale-like	squamous
-stalsis	contraction	peristalsis
stapedi/o	stapes (the stirrup-shaped ear ossicle)/stirrup	stapediotenotomy
staphyl/o	staphylococcus/a grape-like cluster/the uvula	staphylococci
staphylococc/o	staphylococcus	staphylococcal
-stasis	stopping/controlling/cessation of movement	haemostasis (Am. hemostasis)
-stat	an agent/device that prevents change, regulates or stops	cryostat
-static	pertaining to stopping/controlling/standing or without motion	haemostatic (Am. hemostatic)
-staxis	dripping e.g. of blood	epistaxis
stear/i/o	fat	steariform
steat/o	fat	steatoma
sten/o	narrow/constricted	stenocoriasis
-stenosis	abnormal condition of narrowing	urethrostenosis
sterc/o	faeces (Am. feces)	stercolith
ster/e/o	solid/three dimensional	stereoscopic
stern/o	sternum	sternocostal
steth/o	chest/breast	stethoscope
-sthenia	condition of strength/full power	myasthenia
sthen/o	strength/full power	asthenic
-stitial	a space or position/pertaining to standing	interstitial
stomat/o	mouth	stomatitis
stom/o	a mouth/a mouth-like opening	stomal
-stomy	to form a new opening or outlet/a communication/an opening	colostomy
strabism/o	a squint/strabismus	strabismic
strab/o	a squint/strabismus	strabismus
strat/i	layer	stratiform
strept/o	streptococcus/a twisted chain	streptococci
streptococc/o	streptococcus	streptococcal
striat/o	a mark/stripe	striated
styl/o	stake/styloid process (of the temporal bone)	stylomastoid
sub-	beneath/under	subcutaneous
sud/or/i	sweat/perspiration	sudoresis
super/o	superior/above/excess	superolateral

Component	Meaning	Medical Term
supra-	superior/above/excess	**supra**hepatic
sy-	with/together	**sy**stole
sym-	with/together	**sym**melia
sympath/o	sympathetic nervous system/sympathetic nerves	**sympath**olytic
symphysi/o	symphysis (a fibro-cartilaginous joint), e.g. the symphysis pubis	**symphysio**tomy
syn-	together/in association/with	**syn**chronous
synapt-	synapse	**syna**ptic
syncop-	faint/cut off	**syncop**ic
syndesm/o	ligament/connective tissue	**syndesm**ectomy
syndrom/o	running together	**syndrom**ic
-synechia	condition of synechia/adhering together	blepharo**synechia**
synovi/o	synovia/synovial fluid/membranes	**synovi**al
syphil/o	syphilis	**syphil**oma
syring/o	tube/cavity	**syringo**myelia
system/o	system	**system**ic
systol-	systole	**systol**ic
tachy-	fast	**tachy**cardia
tact-	touch	**tact**ile
tal/o	ankle/ankle bone	**tal**ar
tars/o	tarsus, tarsal or tarsal bone/ankle bone/eyelid/connective tissue plate in the eyelid	**tars**algia
-taxia	condition of ordered movement	a**taxia**
tax/o	ordered movement, arrangement or classification	**tax**ology
tectori/o	covering/roof-like	**tectori**al
tel-	tela or web	**tel**angiectasis
-tela	a web-like membrane	epi**tela**
tele-	far away/operating at a distance	**tele**cardiography
telo-	end/complete	**telo**phase
tendin/o	tendon	**tendino**plasty
tend/o	tendon	**tendo**tome
ten/o	tendon	**teno**rrhaphy
tenont/o	tendon	**tenonto**phyma
-tension	pressure	hyper**tension**
ter-	three	**ter**valent
terat/o	monster-like/a deformed embryo or fetus	**terato**genic
testicul/o	testicle/testis	**testicul**ar
test/o	testicle/testis	**testo**sterone
tetra-	four	**tetra**ploid
thalam/o	thalamus (part of cerebral cortex)	**thalamo**tomy
thalass/o	the sea	**thalass**aemia (Am. **thalass**emia)
than/at/o	death	**thanato**phobia
thec/o	sheath	**thec**al
thel/e/o	nipple	**thele**plasty
-therapy	treatment	physio**therapy**
-thermia	condition of heat	hypo**thermia**
therm/o	heat	**thermo**graphy
-thermy	state of heat/process of heating	cystodia**thermy**
thio-	sulphur	**thio**cyanate
thoracico-	thorax	**thoracico**-abdominal
thorac/o	thorax	**thoraco**tomy
-thorax	thorax/chest	pneumo**thorax**
thromb/o	thrombus/clot	**thromb**osis
thrombocyt/o	platelet/thrombocyte	**thrombocyto**penia
thymic/o	thymus gland	**thymico**lymphatic
thym/o	thymus gland	**thym**ic
thyr/o	thyroid gland	**thyro**trophic
thyroid/o	thyroid gland	hypo**thyroid**ism

Component	Meaning	Medical Term
tibi/o	tibia	**tibi**ofibular
-tic	pertaining to	necro**tic**
tine/o	ringworm/like a gnawing worm	*Tinea pedis*
-tion	state or condition/process	resec**tion**
-tocia	condition of birth/labour (Am. labor)	eu**tocia**
toc/o	labour/birth (Am. labor)	**toc**ology
-tome	a cutting instrument	myringo**tome**
tom/o	a slice/section	**tom**ography
-tomy	incision into	laparo**tomy**
-tonia	condition of tension/tone	a**tonia**
ton/o	stretching/tension/tone	**ton**ometer
tonsill/o	tonsil	**tonsill**ectomy
top/o	place/particular area	**top**ology
tort/i	twisted	**tort**icollis
-toxic	pertaining to poisoning	nephro**toxic**
toxic/o	poison	**toxic**ology
tox/i/o	poison	**tox**ic
trabecul/o	trabecula/anchoring strand of connective tissue/the trabecular meshwork of the eye	**trabecul**ectomy
trachel/o	neck/uterine cervix	**trachel**oplasty
trache/o	trachea	**trache**ostomy
trans-	across/through	**trans**urethral
-trauma	injury/wound	baro**trauma**
-tresia	condition of an opening/perforation	a**tresia**
tri-	three	**tri**cuspid
trichin/o	*Trichinella spiralis* (a parasitic nematode worm)	**trichin**iasis
trich/o	hair	**trich**osis
trigon/o	trigone/triangular space e.g. at the base of the bladder	**trigon**itis
-tripsy	act of crushing	litho**tripsy**
-triptor	instrument designed to crush or fragment, e.g. using shock waves	litho**triptor**
-trite	instrument designed to crush or fragment	litho**trite**
-trope	influencing/a cell influencing . . ./influenced by	gonado**trope**
-trophic	pertaining to nourishment/stimulation	adreno**trophic**
troph/o	nourishment/food/stimulation	**troph**oblast
-trophy	nourishment/development/increase in cell size	a**trophy**
-tropia	condition of turning/deviation/heterotropia/strabismus	hyper**tropia**
-tropic	pertaining to affinity for/stimulating/changing in response to a stimulus/turning towards	thyro**tropic**
-tubal	pertaining to a tube	ovario**tubal**
tub/o	Fallopian tube/oviduct/tube/uterine tube	**tub**oplasty
turbin/o	top-shaped/turbinate bone (nasal concha)	**turbin**ectomy
tuss/i	cough	anti**tuss**ive
tympan/o	tympanic membrane/middle ear	**tympan**oplasty
-type	a classification/type of	pheno**type**
typhl/o	caecum (Am. cecum)	**typhl**ocele
-ula	small/little	ling**ula**
ulcer/o	ulcer/sore/local defect in a surface	**ulcer**ogenic
-ule	small	ven**ule**
uln/o	ulna	**uln**oradial
ul/o/e	scar/gingiva (gums)	**ul**oid
ultra-	beyond	**ultra**sonography
-ulum	small	coag**ulum**
-ulus	small	sacc**ulus**
-um	a thing/a structure/noun ending/a name	ov**um**
un-	not/opposite of/release from	**un**differentiated
ungu/o	nail	**ungu**al
uni-	one	**uni**lateral
uran/o	palate	**uran**orrhaphy

Component	Meaning	Medical Term
urat/o	urates/salt of uric acid (found in calculi)	uraturia
urea-	urea	ureapoiesis
ur/o	urine/urinary tract	urology
-uresis	excrete in urine/urinate	lithuresis
ureter/o	ureter	ureterostenosis
urethr/o	urethra	urethroscopy
-uria	condition of urine/urination	polyuria
uric/o	uric acid	uricometer
urin/a/o	urine	urinometer
urticar/i	nettle rash/hives	urticaria
-us	a thing/a structure/noun ending/a name	bronchus
uter/o	uterus	uterotubal
utricul/o	utricle of the inner ear	utriculus
uve/o	uvea (the pigmented parts of the eye)	uveitis
uvul/o	uvula	uvuloptosis
vagin/o	vagina	vaginitis
vag/o	vagus nerve	vagotomy
valv/o	valve	valvotomy
valvul/o	valve	valvulotome
varic/o	varix (a dilated vein)/varicose vein	varicophlebitis
vascul/o	vessel	vascular
vas/o	vessel/vas deferens	vasectomy
vel/o	soft/veil	velopharyngeal
venacav/o	vena cava (a great vein)	venacavography
ven/e/i/o	vein	venesection
vener/o	sexual intercourse	venereal
ventricul/o	ventricle of the heart or brain	ventriculography
ventr/i/o-	ventral/belly side of the body/in front of	ventrodorsal
verm/i	worm	vermicide
-version	turning	retroversion
vertebr/o	vertebra	vertebral
vesic/o	bladder/blister	vesicoprostatic
vesicul/o	seminal vesicle	vesiculitis
vestibul/o	vestibule/vestibular apparatus/a space leading to the entrance of a canal, e.g. in the ear	vestibulotomy
vibri/o	comma-shaped bacterium of the Genus Vibrio	vibriocidal
vibr/o	vibration	vibrocardiogram
vir/o/u	virus/virion	virolactia
viscer/o	viscera/internal organs (esp. of the abdomen)	visceroperitoneal
vit/o	life	vital
vitre/o	glass/the vitreous body of eye	vitreoretinal
viv/i	life	vivisection
vol/o	palm	volar
vulv/o	vulva	vulvitis
xanth/o	yellow	xanthoma
xen/o	strange/foreign	xenograft
xer/o	dry	xerophthalmia
xiph/i/o	xiphoid process	xiphicostal
-y	process/condition/noun ending/a name	apoplexy
-yl-	a substance	butylene
zo/o	animal	zooid
zyg/o	joined	zygodactyly
zygomatic/o	zygomatic arch	zygomaticotemporal
zygot-	zygote/fertilized egg	zygotic
-zyme	enzyme/fermentation	lysozyme
zym/o	enzyme/fermentation	zymosis

INDEX

INDEX

INDEX

INDEX